Core Clinical Competencies in Anesthesiology.

A case-based approach

The core clinical competencies in anesthesiology can be pretty blurry – just how do they apply to real life?

This book answers this question, incorporating the core clinical competencies into an engaging format that anesthesiologists like: case studies. So, far from being a dry and dusty volume of forgotten lore, this book actually makes learning the competencies fun!

Written in the same engaging style as a number of other anesthesia books (specifically, the *Board Stiff* opus) by anesthesiologists from leading medical centers across the United States, this book brings the core clinical competencies to life for residents, attendings, and medical students alike.

Dr. Christopher J. Gallagher is an Associate Professor in the Department of Anesthesiology at Stony Brook University. He is the recipient of teaching awards from Duke University, University of Miami, and Stony Brook University. He was also awarded the Anesthesiology Teaching Recognition Award for Achievement in Education by the International Anesthesia Research Society. Dr. Gallagher is the author of books on oral boards, anesthesia procedures, transesophageal echocardiography, and simulation. Outside of medicine, he has written one book on tennis, one on World War I, and another on learning foreign languages. He is fluent in five languages, conversant in another five, and can ask for the bathroom in an additional five. He has not yet achieved *People* magazine's "50 Most Beautiful People" list, but hope springs eternal in the human breast. He is the father of one and husband of one.

Dr. Michael C. Lewis is a Professor at the Miller School of Medicine at the University of Miami (UM). He has served as chief of anesthesia service at the Miami Veterans Affairs Health Care Center and as its director of medical student teaching. At UM, he has also held the position of chief of academic programs in transplant anesthesia in addition to his capacity as residency program director, chair of the Medical School Faculty Council, and vice chair of the University Senate. Most recently, he was appointed assistant dean for international graduate medical education. Dr. Lewis has been awarded a Hartford Award from the American Society of Geriatrics and was a Fulbright Scholar in 2006. He is active in the Florida Society of Anesthesiologists, presently serving as its president. He is also the current national president of the Israel Medical Association, World Fellowship: USA, and is on two committees of the American Society of Anesthesiologists, while being an active member of the House of Delegates of the American Board of Anesthesiology. He is married to Judy and has three daughters.

Dr. Deborah A. Schwengel is an Assistant Professor in the Department of Anesthesiology at Johns Hopkins School of Medicine and a pediatric anesthesiologist at the Johns Hopkins Children's Center. She is the anesthesiology residency program director and designer of an innovative education program at Johns Hopkins. She is founder and director of the International Adoption Clinic of the Kennedy Krieger Institute and the Johns Hopkins Children's Center. In addition, she is a critical care consultant at St. Agnes Hospital and Mt. Washington Pediatric Hospital, both in Baltimore. Dr. Schwengel's research is focused on clinical studies of the care of children with obstructive sleep apnea. She is also newly involved in educational research, no longer content with the old apprenticeship and lecture hall residency education programs. She has three internationally adopted children who, together with 75 anesthesiology residents, make life a never-ending string of dramatic and humorous tales.

Core Clinical Competencies in Anesthesiology

A case-based approach

Edited by

Christopher J. Gallagher
Stony Brook University

Michael C. Lewis
University of Miami

Deborah A. Schwengel
Johns Hopkins Medical Institutions

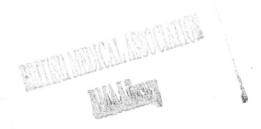

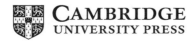
CAMBRIDGE
UNIVERSITY PRESS

CAMBRIDGE UNIVERSITY PRESS
Cambridge, New York, Melbourne, Madrid, Cape Town, Singapore,
São Paulo, Delhi, Dubai, Tokyo

Cambridge University Press
32 Avenue of the Americas, New York, NY 10013-2473, USA

www.cambridge.org
Information on this title: www.cambridge.org/9780521144131

First published 2010

Printed in the United States of America

*A catalog record for this publication is available from the
British Library.*

Library of Congress Cataloging in Publication data

Core clinical competencies in anesthesiology : a case-based
approach / edited by Christopher Gallagher, Michael Lewis,
Deborah Schwengel.
      p. ; cm.
Includes bibliographical references and index.
ISBN 978-0-521-14413-1 (pbk.)
1. Anesthesia – Case studies.   I. Gallagher, Christopher J.
II. Lewis, Michael (Michael C.)   III. Schwengel, Deborah A.
[DNLM: 1. Anesthesia – Case Reports.   2. Clinical
Competence – Case Reports. WO 200 C7965 2010]
RD82.45.C67   2010
617.9′6–dc22   2009036865

ISBN 978-0-521-14413-1 Paperback

To that person who coined the phrase that guides residency directors everywhere: "a residency director should beat the love of learning into his or her residents with a stout stick."

Contents

Contents

Part 2 – Contributions from the University of Medicine and Dentistry of New Jersey under Steven H. Ginsberg

Part 3 – Contribution from the University of Texas M.D. Anderson Cancer Center under Marc Rozner

Part 4 – Contributions from the University of Miami Miller School of Medicine under Michael C. Lewis

Part 5 – Contributions from Johns Hopkins Medical Institutions under Deborah A. Schwengel

Part 6 – Contribution from the Medical College of Wisconsin under Elena J. Holak

Rogues' Gallery of Contributing Authors

The following people allegedly contributed to this book. An insignificant number ($p < .05$) were waterboarded into this admission.

Stony Brook University Medical Center

Ramon Abola, MD, Chief Resident
Rishimani Adsumelli, MD, Associate Professor
Syed Azim, MD, Assistant Professor
Tazeen Beg, MD, Assistant Professor
Helene Benveniste, MD, Professor
Louis Chun, MD, Resident
Ramtin Cohanim, MD, Chief Resident
Dominick Coleman, MD, Resident
Joseph Conrad, MD, Resident
Tommy Corrado, MD, Resident
Jason Daras, DO, Resident
Michelle DiGuglielmo, MD, Chief Resident
Vedan Djesevic, MD, Resident
Andrew Drollinger, DDS, Resident
Kathleen Dubrow, MD, Resident
Brian Durkin, DO, Assistant Professor
Ralph Epstein, DDS, Assistant Professor
Christopher J. Gallagher, MD, Associate Professor
Xiaojun Guo, MD, Assistant Professor
Sofie Hussain, MD, Resident
Ron Jasiewicz, DO, Assistant Professor
Anna Kogan, DO, Resident
Ursula Landman, DO, Associate Professor
Rany Makaryus, MD, Resident
Daryn Moller, MD, Assistant Professor
Tate Montgomery, DDS, Resident
Matthew Neal, MD, Resident
Khoa Nguyen, MD, Resident
Marco Palmieri, DO, Resident
Shaji Poovathor, MD, Assistant Professor
Eric Posner, MD, Resident
Deborah Richman, MB, ChB, FFA(SA), Assistant Professor
Andrew Rozbruch, DO, Resident

Misako Sakamaki, MD, Resident
Joy Schabel, MD, Associate Professor
Bharathi Scott, MD, Professor
Peggy Seidman, MD, Associate Professor
Shiena Sharma, MD, Resident
Vishal Sharma, MD, Resident
Ellen Steinberg, MD, Associate Professor
Neera Tewari, DO, Assistant Professor
Jane Yi, DDS, Resident
Jonida Zeqo, MD, Resident

University of Medicine and Dentistry of New Jersey

Peter Chung, MD, Resident
John Denny, MD, Associate Professor
Steven H. Ginsberg, MD, Associate Professor
Jeremy Grayson, MD, Assistant Professor
Jonathan Kraidin, MD, Associate Professor
Stephen Lemke, DO, Resident
Tejal Patel, MD, Resident
Salvatore Zisa Jr., MD, Fellow

University of Texas M.D. Anderson Cancer Center

Charles Cowles, MD, Instructor
Marc Rozner, MD, PhD, Professor

University of Miami Miller School of Medicine

Shawn Banks, MD, Assistant Professor
Deborah Brauer, MD, Assistant Professor
Lebron Cooper, MD, Assistant Professor
V. Samepathi David, MD, Fellow
Steve Gayer, MD, Associate Professor
Steven Gil, MD, Resident

Eric A. Harris, MD, Assistant Professor
Murlikrishna Kannan, MD, Resident
Michael C. Lewis, MD, Professor
David A. Lindley, DO, Assistant Professor
Carlos M. Mijares, MD, Assistant Professor
Sana Nini, MD, Research Associate
Shafeena Nurani, MD, Resident Physician
Sujatha Pentakota, MD, Resident
Edgar Pierre, MD, Assistant Professor
Amy Klash Pulido, MD, Resident
Michael Rossi, DO, Assistant Professor
Miguel Santos, MD, Resident
Nancy Setzer-Saade, MD, Associate Professor
Adam Sewell, MD, Resident
Omair H. Toor, DO, Fellow
Ashish Udeshi, MD, Resident
Patricia Wawroski, MD, Resident

Johns Hopkins Medical Institutions

Lauren C. Berkow, MD, Assistant Professor
Dan Berkowitz, MD, Professor
Ramola Bhambhani, MD, Resident
Kerry K. Blaha, MD, Resident
Veronica Busso, MD, Resident
Adam J. Carinci, MD, Resident
Paul J. Christo, MD, MBA, Assistant Professor
R. Blaine Easley, MD, Assistant Professor
Ralph J. Fuchs, MD, Assistant Professor
Samuel M. Galvagno Jr., DO, Fellow
Nishant Gandhi, DO, Resident
Andrew Goins, DO, Resident
Robert S. Greenberg, MD, Associate Professor
Sayeh Hamzehzadeh, MD, Resident
Theresa L. Hartsell, MD, PhD, Assistant Professor
Eugenie Heitmiller, MD, Associate Professor

Jeremy M. Huff, DO, Resident
Brijen L. Joshi, MD, Fellow
Sapna Kudchadkar, MD, Fellow
Jennifer K. Lee, MD, Fellow
Ira Lehrer, DO, Resident
Peter Lin, MD, Resident
Justin Lockman, MD, Fellow
Christine L. Mai, MD, Fellow
Christina Miller, MD, Resident
Nanhi Mitter, MD, Assistant Professor
Gillian Newman, MD, Resident
Daniel Nyhan, MD, Professor
Lale Odekon, MD, PhD, Assistant Professor
Rabi Panigrahi, MD, Resident
Melissa Pant, MD, Resident
Alexander Papangelou, MD, Instructor
Mark Rossberg, MD, Assistant Professor
Adam Schiavi, PhD, MD, Instructor
Steven J. Schwartz, MD, Assistant Professor
Deborah A. Schwengel, MD, Assistant Professor
Brandon M. Togioka, MD, Resident
Tina Tran, MD, Assistant Professor
Emmett Whitaker, MD, Resident
Bradford D. Winters, PhD, MD, Assistant Professor
Christopher Wu, MD, Associate Professor

Medical College of Wisconsin

Elena J. Holak, MD, PharmD, Associate Professor
Paul S. Pagel, MD, PhD, Professor

Note on the authors: In their defense, many of these authors were dropped on their heads several times during their formative years. The rumor that others were abducted and raised by wolves has yet to be substantiated.

Core Clinical Competencies in Anesthesiology

A case-based approach

Introduction: "From the mountain"

A long time ago, in a medical galaxy far, far away, medical education was a simple matter of apprenticeship:

- You washed up on the shores of a residency.
- For three years, you did anesthesia.
- The residency released you into the wild, with the admonition, "Go ye forth and minister anesthesia unto the people."

But, alas, as time passed, the educational process grew in complexity.

Enter the Core Clinical Competencies.

Wise men and women gathered themselves together and reconsidered the apprenticeship idea. And thusly they spake, "The doctors know not of what they teach. They are misguided and errant in their ways. For them to teach unto their young charges, they must teach as we, the wise men and women of education, feel you must teach."

And the wise men and women of education climbed a great mountain, to seek commandments. They sought 10, but found they only 6. And these six commandments, they were writ in stone and given unto the wise men and women of education. From the mountain came they down, bearing six commandments with them. And they showed these six commandments to all who would teach doctors the art of healing the halt and lame.

And the teachers of doctors became sore afraid.

And the teachers of doctors asked, "Whence came these commandments, which we of needs must now employ as we teach the young doctors?"

So the wise men and women of education said, "Ye are not put on this earth to question the commandments given from on high. Ye are to obey the six commandments in all your teaching, and ye are to spend all the hours of the day and all the hours of the night documenting that ye are teaching via the commandments. All those who disobey will be cast aside and their residencies shuttered, their hospitals razed unto the ground, so that one brick no longer lies upon another, and the ground thereon to be sown with salt, so nothing there shall ever grow again."

And the teachers of doctors trembled before the men and women of education. And these same teachers rent their garments and gnashed their teeth, crying out, "Woe is us, that the daytime and the nighttime will be filled with documenting all we say and all we do. So great is the fury of the men and women of education that we will live all the years of our lives in fear and loathing and documenting."

Night fell.

The sun rose the next day.

"Ah, what is this on Amazon.com?" a teacher of doctors cried out. "A book, a book which reviews anesthesia cases via the Core Clinical Competencies! As manna from heaven fed those who wandered through the desert, so also this book from three residency directors will feed those who wander through the Core Clinical Competency land. Yea, verily, this is a boon to medical students, residents, and teachers alike."

And great was the happiness.

And now, as you read on, so also will your happiness be great.

For first we shall review the Core Clinical Competencies, and we shall show ye how these selfsame Core Clinical Competencies are viewed through the prism of anesthesia. Then we will leave off the jabber, for we seek not to be as the cackling of hens or the screeching of monkeys. We will go us forth into actual cases, cases we have done ourselves, and we will explain these cases with great and terrible emphasis on the Core Clinical Competencies.

And lo, your understanding will grow mightily. And you will use this knowledge to minister unto those who are afflicted by the thousand and one ills that flesh is heir to.

And when a dark cloud appears upon the horizon, and a great crash of thunder is heard, and the Four Horsemen of the Residency Review Committee

(RRC) Apocalypse come pounding up to your door, you will hold up this selfsame book, and you will have no need to avert your gaze or feel ashamed in your Accreditation Council for Graduate Medical Education compliance nakedness. For you will say, "Look, ye terrible Horsemen of the RRC Apocalypse, and note well. Much have we studied, and all through and with and under the benevolent wing of the Core Clinical Competencies, as we have been commanded by the men and women of education."

And the Four Horsemen of the RRC Apocalypse will rein in their furious mounts, and away they will ride, for no citations will they give, and no complaint will they raise.

For the book is good.

And now you may rest under the shade of the tree.

An anesthetic view of the Core Clinical Competencies

Here are the Core Clinical Competencies with an anesthetic twist. The first two, patient care and medical knowledge, are the traditional things we've always taught. The last four are a bit softer and harder to nail down. But hey, you have to know all six, so let's plow through them.

Patient care

Residents must be able to provide patient care that is compassionate, appropriate, and effective for the treatment of health problems and the promotion of health. Residents are expected to do the following:

- communicate effectively and demonstrate caring and respectful behaviors when interacting with patients and their families
- gather essential and accurate information about their patients
- make informed decisions about diagnostic and therapeutic interventions based on patient information and preferences, up-to-date scientific evidence, and clinical judgment
- develop and carry out patient management plans
- counsel and educate patients and their families
- use information technology to support patient care decisions and patient education
- perform competently all medical and invasive procedures considered essential for the area of practice
- provide health care services aimed at preventing health problems or maintaining health
- work with health care professionals, including those from other disciplines, to provide patient-focused care

The anesthetic take on patient care

This is the most inherently obvious of the clinical competencies. We are patient care people, after all! You can wax dreamy about all the other educational rigmarole,

but if the tube doesn't find the trachea, or the spinal needle doesn't splash down in cerebrospinal fluid, or the central line knifes through the pleura, then we're doing it all wrong.

Patient care means taking care of the patient correctly, and to detail how you take care of a patient correctly, read Miller cover to cover and do a residency. Because it *all* boils down to taking good care of the patient:

- Secure that airway.
- Get the line in.
- Keep an eye on those vital signs.
- Provide good analgesia.
- React to changes and problems.
- Keep those lines open between you and the surgeon, the obstetrician, and the consultants so you don't miss anything.

That is the anesthetic take on patient care, and there's not a lot of room for interpretation.

Medical knowledge

Residents must demonstrate knowledge about established and evolving biomedical, clinical, and cognate (e.g., epidemiological and social-behavioral) sciences and the application of this knowledge to patient care. Residents are expected to do the following:

- demonstrate an investigatory and analytic thinking approach to clinical situations
- know and apply the basic and clinically supportive sciences that are appropriate to their discipline

The anesthetic take on medical knowledge

The anesthetic take on medical knowledge is little removed from the anesthetic take on patient care. You need to *know* the medicine to *care for* the patient:

- Chest pain, ST segment changes? You have to know the components of ischemia, know the latest on beta-blockade (good and bad), and know how best to intervene.

- New device for securing the airway safely? You have to know how to use it to care for the patient.
- New block (say, the transverses abdominalus planar (TAP) block for relieving abdominal pain)? You need to know the landmarks, how you can tell the transverses abdominus on echo, and how to lay the local anesthetic in there.

This is just the knowing behind the doing, so there's not much interpretive wiggle room in this Core Clinical Competency.

So far, so good. Now things get a little mushier.

Practice-based learning and improvement

Residents must be able to investigate and evaluate their patient care practices, appraise and assimilate scientific evidence, and improve their patient care practices. Residents are expected to do the following:

- analyze practice experience and perform practice-based improvement activities using a systematic methodology
- locate, appraise, and assimilate evidence from scientific studies related to their patients' health problems
- obtain and use information about their own population of patients and the larger population from which their patients are drawn
- apply knowledge of study designs and statistical methods to the appraisal of clinical studies and other information on diagnostic and therapeutic effectiveness
- use information technology to manage information, access online medical information, and support their own education

The anesthetic take on practice-based learning and improvement

This means looking at the literature. None of us have enough experience in our own individual practice to draw meaningful demographic conclusions. We tend to stew in our empiric juices and say, "Well, I did this once and somehow the patient survived, so gee whiz, this must be the way to do it!"

This *n* of 1 that we've all leaned on doesn't hold up to statistical scrutiny, so we have to go to the literature. Hillary Clinton told us that "it takes a village"

to raise a child. When it comes to interpreting medical information, it takes the global medical village to guide our therapy. Here's one example that affected our recent thinking:

- Beta-blockers are great! Studies drift out that seem to indicate that one beta-blocker pill given in the perioperative period will stave off death for a thousand years!
- Hey, let's give everyone beta-blockers, and all our patients will live forever.
- This makes inherent sense because slowing down the heart prevents ischemia. Right!

Now, the literature looks at this more rigorously. Out comes the POISE study, looking at 80,000 plus patients and giving them all beta-blockers. And there's a fly in the soup!

- Ischemia is, indeed, down.
- But death and stroke rates are up.
- Oh, no! The sacred cow of perioperative beta-blockade is slain.

Could any *one* of us, in our own experience, have come up with these conclusions? I don't care how fast you turn over a room; you're not going to rack up 80,000 anesthetics in a short time and study this issue – hence practice-based learning and improvement as a Core Clinical Competency.

What's the crucial skill you need in this area? You need to answer the question, is the information in the literature valid? Is it meaningful? Should I change my practice based on what the authors say?

Every month, the journal articles are filled with studies – do you change your practice every time a new paper comes out? Do you snap up every new procedure because it has an "Oh, that looks neat!" air about it? Obviously not. The connoisseur of the literature knows the good stuff from the bad, the Dom Pérignon from the Listerine.

Interpersonal and communication skills

Residents must be able to demonstrate interpersonal and communication skills that result in effective information exchange and teaming with patients, their patients' families, and professional associates. Residents are expected to do the following:

- create and sustain a therapeutic and ethically sound relationship with patients

- use effective listening skills and elicit and provide information using effective nonverbal, explanatory, questioning, and writing skills
- work effectively with others as a member or leader of a health care team or other professional group

The anesthetic take on interpersonal and communication skills

This competency and the next one (professionalism) are damned hard to tease apart. I wish they would have checked with me before they split these into two. Here goes, but, as you will see, there's a lot of overlap here.

You can't be an oaf, dolt, moron, or insensitive clod with the patient, and you have to get ideas *to* them and get ideas *from* them. Same goes for working with nurses, cardiopulmonary bypass techs, doctors, intensive care unit staff, respiratory techs, you name it. Anyone that crosses paths with you in the clinical orbit, you have to work well with them and make sure you get the information right.

Professionalism

Residents must demonstrate a commitment to carrying out professional responsibilities, adherence to ethical principles, and sensitivity to a diverse patient population. Residents are expected to do the following:

- demonstrate respect, compassion, and integrity; a responsiveness to the needs of patients and society that supersedes self-interest; accountability to patients, society, and the profession; and a commitment to excellence and ongoing professional development
- demonstrate a commitment to ethical principles pertaining to provision or withholding of clinical care, confidentiality of patient information, informed consent, and business practice
- demonstrate sensitivity and responsiveness to patients' culture, age, gender, and disabilities

The anesthetic take on professionalism

As noted previously, this goes hand in glove with the competency of interpersonal and communication skills. A professional communicates well with patients, fellow doctors, and all other medical providers. (Core Clinical Competencies force you to use administrato-speak, with stupid phrases like "health care providers" and crap like that.) Part of that communication is registering the different backgrounds your patients have –

different cultures, being sensitive to gender concerns, being sensitive to different disabilities.

This is the Core Clinical Competency that steams most anesthesiologists (and, I suspect, most other specialties, too). Of course, we know to be professional! God all fishhooks, we went through premed and med school and are now in postgraduate training. Do I need the Core Clinical Competencies to tell me that I have to be *ethical*? We all took the Hippocratic oath; our whole life has been geared to taking good care of our fellow human beings. Now some educationo-wonk is telling me I have to be sensitive and appropriate around a person of different background, or a person with a disability?

Gimme a break!

Systems-based practice

Residents must demonstrate an awareness of and responsiveness to the larger context and system of health care and the ability to effectively call on system resources to provide care that is of optimal value. Residents are expected to do the following:

- understand how their patient care and other professional practices affect other health care professionals, the health care organization, and the larger society and how these elements of the system affect their own practice
- know how types of medical practice and delivery systems differ from one another, including methods of controlling health care costs and allocating resources
- practice cost-effective health care and resource allocation that does not compromise quality of care
- advocate for quality patient care and assist patients in dealing with system complexities
- know how to partner with health care managers and health care providers to assess, coordinate, and improve health care and know how these activities can affect system performance

The anesthetic take on systems-based practice

Money makes the world go round, and medicine is no exception. For anesthesiologists, the main idea we glean from systems-based practice is related to money:

- practice cost-effective medicine
- know how you fit into the great big overall picture

- do QA things (they don't call it that anymore – they say *continuous quality improvement* – but we all know that's just more administrato–double talk)

There you have it, the Core Clinical Competencies laid out, complete with the anesthetic take on them. Sound jaded?

Yeah, it's a little jaded. If you pull aside the average resident or attending and ask what he or she thinks about the Core Clinical Competencies, you'll probably get some variant of my barbed comments.

But they're here to stay, and we have to know how to teach them, so that's why this book exists. Rather than sit here and dwell on them and debate their relative merits, let's do what we're best at: clinical anesthesia. We'll lay out a case, then wrap that case around the Core Clinical Competencies. That way, we'll breathe some life and relevance into these bastards. So grab your hat and mask, and let's have at it.

Anesthetic cases through the Core Clinical Competencies looking glass

Without further ado, we launch into the meat of the book – clinical cases with interesting twists (we actually did these cases!). And we'll look at each case through the prism of the Core Clinical Competencies.

The first case, "Pop Goes the Aneurysm," is over the top/overdone/overkill/too much. I have linked aspects of the case to *every single sentence of every single competency*. As you will see, this leads to interesting verbal gymnastics as I struggle to find a connection.

Every case will not be so exhaustive. Slavish adherence to each and every sentence in the Core Clinical Competencies is not the purpose of these cases, nor is it the purpose of this book. Different anesthetic challenges provide different areas of emphasis. As you will see, there will be cases in which all we talk about is two or three of the competencies.

So bear with us on this first one. This will show you how you can take a case, or one horrific moment in midoperation, and wrap it around the Core Clinical Competencies.

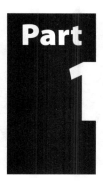

Part 1

Contributions from Stony Brook University under Christopher J. Gallagher

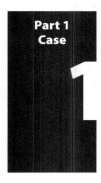

Contributions from Stony Brook University under Christopher J. Gallagher

Pop goes the aneurysm

Christopher J. Gallagher and Tommy Corrado

The case

A previously healthy 45-year-old man developed headaches and blurry vision. Workup revealed a large cerebral aneurysm requiring a heroic procedure. In effect, his face would be taken apart to get at the aneurysm. The lesion itself was extremely large, and the neurosurgeon was quite concerned about whether he'd be able to "get the clamp around the base."

After an initial tracheostomy and 5 hours of dissection, a faint and barely audible *pop!* was heard, followed by a nonfaint and easily audible "oh, shit!" from the surgeon. The patient's blood pressure rose to 260, and his heart rate fell from 90, to 80, to 70, and didn't stop until reaching 40.

A glance over the ether screen revealed a brain ballooning out of the skull. The brain was stretched so taut that there were no sulci present, just "lines on a globe" where the sulci used to be.

Patient care

Residents must be able to provide patient care that is compassionate, appropriate, and effective for the treatment of health problems and the promotion of health.

Communicate effectively and demonstrate caring and respectful behavior when interacting with patients and their families.

No family is in the room, and the patient is under general anesthesia, so we don't have to sweat about caring and respectful behavior in our interaction. We can show the most respect by reacting like lightning to the developing catastrophe.

Gather essential and accurate information about their patients.

Check those monitors; make sure the transducer didn't fall on the floor.

Make informed decisions about diagnostic and therapeutic interventions based on patient information and preferences, up-to-date scientific evidence, and clinical judgment.

It doesn't take a genius to peg this as Cushing's triad stemming from a catastrophic intracerebral bleed. Clinical judgment says that you have to do everything you can to decrease swelling in the brain, and you have about an eighth of a second to do it.

Develop and carry out patient management plans.

Slam in some Pentathol and go with hyperventilation (to hell with concerns about cerebral ischemia – you are in disaster mode).

Counsel and educate patients and their families.

At this point, you'd need to jump into a time machine and go back to the preoperative area to discuss what will be done if things go wrong intraop. Here is a patient who was healthy up to this point, but there is a genuine worry that things may end up very badly (keep in mind that the surgeon himself was extremely concerned, and even getting at the aneurysm required quite an effort).

Does the patient have a living will? Is organ donation (see the later discussion) something the patient and family are willing to discuss and consider?

Use information technology to support patient care decisions and patient education.

Again, this is the sort of thing that is best handled in the preoperative phase of the operation. You look up any studies the patient has had (a chest X-ray or the computed tomograph or magnetic resonance image of the aneurysm) so that you will have knowledge of what the surgeon will be doing.

> Perform competently all medical and invasive procedures considered essential for the area of practice.

At induction, a competent anesthesiologist would skillfully place adequate venous access and a preinduction arterial line (to monitor blood pressure on a beat-to-beat basis during induction and intubation) and would secure the airway appropriately. Later, when the surgeon has placed the tracheostomy (done because the face would be so disrupted by the approach), the anesthesiologist would make sure the switch from oral endotracheal tube to tracheostomy was done well.

> Provide health care services aimed at preventing health problems or maintaining health.

The number-one preventive measure we take during such a case is timing the delivery of prophylactic antibiotics. Current standards dictate that antibiotics be delivered within 1 hour of incision.

Obviously, this aspect of the Core Clinical Competencies seems a bit Pollyannaish at this point – worrying about maintaining health when the patient has just had a massive and potentially life-threatening bleed into the very center of his brain. This is included for the sake of completeness (each case considers all the Core Clinical Competencies, but different competencies receive different emphasis).

> Work with health care professionals, including those from other disciplines, to provide patient-focused care.

Right now, you are *married* to that neurosurgeon – you are joined at the hip, one and the same, because death stalks the land right now. Are you going to work closely with the neurosurgeon and all the other members of the operating room (OR) team to get out of this jam? As Sarah Palin would say, "You betcha!"

Medical knowledge

Residents must demonstrate knowledge about established and evolving biomedical, clinical, and cognate (e.g., epidemiological and social-behavioral) sciences and the application of this knowledge to patient care.

> Demonstrate an investigatory and analytic thinking approach to clinical situations.

On goes your thinking cap – that blood pressure went through the roof for a reason. And that heart rate went down for a linked reason (vagal response to the massive increase in blood pressure). Of course, you do a quick check to make sure nothing else could have caused this insta–pole vault of the blood pressure (syringe swap, patient instantly getting "very light"). You jump to Cushing's triad by putting it all together – complexity of the case; physiology of increased pressure in the brain; your look into the field, confirming a disaster.

> Know and apply the basic and clinically supportive sciences that are appropriate to their discipline.

Before you cross the threshold into the neurosurgery room, you make sure you understand all the physiology that applies to these complex cases: cerebrospinal fluid formation; cerebral autoregulation; function of the blood-brain barrier; intracranial pressure; and cerebral blood flow responses to hypoxemia, hypo/hypercarbia, and potent inhaled agents. The supportive science for neuroanesthesia fills hernia-inducing textbooks.

The quick and dirty physiology that you draw on right now follows:

- the aneurysm popped
- blood is pouring into the "meat" of the brain
- as the brain expands, it attempts to maintain perfusion by increasing the blood pressure
- the heart (which has no way of knowing what's up in the head) "sees" high blood pressure and reacts by slowing down

Practice-based learning and improvement

Residents must be able to investigate and evaluate their patient care practices, appraise and assimilate scientific evidence, and improve their patient care practices.

> Analyze practice experience and perform practice-based improvement activities using a systematic methodology.

Something about the surgeon being spooked about this case and saying "oh, shit!" tells you that you are in deep trouble right now. Call it the world's fastest "analysis of practice experience":

- This surgeon has been working for years.
- He knew this was bad going in.

- He's swearing and the brain is blowing up like a Macy's Thanksgiving Day Parade cartoon character.

There is, unfortunately, no time right now to perform a practice-based improvement activity, but all is not lost as far as this Core Clinical Competency is concerned! The hospital, neurosurgery, and anesthesiology should all have Continuous Quality Improvement committees. Obviously, right this minute, you cannot whip up a committee, but later on, you *should* do just that. Difficult cases, complications, deaths – all these things demand a systematic analysis afterward. You, as the anesthesiologist, should participate in these "after-action reports." Never assume, "we did everything right, so let's not talk about it."

Maybe the case could have been done with coils? Was this case so horrifically complicated that it should have been referred to a better-equipped tertiary center? Should the surgeon have done cardiopulmonary bypass with circulatory arrest to more safely clamp the aneurysm?

> Locate, appraise, and assimilate evidence from scientific studies related to their patients' health problems.

Who are we kidding? This is the gist of practice-based learning and improvement – keeping up with and analyzing the literature. This includes the hefty command, "You need to know what constitutes good literature and what constitutes dreck."

Ooph! In other words, you can't just look at the last sentence of the conclusion and say, "OK, sounds good!" What does the literature say about *this* patient? In a perfect world, each time you did a case, you'd read a timely, scientific article on the very case you're doing. What does the literature say about clipping aneurysms? Keep control of the pressure; be ready to drop the pressure drastically if the surgeon's having trouble getting the clip on; and administer adenosine if you need a heart-stopping (literally, for you and the patient both) few moments, good oxygenation (duh, as if we need to hear that), and eucarbia to avoid cerebral ischemia.

What does the literature say about a disaster like this? It is difficult to do a double-blind, placebo-controlled, multicenter, sufficiently powered study on how best to handle a disastrous and ultimately fatal bleed into the brain. So you're left with your best physiologic guess right now. In the long term, hyperventilation is not a good idea, but right now, you are in the shortest of short terms and need all the help you can get, so you abandon considerations of what's best long term and just do what you can do to try to get a handle on things and save the patient.

> Obtain and use information about their own population of patients and the larger population from which their patients are drawn.

This is another way of saying what was said previously – you draw on your own experience, and you draw on the larger world of experience, that is, the experience described in the literature. In other words, you review and keep abreast of experience with clipping cerebral aneurysms.

> Apply knowledge of study designs and statistical methods to the appraisal of clinical studies and other information on diagnostic and therapeutic effectiveness.

Oh, just kill me now that they've mentioned statistics! Well, there's no getting around it – if you're going to be more than a last-sentence-of-the-conclusion reader, you have to dig in to the guts of the studies and determine whether that last sentence is actually merited.

Back to the cerebral aneurysm literature: let's look at just one aspect of the literature that is worth considering. In the middle of this intracranial Armageddon, you might think, "Maybe we should cool this guy down a little! That will decrease his cerebral metabolic rate and might protect him!"

To the literature!

No soap! Using mild hypothermia to improve neurologic outcome has been examined in the literature and has been found wanting. Although it makes *physiologic sense* that hypothermia would protect the brain, a study looking at that very issue showed that hypothermia does *not* protect the brain. Not only that, but hypothermia causes its own problems (including rhythm disturbances).

So, even in the hurry-up, oh-my-God! atmosphere of an OR emergency, you still have to be able to draw on the literature to guide individual steps.

> Use information technology to manage information, access online medical information, and support their own education.

What did we do before PubMed and all the other online wizardry that brings the world's literature to our fingertips? In this case, you wouldn't be looking things up in the OR, but rather, you'd look up neuroanesthesia updates the night before and make sure you show up prepared. In the OR, you might use an automated record system to keep your hands free while the patient is crashing.

Support your own education with information technology? Of course. Get the latest American Society of Anesthesiologists refresher courses on neuroanesthesia online, or troll the Internet for learning material (different anesthesia programs have the PowerPoint presentations of their lectures online). Surf the Internet and get smart – what a concept!

Professionalism

Residents must demonstrate a commitment to carrying out professional responsibilities, adherence to ethical principles, and sensitivity to a diverse patient population.

> Demonstrate respect, compassion, and integrity; a responsiveness to the needs of patients and society that supersedes self-interest; accountability to patients, society, and the profession; and a commitment to excellence and ongoing professional development.

OK, we're in the middle of big trouble with this intracranial fire hose pouring blood into the middle of the brain. Is there a way to shoehorn this lofty professionalism stuff into the picture? In a practical sense, no, not right this instant. But in terms of your background preparation for the case, yes, there is. (If this sounds like a stretch, I agree, it is.)

Respect and compassion are demonstrated to the patient and family in the preop visit and the holding area. Integrity involves getting enough sleep the night before so you show up alert and ready to work. Check your machine, and do all the things a good, sound anesthesiologist does to provide the best possible care.

Responsiveness to the needs of patient and society, superseding self-interest? If you're on call and this case rolls in, this is no time to check the insurance status and refuse if you're not going to get paid. Accountability? Are your continuing medical education credits, your licensing requirements, and your hospital privileges all up to date? That is part of accountability and, hence, professionalism. Commitment to excellence and your development? Attend hospital and teaching rounds, go to meetings, and get the latest on medical practice.

> Demonstrate a commitment to ethical principles pertaining to provision or withholding of clinical care, confidentiality of patient information, informed consent, and business practice.

Before the case, make sure that informed consent, site of surgery, and all the paperwork are in order. Observe all HIPAA regulations (don't talk about the case where others can overhear, and don't reveal any confidential patient information). When filling out your billing slips, be ethical. Bill for what you did and nothing more. As noted previously, this is background behavior that applies to all cases.

> Demonstrate sensitivity and responsiveness to patients' culture, age, gender, and disabilities.

Say this patient were not a 45-year-old man with a generic suburban lifestyle. You would make a note of each aspect of the patient's background and hold it up for mock and ridicule to crack everyone up in the holding area, right?

Uh, no.

You could call this aspect of professionalism the "Eagle Scout mandate." Behave like an Eagle Scout around your patients, with appropriate deference and respect for everything that they are:

- Sexist comments to make someone feel uncomfortable about his or her gender? No, an Eagle Scout wouldn't do that.
- Disparaging comments about a patient's national identity? No, an Eagle Scout wouldn't do that.
- Poke fun at the elderly? Point and stare at the mentally or physically challenged? Of course not – if our imaginary Eagle Scout wouldn't do it, then neither should we.

(Truth to tell, mandates like these set my teeth on edge. Just what is the reason for laying this obvious commandment out there? Is the implication that, before the Core Clinical Competencies came along, doctors were taught to make fun of their patients and treat them impolitely? The wise men and women of education may find this hard to believe, but before the Core Clinical Competencies became the law of the land, we were taught to be respectful.)

Interpersonal and communication skills

Residents must be able to demonstrate interpersonal and communication skills that result in effective information exchange and teaming with patients, their patients' families, and professional associates.

Create and sustain a therapeutic and ethically sound relationship with patients.

Back in our time machine, fly back to yesterday during the preop visit as well as this morning's preinduction. Part of building up a sound and therapeutic relationship starts with hand washing! Wash those hands before you go in to shake the patient's hand. Introduce yourself, look professional, and give the patient your undivided attention.

Use effective listening skills and elicit and provide information using effective nonverbal, explanatory, questioning, and writing skills.

As an anesthesiologist, your job is to get the information you need – a directed history and physical. In the case of this 45-year-old man, you would pick up clues as to the man's level of understanding and gear your interaction appropriately. University professor in the neurosciences? Your explanation can be technical. Blue-collar worker who never finished high school? Different tack on the explanation, of course.

Your preop note will demonstrate your writing skills. The rule here is simple: if, for some reason, you can't do the case (say, e.g., you get shot by a jealous husband between the preop visit and doing the case), then make sure all the information is there. In this particular case, you would want to make sure that your notes include the surgeon's concerns (big aneurysm, possibility of rupture is real), the plans for the airway (intubation followed by trach because of extensive dissection in the facial area), and the patient's understanding of the risks.

Work effectively with others as a member or leader of a health care team or other professional group.

Aha! Now there's some actual relevance, and we can get away from Eagle Scout discussions! (You will see this same pattern in subsequent cases discussed in this book – different areas of the Core Clinical Competencies merit emphasis in different cases.)

Back to the case, what happened, and what we did.

It became evident, after just a few minutes, that the bleed into the brain was unstoppable and the brain damage was irreversible. There was no way to salvage this man. Frantic medical attempts to drive down the pressure (whole sticks of Pentathol, Nipride wide open) as well as attempts to decrease intracranial pressure (hyperventilation, more head up, mannitol bolus) were all futile. The bleed into the brain from the burst aneurysm was too much. The swollen and expanding brain looked like a scene from a science fiction movie. We all suspected (and we later demonstrated) that the man was effectively brain-dead.

What now? Turn off the ventilator and call it a day?

No. Here's how the discussion among the team went:

- We had to notify the family.
- We now had an "otherwise healthy" man with intact kidneys, liver, heart, and lungs.
- Efforts should now focus on keeping all organs viable for possible donation.

Clergy was brought into the discussion, along with organ procurement and surgical teams – a host of different members of the health care team joined in the process.

Systems-based practice

Residents must demonstrate an awareness of and responsiveness to the larger context and system of health care and the ability to effectively call on system resources to provide care that is of optimal value.

Understand how their patient care and other professional practices affect other health care professionals, the health care organization, and the larger society and how these elements of the system affect their own practice.

This first aspect of systems-based practice segues with the last aspect of professionalism just stated. (These damned competencies overlap all over the place – it's hard to draw a line where one ends and another begins.)

This neurosurgical patient has suffered a life-ending hemorrhage, but his organs may save the lives of others in society. Thus your responsibility has, in a sense, shifted to the concerns of the larger society. You are to take the best possible care of this patient to ensure that his organs are best preserved. That means maintaining hemodynamic stability, keeping fluids to a minimum (to avoid pulmonary edema, thus ruining the lungs for transplant), avoiding vasoconstrictors (harmful to kidneys and liver), and keeping the patient heart healthy (monitoring, preventing, and treating any ischemia) – all the considerations that go into providing anesthesia care for an organ donor.

Know how types of medical practice and delivery systems differ from one another, including methods of controlling health care costs and allocating resources.

The primary resource of interest here is the healthy organs of the soon-to-be donor. As an anesthesiologist, you should be aware of the hospital's policy on notifying the organ procurement team and how much lead time they need (including, of course, the all-important discussion with family). Allocation will be up to the organ team, but you should at least know how the system works (organ recipients are kept on call and are notified when an organ becomes available; extensive blood work is required from the donor to make sure complex cross-match studies are performed). Different areas of the country have different teams. Sometimes a harvest team is flown in, whereas sometimes surgeons at the hospital do the harvesting for them.

Practice cost-effective health care and resource allocation that does not compromise quality of care.

High flow of oxygen? Most expensive potent inhaled agent? No and no. Responsible care of the patient at this point mandates standard cost-effective maneuvers: low flows of oxygen; no need for expensive desflurane, can use isoflurane; muscle relaxant – pancuronium. Because a quick wake-up is not exactly in the cards here, you shift gears to the least expensive regimen, while always maintaining the optimal physiologic environment for organ preservation.

Advocate for quality patient care and assist patients in dealing with system complexities.

The primary people who need assistance in system complexities at this point are the family members, who are wrestling with the heartrending consequences of the operation and the decision to donate organs. Your advocacy for quality patient care is manifested as you continue to take good care of all the physiologic variables (which can be tough, as the brain-dead patient can develop all kinds of instability).

Your assistance with the family may be required. A few points (which we all know, and this is insulting your intelligence) follow:

- Get everyone in a private room – this is no hallway conference.
- Turn your beeper and cell phone off – this is no time for interruptions.
- Allow time for family members to vent their emotions.
- Repeat information as necessary – this is difficult material to process.

Know how to partner with health care managers and health care providers to assess, coordinate, and improve health care, and know how these activities can affect system performance.

This is another aspect of the case that is handled afterward. Keep in touch with hospital administration about where the organs went. A lot of times, the organ procurement people will send letters to the OR team letting them know, for example, that the "kidney went to a 34-year-old woman, who was so happy to get off dialysis" and the "liver saved a man with idiopathic cirrhosis." The whole team in the OR should maintain that link with the team outside the OR that was involved in this patient's care and, ultimately, his donation to other people's lives.

The first case (gloomy, admittedly) wrestles with just what is brain death. An article on brain death is included in Additional Reading.

You will notice that in this, the first case, we wrote something for each sentence of each competency. We won't be doing that for all the rest of the cases because different cases will emphasize different competencies.

Additional reading

1. Wijdicks EFM. The diagnosis of brain death. Neurosurgery 2001;344:1215–1221.

2. Qureshi AI, Suri MF, Khan J, et al. Endovascular treatment of intracranial aneurysms by using Guglielmi detachable coils in awake patients: safety and feasibility. J Neurosurg 2001;94:880–885.

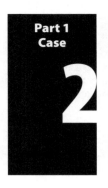

Contributions from Stony Brook University under Christopher J. Gallagher

2 No Foley, no surgeon; what now?

Christopher J. Gallagher and Khoa Nguyen

The case

A 70-year-old man is scheduled for coronary artery bypass surgery in the usual way on the usual day with the usual people. Ho hum, what could go wrong? Induction is carried out in the (what else?) usual fashion, and the airway is secured. Invasive lines are placed, while the nurse attempts to place a Foley catheter.

No luck!

The catheter won't pass for love or money. Speculation arises as to prostatism or, perhaps, just perhaps, some kind of a urethral stricture (the hang-up is early on and not later on, pointing to the urethra as the culprit). Of course, a urethral stricture could arise from any number of things, but one subject of intense speculation is this patient's early dalliances in the romantic realm. Could this Foley-not-passing be evidence of looking for love in all the wrong places?

The cardiac surgeon is summoned because this looks like a tough Foley placement. Consideration is also given to summoning clergy so that the patient can receive a stern admonition as to wayward conduct/the sins of the flesh/eternal damnation and related topics of the ecclesiastic bent. (This latter idea is quashed, more's the pity.)

The surgeon doesn't answer the call. Still, the Foley won't pass, and now there's blood in the tip of the organ of interest. Now what?

Patient care

Residents must be able to provide patient care that is compassionate, appropriate, and effective for the treatment of health problems and the promotion of health.

Communicate effectively and demonstrate caring and respectful behaviors when interacting with patients and their families.

The patient is under anesthesia, so we can't be talking to the patient or family. To instill a little more respect in the room, consider smacking the people who made the snippy comments about looking for love in all the wrong places. (Oops, that was me. Forget that.)

Gather essential and accurate information about their patients.

Review the chart – have they had trouble placing a Foley before? Does the patient have a history of prostatism or urethral stricture?

Make informed decisions about diagnostic and therapeutic interventions based on patient information and preferences, up-to-date scientific evidence, and clinical judgment.

At this point, the question is whether to get a genitourinary (GU) consult or not to place the Foley. They'll likely need their fancier kinds of probes, perhaps going all the way to checking things out with a scope. In the last word on this, with no way at all to place a Foley, the next step is a suprapubic catheter.

Develop and carry out patient management plans.

God, how I hate phrases like *patient management plan*. It has an air of the administrator who calls patients "clients" and junk like that.

The current best (gag) patient management plan in the cardiac realm is to use the common sense that all anesthesiologists have when watching *any* patient:

- keep the myocardial oxygen supply–demand ratio favorable
- fast-tracking makes sense – get the patient off the ventilator and breathing on his own as soon as safe and practical
- to minimize the time on the table, call the GU consult right away and get that Foley in
- give gram-negative antibiotic coverage; all this digging around in the urethral area may well be seeding the bloodstream with gram-negative bacteria, and the last thing you need is a perioperative infection in a cardiac patient

Perform competently all medical and invasive procedures considered essential for the area of practice.

No real thinking here – get your art line and central line in competently.

Provide health care services aimed at preventing health problems or maintaining health.

Be sure to follow the current guidelines to minimize the possibility of central line infection:

- wash hands ahead of time
- gown and glove
- full body drape

Work with health care professionals, including those from other disciplines, to provide patient-focused care.

If that cardiac surgeon doesn't show up, then you have to assume the role of consultant getting a consultant and do what's right for the patient. Tell the GU doc what's going on and get him or her whatever equipment is necessary for the funky Foley placement.

Medical knowledge

Residents must demonstrate knowledge about established and evolving biomedical, clinical, and cognate (e.g., epidemiological and social-behavioral) sciences and the application of this knowledge to patient care.

Demonstrate an investigatory and analytic thinking approach to clinical situations.

It doesn't take Sherlock Holmes or Albert Einstein to analyze this situation. The case is at a standstill and the surgeon is AWOL. Nothing can happen until the urine drainage situation is addressed, so have at it.

Know and apply the basic and clinically supportive sciences that are appropriate to their discipline.

Basic science tells us that a cardiac case involves a lot of fluid administration, including lots of fluids containing mannitol (from the cardiopulmonary bypass machine). This will fill the bladder with lots of urine, so proceeding without a Foley invites problematic bladder overdistension, or even rupture.

Practice-based learning and improvement

Residents must be able to investigate and evaluate their patient care practices, appraise and assimilate scientific evidence, and improve their patient care practices.

Analyze practice experience and perform practice-based improvement activities using a systematic methodology.

In the middle of a difficult situation with a bleeding urethra and no surgeon, this is not the optimal time to get a committee together to discuss how we can improve on the situation and possible future situations like it. That would best be discussed after the Foley was placed and the case went off without a hitch. Possible discussion topics could include a more detailed medical and social history, an array of different catheters to fit the various different anatomical specimens seen in the operating room (OR), and an alternative method to drain urine with the help of our urology colleagues.

Locate, appraise, and assimilate evidence from scientific studies related to their patients' health problems.

Since you were prepared for anything that might occur with your patient, you did your research into difficult Foley placement. You read several case studies of the effects of traumatic Foley placements, including urethral strictures postoperatively to even (gasp!) a venous air embolism in the vena cava. There are not a great deal of scientific data regarding the placement of Foleys. The gist of the available data shows that educating the people who place Foleys (i.e., nurses and physicians) about the anatomy and proper technique reduces the incidence of iatrogenic injury. The moral of story is that you hope the nurse who tried to place the Foley has been properly trained and educated about the anatomy; otherwise, he or she should defer to someone who has more experience placing a difficult Foley such as our urology colleagues.

Apply knowledge of study designs and statistical methods to the appraisal of clinical studies and other information on diagnostic and therapeutic effectiveness.

Again, not many studies have looked at difficult Foley placement as they are usually unanticipated cases; otherwise, we could prepare for them and make them not so difficult.

> Use information technology to manage information, access online medical information, and support their own education.

With the Internet at our fingertips these days, there is a wealth of knowledge waiting to be obtained. PubMed is always available for finding articles related to your desired topics. Having our urology colleagues give the OR department a refresher on tips and tricks to placing a Foley may not be a bad idea, as well.

Interpersonal and communication skills

Residents must be able to demonstrate interpersonal and communication skills that result in effective information exchange and teaming with patients, their patients' families, and professional associates.

> Create and sustain a therapeutic and ethically sound relationship with patients.

This should have been done during the preoperative visit, and again that morning, prior to entering the OR. Make sure that all questions are answered and everyone is on the same page. Also, make sure you look and act professional, and that includes being on time.

> Use effective listening skills and elicit and provide information using effective nonverbal, explanatory, questioning, and writing skills.

This was mentioned previously as part of developing a sound relationship with the patient. Listen to what the patient has to say and provide all explanations effectively using whatever methods work best for the patient. Hone your writing skills as you write your updated history and physical in the patient's chart as well as your possible plan for the case.

> Work effectively with others as a member or leader of a health care team or other professional group.

With no surgeon to be found, you as the anesthesiologist must take the lead in the OR. Communicate with those in the room and start to delegate responsibility to the other team members about a plan of action. One person should be calling for a urology consult, while another person should be continuing to contact the surgeon. If possible, a nurse or technician may start to look for alternative Foley catheters and prepare for suprapubic placement of a catheter, if necessary.

Systems-based practice

Residents must demonstrate an awareness of and responsiveness to the larger context and system of health care and the ability to effectively call on system resources to provide care that is of optimal value.

> Understand how their patient care and other professional practices affect other health care professionals, the health care organization, and the larger society and how these elements of the system affect their own practice.

Our current dilemma with the Foley may involve other services, such as urology, but should not affect the larger society per se. How we handle this situation may affect patients who face similar problems in the future and, it is hoped, affect them in a positive way as we determine the best course of action, having been through this once already.

> Practice cost-effective health care and resource allocation that does not compromise quality of care.

Cost-effective health care, at this point, may include not opening every Foley catheter that the OR has stocked and waiting for our urology associates to determine what they need and have those tools available.

> Advocate for quality patient care and assist patients in dealing with system complexities.

During the case, you can advocate for the least invasive but safest method for placement of the Foley catheter, but if you called a urology consult for expert advice, it would probably be smart to follow that advice. There are not a great deal of complexities in the system about Foleys.

> Know how to partner with health care managers and health care providers to assess, coordinate, and improve health care and know how these activities can affect system performance.

This can be done once the case is completed. A multidisciplinary team of nurses and physicians can sit down to determine the best way to prevent trauma during difficult Foley placements and what do to in the event of such an event in the middle of an OR case. Our urology colleagues can also, at that time, give us a refresher on the anatomy and proper technique of placing a Foley catheter to help improve the outcomes of future placements and reduce cost from lost OR time as well as complications.

Additional reading

1. Chavez AH, Reilly TP, Bird ET. Vena cava air embolism after traumatic Foley catheter placement. Urology 2009;73(4):748–749.

2. Kashefi C, Messer K, Barden R, Sexton C, Parsons JK. Incidence and prevention of iatrogenic urethral injuries. J Urol 2008;179:2254–2257; discussion 2257–2258.

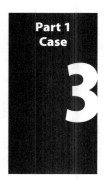

Contributions from Stony Brook University under Christopher J. Gallagher

3 Bad airway in the Andes

Christopher J. Gallagher and Khoa Nguyen

The case

"They don't have electricity up there, in the mountains," the plastic surgeon told me. "It's all oil lamps. Kerosene. And then the kids, you know, they're crawling around, pulling on things, so they pull on the blanket that's hanging down, and everything comes down on them. The lamp, too. That's how they get burned."

And did they get burned. Maria Luisa was the worst of all.

"But the scarring?" I asked. "We get burns in America all the time, but you don't see scarring like this."

"No," the surgeon said, "you don't."

Maria Luisa's lip was fused to her chest, her 13-year-old head bent straight down, forcing her to be forever straining her eyes upward to see forward. Drool ran down her chest. She dabbed at it every few minutes.

Maria Luisa looked up/forward at us. With her lip fused to her chest, she was in the exact *wrong* position for placing the endotracheal tube. And we were standing in Loja, Ecuador, high in the Andes, at a small hospital. They didn't have any fiber-optic equipment here. How was I going to get that tube in?

Patient care

Residents must be able to provide patient care that is compassionate, appropriate, and effective for the treatment of health problems and the promotion of health.

Communicate effectively and demonstrate caring and respectful behaviors when interacting with patients and their families.

This is an extremely important issue, especially when dealing with a difficult situation in a foreign country. First, if one does not speak Spanish (or the local language) fluently, then make sure that someone who does is in the room to translate. As a part of being respectful and caring, every effort should be

made to make sure the patient and her family understand everything that is being discussed. Make sure to answer all questions asked by the patient and family after listening to all their concerns. Having a local translate may also be helpful in that he or she could give you an idea of what may be considered appropriate and disrespectful behavior in this region of the world, as I am sure that there are differences between this region and the United States.

Gather essential and accurate information about their patients.

As accurately as possible, get a detailed history from the patient and her family regarding the injury and her general state of health. Make sure a full physical exam is done to best determine physical health, but obvious attention should be placed on the head and chest exam, considering that that is our area of expertise.

Make informed decisions about diagnostic and therapeutic interventions based on patient information and preferences, up-to-date scientific evidence, and clinical judgment.

Considering the obvious limitations due to lack of resources in our current location and the severity of her injuries, the patient and her family should be given a detailed explanation of all the risks, benefits, and alternatives to make the best informed decision they can about the upcoming surgery. The glaring risk for her surgery is loss of her airway, as she would be considered a "difficult airway" in my book. Regional anesthesia is definitely not an option here. Do we have any equipment to aid in obtaining the airway? Is the surgeon prepared to perform an emergency surgical airway maneuver? In addition, if and when we secure the airway, what if we cannot extubate? Can the facility handle such a patient postoperatively? Laryngeal mask airways seem to work well in these types of patients, per our colleagues in India and the Middle East, as their case reports seem to show, though some imagination is required for their placement. If none of the necessary tools that may be required are at our disposal, then would postponing this case and transferring her to a larger, more well-equipped facility that can handle her delicate situation be a better choice?

Develop and carry out patient management plans.

The patient and the family are desperate and do not have the means to travel to another hospital, so we are moving forward here. Luckily, we have brought variously sized laryngeal mask airways (LMAs), endotracheal tubes (ETs), and stylets. The patient is topicalized with 1% lidocaine, which we happened to have, through a syringe attached to a 20-gauge angiocatheter. She can barely open her mouth, but there is enough wiggle room for us to work. We induce with some inhaled halothane from the local anesthesia machine and then hold our breaths as we try to secure the airway. She is spontaneously breathing well, so minimal assistance is required for mask ventilation.

Counsel and educate patients and their families.

The patient and her family are made aware of our concerns regarding her surgery, and all questions are answered as thoroughly as possible with the help of our trusty translator.

Use information technology to support patient care decisions and patient education.

Not many people in the Andes have Internet capabilities, including the hospital, so information technology is not so helpful here.

Perform competently all medical and invasive procedures considered essential for the area of practice.

Place all available monitors that we have (our portable pulse oximeter, electrocardiogram machine, and blood pressure cuff) and obtain intravenous access in the event that trouble finds us.

Work with health care professionals, including those from other disciplines, to provide patient-focused care.

Make sure that the plastic surgeon is in the room at all times if a surgical airway is required. The rest of your staff in the operating room (OR) should also be observant of what is transpiring to be ready to jump into action at the drop of a hat.

Medical knowledge

Residents must demonstrate knowledge about established and evolving biomedical, clinical, and cognate (e.g., epidemiological and social-behavioral) sciences and the application of this knowledge to patient care.

Demonstrate an investigatory and analytic thinking approach to clinical situations.

You knew things were bad as soon as you saw the patient, and immediately, you went into difficult airway mode. The first thing that came to mind was awake fiber optics, but that is just not an option, especially when you do not have a fiber-optic scope handy. You performed a thorough history, and after speaking to the surgeon, you made the patient and her family aware of the situation. Using the resources available, you made the best plan you could to secure the airway.

Know and apply the basic and clinically supportive sciences that are appropriate to their discipline.

The difficult airway algorithm runs through your head over and over, and you regret not buying that handheld fiber-optic scope you saw on eBay. Nonetheless, you adhere as closely to the algorithm as possible with what you have, and fortunately, it works.

Practice-based learning and improvement

Residents must be able to investigate and evaluate their patient care practices, appraise and assimilate scientific evidence, and improve their patient care practices.

Analyze practice experience and perform practice-based improvement activities using a systematic methodology.

Not often are you put in a situation in which you have such an unusually difficult airway with no real equipment, as in this case, so this is the perfect time to analyze the experience. If you plan to travel to exotic destinations and perform anesthesia on any patient that may come, then consider investing in a small arsenal of equipment such as portable fiber-optic scopes, intubating LMAs, and other such emergency devices. Do some research into the area of travel to learn more about the health care system and the larger hospitals in the area, if needed, to better acquaint yourself with what you're getting yourself into.

> Locate, appraise, and assimilate evidence from scientific studies related to their patients' health problems.

Not a great many studies exist on cases, but it is always helpful to read case studies on how others obtained the airway and performed anesthesia on such difficult cases.

> Use information technology to manage information, access online medical information, and support their own education.

After returning from the trip, make an effort to write up the case with all the details and cross reference them with the current case reports. The more information we have on a subject, the better, as these case reports may give someone an idea in the future about how to handle a difficult airway in a remote area.

Professionalism

Residents must demonstrate a commitment to carrying out professional responsibilities, adherence to ethical principles, and sensitivity to a diverse patient population.

> Demonstrate respect, compassion, and integrity; a responsiveness to the needs of patients and society that supersedes self-interest; accountability to patients, society, and the profession; and a commitment to excellence and ongoing professional development.

Demonstrate respect, compassion, and integrity by being honest about the whole situation, providing a translator to make sure the patient and her family fully understand all that was discussed, and provide the best care that you can with the available instruments.

> Demonstrate a commitment to ethical principles pertaining to provision or withholding of clinical care, confidentiality of patient information, informed consent, and business practice.

You obtained informed consent prior to the operation and confirmed the site with your eyes. Confidentiality is not really possible as everyone in the village knows that Maria is going to surgery, but keeping the details of the operation private may provide some level of privacy.

> Demonstrate sensitivity and responsiveness to patients' culture, age, gender, and disabilities.

You made sure that you asked the translator several times what not to do so that you would not offend the people of region. You tried your best to make Maria feel comfortable, even though she was severely deformed, by looking her in the eyes when you spoke to her and even offering to dab the saliva from her chest.

Interpersonal and communication skills

Residents must be able to demonstrate interpersonal and communication skills that result in effective information exchange and teaming with patients, their patients' families, and professional associates.

> Create and sustain a therapeutic and ethically sound relationship with patients.

This was addressed earlier with a local translator, as we made sure that the patient and her family fully understood everything that was involved in the case. Part of sustaining a sound relationship entails obtaining the patient's trust, which we do by answering all her questions as honestly and compassionately as possible.

> Use effective listening skills and elicit and provide information using effective nonverbal, explanatory, questioning, and writing skills.

Having the local translator there is the most effective skill we have. We make sure to listen attentively as the patient, her family, and the translator speak, although we can only catch bits and pieces of their mile-a-minute Spanish. Then we listen attentively again as the translator explains the answers in English.

> Work effectively with others as a member or leader of a health care team or other professional group.

As the anesthesiologist, you make the effort to be a team leader in the OR. Coordinating duties between surgeons, nurses, and aids in the OR is no easy task, but you do what is necessary for the patient, especially one with special needs.

Systems-based practice

Residents must demonstrate an awareness of and responsiveness to the larger context and system of health care and the ability to effectively call on system resources to provide care that is of optimal value.

Understand how their patient care and other professional practices affect other health care professionals, the health care organization, and the larger society and how these elements of the system affect their own practice.

Our actions in a foreign country represent those of our home country, so we must act and perform to best represent our superb training and ourselves. Having experiences like this under our belt helps us realize how fortunate we are to have the tools we do and gives us more knowledge to handle difficult situations with the tools at hand.

Practice cost-effective health care and resource allocation that does not compromise quality of care.

Not much choice here. We never compromise the quality of care we provide, but cost is not an issue as we don't have many options to choose from.

Advocate for quality patient care and assist patients in dealing with system complexities.

If we can teach the local physicians how to use their present tools more effectively and introduce them to new tools in anesthesia, we can advocate for better quality patient care and thus assist the most important piece of the health care system: the patients.

Additional reading

1. Rutledge C. Difficult mask ventilation in 5-year-old due to submental hypertrophic scar: a case report. AANA J 2008;76:1778.

2. Khan RM, Verma V, Bhradwaj A, et al. Difficult laryngeal mask airway placement in a pediatric-burned patient: a new solution to an old problem. Paediatr Anaesth 2006;16:360–361.

3. Karam R, Ibrahim G, Tohme H, Moukarzel Z, Raphael N. Severe neck burns and laryngeal mask airway for frequent general anesthetics. Middle East J Anesthesiol 1996;13:527–535.

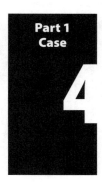

Contributions from Stony Brook University under Christopher J. Gallagher

4 Wedge is 18; he *must* be full

Christopher J. Gallagher and Dominick Coleman

The case

A 72-year-old vasculopath goes to the operating room (OR) for endovascular repair of a thoracoabdominal aortic aneurysm. At first, all seems well, the stent deploys in the OR, and the patient seems all better.

Alas, things take a turn. The stent causes a leak in the aorta and the patient bleeds like nobody's business, requiring a heroic trip back to and through the OR. Blood, factors, packing the abdomen, reexploration – the whole shooting match.

Now the patient is back in the intensive care unit (ICU), urine output is down, and someone has floated the almighty pulmonary artery (PA) catheter. Wedge is 18, and the renal service advises furosemide. "The wedge is 18; he *must* be full," they say.

A furosemide drip is started. The next day, the patient is started on continuous venovenous dialysis.

Patient care

Residents must be able to provide patient care that is compassionate, appropriate, and effective for the treatment of health problems and the promotion of health.

> Communicate effectively and demonstrate caring and respectful behaviors when interacting with patients and their families.

Assuming that the patient is intubated and the surgeon has communicated with the family the events in the OR, at this point, the family would need to be updated as to the current state of the patient, including concerns regarding the low urine output. It would be appropriate to explain why the patient is still intubated and answer the family's questions truthfully, without omission. This would likely involve answering questions about pain, death, and length of stay in the ICU.

> Gather essential and accurate information about their patients.

These include the vitals from the monitor, PA numbers, intravenous (IV) fluid/nutritionals or drips the patient may be on to maintain hemodynamic stability, and also output such as urine and drains. In addition, it would be important to know the hematocrit and coagulation status.

> Make informed decisions about diagnostic and therapeutic interventions based on patient information and preferences, up-to-date scientific evidence, and clinical judgment.

The patient is s/p (status post) endovascular aneurysm repair (EVAR) with hemorrhage from an aortic puncture, which was explored intraop and controlled. Although the patient was aggressively resuscitated with blood products and factors in the OR, intercompartmental fluid shifts would warrant ongoing resuscitation to ensure adequate perfusion. It would be necessary to monitor for ongoing bleeding and also be aware of the complications related to EVAR and also those related to the repair that was necessary to control the bleeding (e.g., were any vessels ligated that could lead to bowel ischemia?). Also, the patient is in renal failure, which is assumingly inadequately responsive to a lasix drip, thus requiring continuous veno venous hemodialysis (CVVHD).

> Develop and carry out patient management plans.

At minimal, a CVP would be necessary, along with appropriate colloid, crystalloid, and factor replacement. Fluid replacement would be guided by lab values, blood pressure, and urine output. Use of a PA catheter (PAC) in the acutely ill patient, as in this case, is useful for determining the CO, pulmonary filling pressures, and mixed venous O_2 saturation.

> Counsel and educate patients and their families.

As stated previously, honest and open discussions with the family regarding the patient's status are important to help minimize stress. They should be informed of the efforts being taken to get the patient better and also be made aware that there is a possibility that the patient may expire.

Use information technology to support patient care decisions and patient education.

At some point, the patient may need a computed tomography (CT) angiogram to assess the repair. Also, depending on kidney function, a renal ultrasound may be warranted in the future.

Perform competently all medical and invasive procedures considered essential for the area of practice.

A PAC was placed in this patient, which may not have been necessary; however, an arterial (CVP) line would be appropriate, as would an ALine.

Provide health care services aimed at preventing health problems or maintaining health.

Aseptic technique when placing all invasive lines is paramount. The patient should be on broad-spectrum IV antibiotics. It is important to perform frequent suctioning of the endotracheal tube (ETT) while on the ventilator and chest physical therapy (PT) as the chance for ventilator-associated pneumonia is high. Also, turning the patient at least every 2 hours would help with preventing decubitus ulcers, and placing sequential compression devices (SCDs) would ward off acute deep venous thromboses (DVTs) with resultant pulmonary embolus (PE).

Work with health care professionals, including those from other disciplines, to provide patient-focused care.

Efficient and appropriate consults are important. As in this case, the renal service was consulted due to low urine output and the appropriate management was implemented. However, consults are not golden, and so their recommendations should be factored into the equation. Their concern with the wedge of 18 is possibly inconsequential as the patient may be developing acute lung injury/acute respiratory distress syndrome (ALI/ARDS) due to the amount of transfusions and fluid replacement. Furthermore, questions regarding if or when to start IV anticoagulation would need to be answered by the surgeon.

Medical knowledge

Residents must demonstrate knowledge about established and evolving biomedical, clinical, and cognate (e.g., epidemiological and social-behavioral) sciences and the application of this knowledge to patient care.

Demonstrate an investigatory and analytic thinking approach to clinical situations.

Currently the patient is being treated for low urine output, which could be prerenal (low intravascular volume or blockage of one or both of the renal arteries by the graft), renal (acute tubular necrosis or ATN), or postrenal (kinked Foley). Also, there is concern regarding the elevated wedge of 18, which could be due to pulmonary (evolving ALI/ARDS) or cardiac causes (valvular disease). Knowing that the patient is a vasculopath almost always implies the presence of coronary artery disease (CAD), and possibly even cerebrovascular disease (CVD) and/or peripheral vascular disease (PVD). Therefore sustaining a myocardial infarction (MI) or stroke in the immediate future is a real possibility.

Know and apply the basic and clinically supportive sciences that are appropriate to their discipline.

The patient has sustained a hemorrhage requiring both crystalloid and colloid resuscitation. Being aware of the fluid shifts and hemodynamic changes and their consequences is important. The low urine output implies decreased perfusion of the kidneys but could also be the result of damage caused by the kidneys being hypoperfused previously. Giving diuretics intravenously on an as-needed basis or as an infusion should stimulate the kidneys to make urine, provided that perfusion is adequate. However, if there is significant damage, dialysis is necessary.

Wedge pressure is an indirect measure of left-side atrial pressure, normal being approximately 6–12. Elevation would be due to either a cardiac or pulmonary cause. When interpreting the data, understanding the Startling curve is helpful. A wedge of 18 may be present in someone who has had an MI or long-standing cardiac disease and needs a high wedge to maintain CO. In the absence of significant cardiac disease, the elevated wedge would be due to fluid overload or pulmonary pathology. When giving massive transfusions, it is important to remember the sequelae that can result, including fluid overload and/or ARDS.

Practice-based learning and improvement

Residents must be able to investigate and evaluate their patient care practices, appraise and assimilate scientific evidence, and improve their patient care practices.

Analyze practice experience and perform practice-based improvement activities using a systematic methodology.

With regard to improvements, the sentinel event in this case is a known complication related to the procedure. There should be a discussion at some point to determine what might have gone wrong to cause such a big leak. Was it a flaw with the equipment being used, or was it a technical error on the part of the surgeon?

Locate, appraise, and assimilate evidence from scientific studies related to their patients' health problems.

Abdominal aortic aneurysms (AAAs) can be repaired either open (i.e., laparotomy) or endovascularly. Patients are selected for EVAR based on various factors, including body habitus, anatomy of the AAA, and comorbidities. It is known that EVAR offers a slight survival benefit as it relates to the aneurysm itself; however, EVAR is associated with more complications than an open repair. These complications include having to reoperate for bleeding secondary to endoleaks around the stent. As with any major bleed, prompt resuscitation with crystalloid and blood products is key to maintain hemodynamics and adequate end-organ perfusion. The use of a central venous pressure (CVP) catheter or PA catheter to help assess adequacy of resuscitation is determined on an individual basis.

Obtain and use information about their own population of patients and the larger population from which their patients are drawn.

This is an elderly patient with vascular disease undergoing an AAA repair. One can assume that the patient has CAD and possibly some degree of renal insufficiency. Prior to going to the OR, the patient would have been medically optimized and assessed for appropriateness to undergo an EVAR procedure.

Apply knowledge of study designs and statistical methods to the appraisal of clinical studies and other information on diagnostic and therapeutic effectiveness.

As stated, it is known that EVAR offers an aneurysm-related survival benefit over an open repair. One multicenter randomized control study (RCT) demonstrated this benefit to be approximately 3%. However, the postoperative complications for up to 4 years postprocedure were significantly higher with the EVAR group. Furthermore, there is no difference between EVAR and open as it relates to all-cause mortality.

Use information technology to manage information, access online medical information, and support their own education.

Familiarity with literature using such databases as PubMed is most beneficial when addressing issues such as those presented in this case. For a more comprehensive review of specific topics, information resources like UpToDate are helpful.

Professionalism

Residents must demonstrate a commitment to carrying out professional responsibilities, adherence to ethical principles, and sensitivity to a diverse patient population.

Demonstrate respect, compassion, and integrity; a responsiveness to the needs of patients and society that supersedes self-interest; accountability to patients, society, and the profession; and a commitment to excellence and ongoing professional development.

Respect and compassion, while caring for this and any other patient in the ICU, are important. When the patient is unable to communicate for himself or herself, at least one family member is usually available to inform the service of the patient's wishes, including whether the patient would not want blood products due to religious beliefs or personal preference. This would have also been addressed with the patient preoperatively as part of the informed consent. Also, depending on the patient's prognosis, at some point, there may need to be a discussion with the family about do not resuscitate/do not intubate (DNR/DNI) status.

Integrity would be demonstrated by ensuring that everything is being done for the patient, and by doing so in a timely fashion. For example, if a CT scan is scheduled but there are delays, going the extra step to discuss the matter with the CT tech to have the scan done faster would demonstrate integrity and commitment to the patient.

> Demonstrate a commitment to ethical principles pertaining to provision or withholding of clinical care, confidentiality of patient information, informed consent, and business practice.

Again, discussion of care-related issues with the family of an intubated patient is usually done with a designated next of kin or health care proxy. It is important to be up front with any information that is known. At the same time, care for every patient should be optimal and not determined by social class, race, or ability to pay for the service. In addition, prior to the initial surgery, all patients should have informed consent regarding the procedure and its potential complications, including bleeding, infection, pain, and the need for additional surgery.

> Demonstrate sensitivity and responsiveness to patients' culture, age, gender, and disabilities.

An integral part of being professional is being able to deal with individuals from many different backgrounds with various beliefs and disabilities. Simply being dedicated to the patient and his or her well-being, without bias, fulfills this requirement.

Interpersonal and communication skills

Residents must be able to demonstrate interpersonal and communication skills that result in effective information exchange and teaming with patients, their patients' families, and professional associates.

> Create and sustain a therapeutic and ethically sound relationship with patients.

Developing a trustworthy relationship with the patient begins at the very first meeting; first impressions are lasting impressions. If the patient feels that you care, are approachable, and are open in your discussions with him or her, you will have effectively developed a sound relationship.

> Use effective listening skills and elicit and provide information using effective nonverbal, explanatory, questioning, and writing skills.

Allowing the patient to talk and ask questions is the best way to determine how much the patient understands about his or her condition, his or her beliefs related to health care in general, and his or her level of anxiety. Communicating effectively, both nonverbally and verbally, would be done by responding to any issues that may arise during the conversation. Again, this is building trust between you and the patient.

> Work effectively with others as a member or leader of a health care team or other professional group.

Working in the ICU implies work with a team, which includes doctors, nurses, social workers, a pharmacist, and a respiratory therapist. Effectively communicating within this multidisciplinary system optimizes care for the patient and thus again demonstrates integrity.

Systems-based practice

Residents must demonstrate an awareness of and responsiveness to the larger context and system of health care and the ability to effectively call on system resources to provide care that is of optimal value.

> Understand how their patient care and other professional practices affect other health care professionals, the health care organization, and the larger society and how these elements of the system affect their own practice.

The patient was taken to surgery for a minimally invasive procedure to repair an AAA and was taken back promptly for bleeding. In the recovery period, resuscitation with transfusions, while at the same time properly diagnosing and managing any other issues, such as low urine output or transfusion reactions, have implications for length of stay in the hospital. The same is true with regard to appropriately ordering diagnostic studies.

> Practice cost-effective health care and resource allocation that does not compromise quality of care.

Again, an example of this would be appropriately ordering diagnostic studies. Also, placing the PA catheter could compromise quality of care due to misinterpretation of the data gathered. Inappropriately bolusing the patient or starting pressors or vasodilators could lead to compromised care and also incur costs due to prolonged hospitalization and potential compounding complications.

> Advocate for quality patient care and assist patients in dealing with system complexities.

The multidisciplinary team approach in the ICU setting is set up to specifically deal with quality of care and also with helping the patient and his or her family deal with social issues in the hospital and at home. If a social worker is not involved, contacting the social work service and communicating with them throughout the patient's stay in the hospital is important. This would be useful especially if the patient has limited insurance but requires extensive and prolonged treatment. In addition, when the patient leaves, if there is a need for equipment in the home, working with the social services workers would ensure that these things are available.

> Know how to partner with health care managers and health care providers to assess, coordinate, and improve health care and know how these activities can affect system performance.

Again, communicating with the team members effectively, letting everyone know the plan for the day, and keeping abreast of any changes that may have occurred will help to optimize care. When everyone is informed and ideas are shared, the patient is better cared for and unforeseen problems are better managed.

A final word – I felt that they should have placed a transesophageal echocardiograph (TEE) to see if he really *was* overloaded at a wedge of 18. He may have been empty, with the wedge falsely elevated by the extensive abdominal packing.

I strongly advocated for the ICU to incorporate TEE into their evaluations rather than placing faith in the (ever controversial) PA catheter.

Additional reading

1. Barkhordarian S, Dardik A. Preoperative assessment and management to prevent complications during high-risk vascular surgery. Crit Care Med 2004; 32: S174–S185.

2. Ferguson ND, Meade MO, Hallett DC, Stewart TE. High values of pulmonary artery wedge pressure in patients with acute lung injury and acute respiratory distress syndrome. Intensive Care Med 2002;28: 1073–1077.

3. Greenhalgh RM, Brown LC, Epstein D, et al. Endovascular aneurysm repair versus open repair in patients with abdominal aortic aneurysm (EVAR trial 1): randomised controlled trial. Lancet 2005;365:2179–2186.

4. Vincent J-L, Pinsky MR, Sprung CL, et al. The pulmonary artery catheter: in medio virtus. Crit Care Med 2008;36:3093–3096.

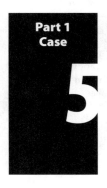

**Contributions from Stony Brook University under
Christopher J. Gallagher**

5 Calling across specialties

Christopher J. Gallagher and Kathleen Dubrow

The case

A 59-year-old woman is having a transhiatal esopha-gectomy. She suffers from malnutrition (she has not been able to eat well for many months), chronic obstructive pulmonary disease (COPD), and coronary artery disease (CAD). The general surgeon is having a hard time during the reach-up part of the operation, and the anesthesiologist must remind him several times that he is compressing the mediastinum and forcing the blood pressure down.

A distinct "oops" is heard coming from his lips as he tries to wedge free the esophagus way up by the neck. Bright blood is seen filling up the neck, and the blood pressure drops to the 50s.

Patient care

Residents must be able to provide patient care that is compassionate, appropriate, and effective for the treatment of health problems and the promotion of health.

> Communicate effectively and demonstrate caring and respectful behaviors when interacting with patients and their families.

When evaluating this patient preoperatively, we can show caring and respect by explaining the anesthesia management in terms that the patient can understand and by answering any questions that the patient or family member may have. As anesthesiologists, we should continue this behavior in the postoperative period, as well. During this particular situation, we would not have any family members around, but an anesthetized patient who has become acutely critical needs our quick attention.

> Gather essential and accurate information about their patients.

This patient needs quick action to attempt to reach the best possible outcome. The anesthesiologist needs to quickly check all the monitors and recycle the manual blood pressure cuff. If an arterial line is in place, then double-check the transducer location. This patient will likely need blood; ask the nurse in the room to make sure that this patient has a current type and cross and to get cross-matched blood in the room as soon as possible.

> Make informed decisions about diagnostic and therapeutic interventions based on patient information and preferences, up-to-date scientific evidence, and clinical judgment.

It is likely that the surgeon has avulsed or ruptured an artery (descending aorta?) while manipulating the esophagus. This patient is becoming hypovolemic from the rapid blood loss, and the anesthesiologist needs to hang blood on the patient as soon as possible. While waiting for the blood, the patient needs to be given crystalloid/colloid for fluid replacement. If necessary, further intravenous (IV) access needs to be established, and supportive vasoactive medications need to be administered, if necessary. While the anesthesiologist is trying to save the patient, the surgeon, it is hoped, will be trying to stop the source of bleeding, and the circulating nurse will be calling the cardiothoracic surgeon for a sideline consult.

> Develop and carry out patient management plans.

The anesthesia team needs to hang blood, open up fluids, start an arterial line if one is not already in place, and obtain further peripheral and central IV access. All these things need to be done immediately and basically all at the same time. The anesthesia team may need to expand.

> Counsel and educate patients and their families.

At this point, it may be difficult to consider the patient's family. If and when the patient becomes more stable, a conversation could be held with the family regarding the patient's status. If the outcome is poor with this patient, the wishes of the patient and the family regarding end-of-life care, further resuscitation, and possible organ donation need consideration. Even if the patient and family were educated regarding all possible risks of the surgery prior to the procedure, a poor outcome will necessitate counsel and support from the surgical and anesthesia team.

Use information technology to support patient care decisions and patient education.

This patient may have computed tomography scans of the chest preoperatively that will show his or her anatomy. The use of ultrasound-guided line placement may be helpful.

Perform competently all medical and invasive procedures considered essential for the area of practice.

Given this patient's current critical condition, an arterial line and central line are a necessity. This patient needs multiple large bore IVs and possible Cordis placement. Conversation between the anesthesiologist and surgeon will need to take place because this patient is likely in the lateral position, which may make line placement extremely difficult. Cross-matched blood and fluids need to be run wide open in this patient. The use of a rapid fluid infuser would be very helpful.

Provide health care services aimed at preventing health problems or maintaining health.

In between checking and hanging blood, placing lines, and praying, the anesthesiologist should ask the circulating nurse to page the primary care doctor stat to find out when this patient last had the flu shot and his most recent colonoscopy. (Just kidding!)

Prior to this catastrophic event, antibiotics should be given prior to incision within an hour. Assessment of need and continuation of beta-blockers should also be established.

Work with health care professionals, including those from other disciplines, to provide patient-focused care.

This patient is in an extremely critical situation. To realize the best possible outcome for the patient, it will be absolutely necessary to have rapid and fluid teamwork between the anesthesia, surgical, and nursing personnel. Morbidity and mortality will be reduced if patient care is a team effort

Medical knowledge

Residents must demonstrate knowledge about established and evolving biomedical, clinical, and cognate (e.g., epidemiological and social-behavioral) sciences and the application of this knowledge to patient care.

Demonstrate an investigatory and analytic thinking approach to clinical situations.

In addition to acting quickly to improve the outcome for this patient, it is vital to determine the cause of this drastic change. The patient is having an esophagectomy, possibly likely secondary to cancer. While manipulating the esophagus, the surgeon likely ruptured or avulsed the aorta, which is obvious given the immediate rush of bright red blood and the dramatic drop in blood pressure.

Know and apply the basic and clinically supportive sciences that are appropriate to their discipline.

This patient is having this procedure likely because of esophageal cancer. Understanding a basic pathophysiology is helpful to an anesthesiologist in perioperative management. Esophagectomies performed for esophageal cancer are associated with increased morbidity and mortality.

Anesthetic considerations regarding a patient with esophageal cancer include the following:

- chronic alcohol use (increase MAC)
- liver disease (drug metabolism)
- significant smoking history (ventilatory difficulties, COPD)
- emaciation, malnutrition (decreased reserve, decreased preload and intravascular volume, hemodynamic instability)

Knowledge of these factors will help the anesthesiologist to better care for this specific patient. Perioperative problems may be prevented from an anesthesia perspective through anticipation and vigilance to patient care.

Practice-based learning and improvement

Residents must be able to investigate and evaluate their patient care practices, appraise and assimilate scientific evidence, and improve their patient care practices.

> Analyze practice experience and perform practice-based improvement activities using a systematic methodology.

An esophagectomy is an invasive surgery that must be performed by a well-trained surgeon. Even in clinical situations where every manipulation is done correctly by a world-class surgeon, complications or adverse outcomes may occur.

Regardless of the outcome for this unfortunate soul, a discussion should be held, possibly in the form of a mortality and morbidity conference. A conversation among a group of professionals in the surgical and anesthesia field may improve outcomes for future patients:

- What went wrong? How was it handled? Did all parties act accordingly? What could have been done differently? What will be done next time?
- Was there enough surgical exposure? Should cardiopulmonary bypass (CPB) have been more readily available?

> Locate, appraise, and assimilate evidence from scientific studies related to their patients' health problems.

What does the literature say about handling complications of esophagectomies? Esophagectomies are usually performed in a minimally invasive laparoscopic approach with possible conversion to a more invasive, open approach. Either approach may be effective in achieving a successful anastomosis, but differences exist in postoperative outcomes.

> Obtain and use information about their own population of patients and the larger population from which their patients are drawn.

The anesthesiologist will provide better care to patients by being well read on esophagectomies, differences in surgical approaches, potential complications, and considerations of anesthetic management (laparoscopic vs. open, CPB, one-lung ventilation).

> Use information technology to manage information, access online medical information, and support their own education.

The torture of the Dewey Decimal System is over. Feel free to Google away, but be aware of inaccurate sources. Look for respectable medical journals and review articles for quick references.

Professionalism

Residents must demonstrate a commitment to carrying out professional responsibilities, adherence to ethical principles, and sensitivity to a diverse patient population.

> Demonstrate respect, compassion, and integrity; a responsiveness to the needs of patients and society that supersedes self-interest; accountability to patients, society, and the profession; and a commitment to excellence and ongoing professional development.

Professionalism is the easy part. Respect and compassion were obvious with the preoperative discussion held with the patient and the patient's family. As physicians, we must act with integrity at all times by keeping the patient's safety and best interests in mind. Prepare accordingly for each case and show up ready to work and take care of each specific patient.

> Demonstrate a commitment to ethical principles pertaining to provision or withholding of clinical care, confidentiality of patient information, informed consent, and business practice.

Prior to surgery, as an anesthesiologist providing care to an anesthetized patient, it is our responsibility to make sure that the patient has been fully consented regarding risks, benefits, and alternatives to surgery. The patient also needs to be aware of potential blood loss and the need for blood products intraoperatively.

As part of the health care team, we need to respect confidentiality of patients. A simple act like placing the chart in the appropriate area is important. When talking to and examining patients, we should pull curtains and speak in appropriate tones to respect the privacy of patients.

> Demonstrate sensitivity and responsiveness to patients' culture, age, gender, and disabilities.

Patients come from all different backgrounds, and this must be considered in a preoperative evaluation of patients. Addressing patients as "Mr." or "Mrs." shows a great deal of respect. Maybe a female's religion prohibits men from seeing her exposed, and a different operative team may need to be assembled.

Showing respect to patients isn't just for health care professionals. Being respectful to people in general makes someone a good human being!

Interpersonal and communication skills

Residents must be able to demonstrate interpersonal and communication skills that result in effective information exchange and teaming with patients, their patients' families, and professional associates.

> Create and sustain a therapeutic and ethically sound relationship with patients.

Build a relationship with the patient during the preoperative evaluation and postoperative follow-up. Explain the procedure in terms the patient will understand. Let the patient know of possible complications and adverse outcomes, and discuss his or her wishes with the patient should extremely poor outcomes occur. As physicians, we need to both act and look the part. Looking professional and exuding confidence will help to instill confidence in their physicians in the patient. Showing up with rumpled, day-old scrubs and bleary eyes will not help treat preoperative anxiety.

> Use effective listening skills and elicit and provide information using effective nonverbal, explanatory, questioning, and writing skills.

Speak to patients and their families in a language that they can understand, including about all risks, benefits, alternatives to the surgery, and anesthetic management. This will need to be done with the cooperation of the surgeon. Proper documentation of these discussions should be made in the medical record. Invasive procedures with a high risk of morbidity and mortality need proper explanations to patients, and documentation reflects completeness of patient care.

> Work effectively with others as a member or leader of a health care team or other professional group.

When these critical events are happening with this patient, the operative team must act together quickly. The surgeon must control the bleeding; the anesthesiologist must treat hemodynamic instability; and nursing must be ready to run for supplies and make calls for help, make a crash cart available, and be ready to give report to the intensive care unit (ICU). The cardiothoracic surgeon and CPB team need to be immediately aware of this patient. The blood bank needs to be called to make available a full supply of blood products. If the patient is able to make it out of the operating room, then respiratory therapy should be available for ventilatory management. Pharmacy needs to know about this patient to make sure plenty of vasopressors are made available for inotropic support.

Systems-based practice

Residents must demonstrate an awareness of and responsiveness to the larger context and system of health care and the ability to effectively call on system resources to provide care that is of optimal value.

> Understand how their patient care and other professional practices affect other health care professionals, the health care organization, and the larger society and how these elements of the system affect their own practice.

This patient needs quick action to realize the best outcome. Despite best efforts by all parties involved, it is likely that this patient will go into hypovolemic shock, suffer cardiac arrest, and die. Once efforts become futile, and any possibility for a good quality of life no longer exists, resources should no longer be used for this patient. Blood products are a limited resource and will no longer benefit this patient. ICU care in hospitals is expensive and is sometimes used as a wasted resource.

> Practice cost-effective health care and resource allocation that does not compromise quality of care.

Every effort must be made to save this patient, using all the resources possible, until efforts become futile, which is extremely likely with this patient. Blood products, medical supplies, and ICU care should not be used on a patient who has undergone hours of CPR and hemodynamic instability. It is also possible to care for this acutely critical patient by practicing cost-effective anesthesia. Expensive anesthetic agents like Precedex for sedation wouldn't be indicated in this patient. It is likely that minimal anesthetic agents would be needed in a patient who is so unstable.

Advocate for quality patient care and assist patients in dealing with system complexities.

Prior to officially "calling" this patient, the family should be informed of the critical nature of the patient. CPR could be continued until the patient arrives in the ICU so that the family is able to see the patient prior to passing. Once the patient has died, the family will need assistance from the operative team and the hospital in handling the emotional aspect of the death as well as the administrative duties they will have prior to releasing their family member.

Know how to partner with health care managers and health care providers to assess, coordinate, and improve health care and know how these activities can affect system performance.

End-of-life issues will affect anesthesiologists working with critically ill patients. We should be familiar with our hospitals' policies and the methods for dealing with the death of a patient. This knowledge will help to expedite the process for the family and allow the grieving period to continue outside the hospital.

Additional reading

1.   Nguyen NT, Hinojosa MW, Smith BR, Chang KJ, Gray
      J, Hoyt D. Minimally invasive esophagectomy: lessons
      learned from 104 operations. Ann Surg
      2008;248:1081–1091.

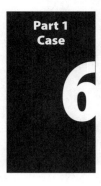

Part 1
Case

Contributions from Stony Brook University under Christopher J. Gallagher

6 Extubation wrecking a perfectly good Sunday

Christopher J. Gallagher and Eric Posner

The case

A great hue and cry arises from the neuro intensive care unit (ICU). A patient has summoned sufficient guff and moxie to extubate herself, in spite of a rich array of clinical and laboratory signs that such a move is detrimental to her health. Much to your dismay, on arrival at said neuro ICU, you see a note above her bed saying, "Extremely difficult intubation, took 1 hour with a fiber optic."

Respiratory therapy is mask ventilating the patient. You see the world's shortest chin and neck. You are alone in this setting as it's Sunday afternoon.

Patient care

Residents must be able to provide patient care that is compassionate, appropriate, and effective for the treatment of health problems and the promotion of health.

Communicate effectively and demonstrate caring and respectful behaviors when interacting with patients and their families.

Because of the urgency involved, it would be best to tell the family, if they are present, that this is an emergency and that their loved one needs to be reintubated immediately, and I would ask them to step out and then I will speak to them after.

Gather essential and accurate information about their patients.

The information that I need seems to be there. The writing is on the wall, literally.

Make informed decisions about diagnostic and therapeutic interventions based on patient information and preferences, up-to-date scientific evidence, and clinical judgment.

The patient needs to be intubated.

Develop and carry out patient management plans.

The plan would be to call for help from my colleagues and from surgery.

Counsel and educate patients and their families.

In this case, it would be best to speak to the family at length after the intubation is complete; however, I would briefly explain to them that their family member needs to be intubated and possibly may need a surgical airway.

Perform competently all medical and invasive procedures considered essential for the area of practice.

Wise counsel would indicate that the trachea is the intubation target of choice because the esophagus has done poorly in several attempts at being a respiratory organ.

Provide health care services aimed at preventing health problems or maintaining health.

This is not immediately applicable; however, restraints may be needed after the patient is intubated.

Work with health care professionals, including those from other disciplines, to provide patient-focused care.

In this case, I would need help from my anesthesia colleagues as well as surgeons and nursing and respiratory therapy.

Medical knowledge

Residents must demonstrate knowledge about established and evolving biomedical, clinical, and cognate (e.g., epidemiological and social-behavioral)

40

sciences and the application of this knowledge to patient care.

> Demonstrate an investigatory and analytic thinking approach to clinical situations.

As this is an emergency, I would need to quickly formulate a plan with the help of others and carry out that plan as safely as possible. If the patient's vital signs are stable, I would attempt to reintubate, with the surgeons standing by to perform a surgical airway.

Practice-based learning and improvement

Residents must be able to investigate and evaluate their patient care practices, appraise and assimilate scientific evidence, and improve their patient care practices.

> Analyze practice experience and perform practice-based improvement activities using a systematic methodology.

> I would use the difficult airway algorithm.

> Obtain and use information about their own population of patients and the larger population from which their patients are drawn.

This patient is of the difficult intubation population; therefore I would apply my knowledge of this and be prepared for what could be a very difficult situation.

Systems-based practice

Residents must demonstrate an awareness of and responsiveness to the larger context and system of health care and the ability to effectively call on system resources to provide care that is of optimal value.

> Practice cost-effective health care and resource allocation that does not compromise quality of care.

It would be cost-effective to intubate this patient as quickly as possible to prevent any further damage to the patient.

So you see, some cases require prolonged discussions of all the core clinical competencies. But others, such as this airway emergency, require only the briefest treatment of the competencies.

Additional reading

1. Williams WB, Jiang Y. Management of a difficult airway with direct ventilation through nasal airway without facemask. J Oral Maxillofac Surg 2009;67(11):2541–2543.

2. Djabatey EA, Barclay PM. Difficult and failed intubation in 3430 obstetric general anaesthetics. Anaesthesia 2009;64(11):1168–1171.

3. Huang YT. Factors leading to self-extubation of endotracheal tubes in the intensive care unit. Nurs Crit Care 2009;14(2):68–74.

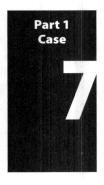

7

Contributions from Stony Brook University under Christopher J. Gallagher

The sin of pride after an awake intubation

Christopher J. Gallagher and Eric Posner

The case

A 320-pound man with an ego to match attempts to lift a 700-pound refrigerator. *Rrrrip*! His biceps tendon peels off its attachment to the bone and goes fip-fip-fip up his arm like an old window shade.

Clever you, you see that he will be a difficult intubation (thick, muscular neck; Mallampati class IV view; big teeth), so you do an awake intubation.

The case goes well, and now it's time to extubate. You do all the cautious stuff – sitting him up, making sure he's wide awake. You extubate, and within roughly 6 nanoseconds, you see that this was *not* the brightest idea of your life. He starts to obstruct, arterial saturation drops to the middle to low 80s, and his color looks less than reassuring. He has neither lost weight nor improved his airway since last you intubated him, which was approximately 2 hours ago.

Patient care

Residents must be able to provide patient care that is compassionate, appropriate, and effective for the treatment of health problems and the promotion of health.

Communicate effectively and demonstrate caring and respectful behaviors when interacting with patients and their families.

This is an emergency, and because there will be no family around, the best thing would be to reintubate this patient as quickly and safely as possible. When the patient is in the recovery room, I would then explain to the family members what is going on.

Gather essential and accurate information about their patients.

I already know that this patient is a difficult intubation.

Develop and carry out patient management plans.

The plan is to reintubate this patient.

Counsel and educate patients and their families.

After all is said and done, I would counsel the patient about his difficult intubation and that he should inform his anesthesiologists in the future about this problem.

Provide health care services aimed at preventing health problems or maintaining health.

To prevent future problems, I would counsel this patient to lose weight and also to keep his doctors informed about the fact that he is a difficult intubation.

Work with health care professionals, including those from other disciplines, to provide patient-focused care.

I would refer the patient to his primary care physician to get help losing weight.

Medical knowledge

Residents must demonstrate knowledge about established and evolving biomedical, clinical, and cognate (e.g., epidemiological and social-behavioral) sciences and the application of this knowledge to patient care.

Demonstrate an investigatory and analytic thinking approach to clinical situations.

This is a situation that would call for immediate action using the difficult airway algorithm.

Practice-based learning and improvement

Residents must be able to investigate and evaluate their patient care practices, appraise and assimilate scientific evidence, and improve their patient care practices.

43

Locate, appraise, and assimilate evidence from scientific studies related to their patients' health problems.

I would not be able to look up any studies for the immediate care of this patient, but I would be expected to be aware of the current literature regarding airway management.

Obtain and use information about their own population of patients and the larger population from which their patients are drawn.

This patient is obese and has a difficult airway, so I would draw on my knowledge of this population to treat this patient.

There! We've made the point twice. Brief cases with focused problems result in a brief brush on the core clinical competencies, no more.

Additional reading

1. Kheterpal S, Martin L, Shanks AM, Tremper KK. Prediction and outcomes of impossible mask ventilation: a review of 50,000 anesthetics. Anesthesiology 2009;110:891–897.

2. de Almeida MC, Pederneiras SG, Chiaroni S, de Souza L, Locks GF. Evaluation of tracheal intubation conditions in morbidly obese patients: a comparison of succinylcholine and rocuronium (in Spanish). Rev Esp Anestesiol Reanim 2009;56:3–8.

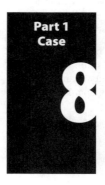

Contributions from Stony Brook University under
Christopher J. Gallagher

8 Brown-Sequard and the orthopedic knife extraction

Christopher J. Gallagher and Tommy Corrado

The case

Love is many things, earning the sobriquet "a many-splendored thing" among others. But Cupid's arrows may sometimes be *too* barbed, as one 32-year-old man learned too late.

Lover boy's lover took a steak knife in her right hand and registered her displeasure with events by burying this knife to the hilt, right in the middle of the man's back. Perfect precision was the order of the day, as she created a perfect Brown-Sequard syndrome.

The knife is still sticking out of his back, and he's going to the operating room (OR) for removal. He can't lie on his back, and angiography shows the knife inside the aorta, with the perfect position of the knife acting as a tamponade.

Patient care

Residents must be able to provide patient care that is compassionate, appropriate, and effective for the treatment of health problems and the promotion of health.

> Communicate effectively and demonstrate caring and respectful behaviors when interacting with patients and their families.

Effective communication may not be this gentleman's strong suit (the overwhelming majority of lovers' quarrels fortunately don't end up in a stabbing), but it's our duty to tactfully and efficiently gather as much information about this situation as possible. If the patient is awake and responsive, we can first reassure him that we will do everything we can to help him (he's probably having a pretty rough day as it is) and then get a quick history (allergies, last meal, medical conditions and medications, assess airway, etc.). If he came in accompanied by someone, it may be worthwhile talking to that person, as well (the same person who stuck him in the back may be the one who pushes his insulin every morning).

> Gather essential and accurate information about their patients.

A protracted and extensive medical and social history may seem contraindicated in the case of a patient who is having his intravascular volume maintained by a knife now acting as a wine cork. First and foremost, think the ABCs. Is he acutely stable (relatively) or unstable? Does he have an airway? Is he actively hemorrhaging buckets, or is his bleeding relatively controlled? Do we have good access, or are we working off a 22 Ga in the scalp? As mentioned before, if the patient is able to communicate, we can speak directly to him (while being mindful not to move or agitate him – stability is not this guy's strong suit). If not, we would like to hear from the trauma team that is caring for him and the emergency medical service (EMS) responders, and the results of the studies taken.

> Make informed decisions about diagnostic and therapeutic interventions based on patient information and preferences, up-to-date scientific evidence, and clinical judgment.

Now that we know what we can about this patient, we have to get him to the OR (this isn't a wait-and-see type of injury). The big hurdles we are looking at here are going to be smoothly securing the airway of a patient who cannot be moved and maintaining hemodynamic stability in a patient with a major vascular injury and an acute spinal cord injury.

> Develop and carry out patient management plans.

Like any good Boy Scout could tell you, being prepared is going to be key for this patient's survival. This means appropriate equipment, primary and ancillary services, and sufficient personnel. Blood bank should be made aware, with matched blood obtained, if available, and O negative, if necessary, as well as sufficient other products (fresh frozen plasma [FFP], platelets, factor VII, etc.). Ideally, we would like to be able to isolate the lungs to aid the surgeons, but all our plans need contingencies – a surgical airway if we fail; perfusionists ready for partial cardiopulmonary bypass (CPB), if necessary. Appropriate intensive care unit (ICU) care should be arranged for the patient to ensure the smooth transfer of care.

Counsel and educate patients and their families.

Acutely, the family should be made aware of the severity of the situation and should be provided with whatever support is available (e.g., a chaplain should be made available should they request one).

Use information technology to support patient care decisions and patient education.

While the time for an in-depth literature review is not at hand, information technology may still play a role. Many hospitals now have integrated computer systems, which allow the practitioner to view radiological studies, access old records, and so on. A quick look at the patient's angiogram and any other studies he may have had will certainly help direct anesthetic care.

Perform competently all medical and invasive procedures considered essential for the area of practice.

Now we have to use our clinical knowledge and skill. For all intents and purposes, we are living an oral boards stem. Airway issues will be paramount here. Not only can we not lay this guy on his back, but with any movement, we run the risk of him bucking and dislodging the knife that is, at present, holding the blood in him. While we are going to ensure that the patient is adequately anesthetized and will have a fiber optic ready, with support to help us use it, as well as rescue equipment (maybe intubating laryngeal mask airway (LMA), direct laryngoscope (DL) in a weird position in a pinch), we are also going to want surgery to have open and ready everything necessary to do an emergent tracheostomy or cricothyrotomy should the need arise. Apart from appropriate American Society of Anesthesiologists (ASA) monitors, we would need invasive monitoring such as ALine (both right arm and femoral monitoring would be nice to monitor perfusion pressures both above and below the aortic lesion) as well as central access for both fluids and medications. Perfusionists may want to prepare for partial CPB, if necessary. When the knife is finally

removed, we have to be ready for the inevitable change in hemodynamics (huge fluid shifts; the potential need for cross-clamping, requiring the use of sodium nitroprusside (SNP), nitroglycerin, or esmolol, as seen in aortic aneurysm repair, etc.).

Not only do we have to worry about the knife in the aorta, but we also have the spinal cord injury to worry about. While the loss of sensation contralateral and loss of motor function ipsilateral to and below the lesion in Brown-Sequard syndrome may not affect us much now, the possible decrease in spinal cord reflexes and the potential drop in SBP may complicate issues intraoperatively. Also, we have to be mindful of the likelihood of a growing hematoma in a patient at severe risk for coagulopathy.

Provide health care services aimed at preventing health problems or maintaining health.

Not only should we be aware of the immediate issues, but also, we should be thinking about optimizing long-term outcomes. Things like dosing and redosing of antibiotics, steroid administration for spinal cord injury, and maintaining euthermia all play a role in positive patient outcome.

Work with health care professionals, including those from other disciplines, to provide patient-focused care.

Eventually, this patient is going to have significant needs that may require the assistance of many different services (appropriate surgical follow-up, neurology and physical and occupational therapy for his neurological deficits, pain management issues, and psych and social work, to name a few).

Medical knowledge

Residents must demonstrate knowledge about established and evolving biomedical, clinical, and cognate (e.g., epidemiological and social-behavioral) sciences and the application of this knowledge to patient care.

Demonstrate an investigatory and analytic thinking approach to clinical situations.

In this very complicated case, it was extremely important to break things down into recognizable and manageable pieces that the resident had likely seen before. Understanding that airway management would be difficult and being prepared with knowledge of the difficult airway algorithm were key. Recognizing the similarity between this case and aortic dissection/rupture helped give direction to managing this patient from a hemodynamic perspective. Being aware that the spinal cord injury not only played an acute role in this patient's management, but also had the potential to worsen throughout the case helped the resident maintain focus on the entire patient, not just on the obvious and acute vascular wound.

Practice-based learning and improvement

Residents must be able to investigate and evaluate their patient care practices, appraise and assimilate scientific evidence, and improve their patient care practices.

> Analyze practice experience and perform practice-based improvement activities using a systematic methodology.

Like many traumas, there is less time for evaluation than action. After the case is done, however, a tremendous amount can be learned from it. An interdisciplinary debriefing would be hugely valuable. All too often, when a case is done, the team members line up to shake hands like a Little League baseball team and then retire to their respective dugouts. Taking the time to go over the critical events and reviewing, in a nonjudgmental way, what was done can help improve efficiency and safety. For example, points to address could include the following:

- What was done right: take note of things that were done properly, which facilitated the case. Was the OR notified ahead so they had sufficient equipment ready? Were appropriate team members present? Were adequate resources available?
- What could be improved: was the transfer of the patient efficient and thorough? Did anesthesia notify surgery of changes in patient status (trending changes in pressure, urine output [UO], etc.)? Did surgery notify anesthesia before any major interventions (cross-clamping, placing or removing shunts, etc.)? Was paper work properly filled out and returned? Was the patient adequately followed up by services other than primary services? For example, if the patient began to decompensate, were OR and anesthesia notified in advance about the possibility of a bring-back?

- If any adverse events took place, at what point did they occur? Where was there a deviation from the standard of care, if any, and what policies can be enacted to prevent a repeat of this deviation in the future?

> Locate, appraise, and assimilate evidence from scientific studies related to their patients' health problems.

As we mentioned before, this is no time for a literature search; rather, this looks like a case study waiting to be written up (not an M&M, it is hoped, should things go badly). It is possible, however, to extrapolate information from related cases and apply that knowledge where appropriate. Keeping up to date with the current recommendations for managing a ruptured aortic aneurysm, for example, would likely be applicable to the patient who has recently had his or her aorta redesigned at knifepoint.

A quick literature search after the case, when the details are still fresh, would be a great idea. Doing this would allow the resident to reevaluate what was done and possibly see how management of a similar case could be improved in the future.

> Obtain and use information about their own population of patients and the larger population from which their patients are drawn.

It's hard to think of a case for which this competency is more relevant. While it's unlikely that many people will see this exact case on a regular basis, the basic components are much more common. Major vascular injury (as a result either of trauma or aneurysm rupture), penetrating trauma, spinal cord injury (either total or partial), and difficult airway are all entities most practitioners have seen at some point in their careers. What is required here is the ability to extract relevant information about the care of each of these patients and combine it into a reasonable care plan for this case in particular.

> Apply knowledge of study designs and statistical methods to the appraisal of clinical studies and other information on diagnostic and therapeutic effectiveness.

Obviously, this sort of case doesn't lend itself to the randomized, prospective, double-blind study design. Individual case studies or retrospective analyses may be the only reasonable way to effectively evaluate this type of patient.

> Use information technology to manage information, access online medical information, and support their own education.

In the age of Medline, most people can string together enough Booleanisms to do a decent literature search, and this should certainly be the backbone of any significant clinical investigation. Other resources, however, can add some depth and perspective to a resident's education. Plugging a term into a search engine like Google is bound to return a host of places to begin to get information, as is doing a wiki search. While many of these sources aren't peer reviewed and their information may be flawed, they frequently have good references and can help focus your efforts. Many sites have message boards or forums, in which people post information about cases they have done and novel ways they approached various problems.

Professionalism

Residents must demonstrate a commitment to carrying out professional responsibilities, adherence to ethical principles, and sensitivity to a diverse patient population.

> Demonstrate a commitment to ethical principles pertaining to provision or withholding of clinical care, confidentiality of patient information, informed consent, and business practice.

This is likely the case everyone is going to want to talk about. When everyone has finally scrubbed out, you'll want to tell a coresident and the nurses and maintenance and that nice lady in the cafeteria and…Long story short: while there is definitely validity to discussing a case for the sake of education, sensitivity for the patient and his family and loved ones is as much our responsibility as placing a tube. Patient information should never be discussed in a public place (the elevator opens more mouths than Mac and Miller combined), and identifiers like names or dates of birth shouldn't be included when referring to the case for educational purposes.

> Demonstrate sensitivity and responsiveness to patients' culture, age, gender, and disabilities.

Sensitivity can be an issue in such an acute case, but there are still a few things we can do to soften the situation a little. While chaos tends to follow this type of case, and a whirlwind of people are going to be surrounding the patient, we can still do our best to maintain some semblance of modesty. This can include simple measures like closing curtains and moving bystanders along. (The same people who stop to look at a car crash will want to watch something like this. If they aren't involved in the care of the patient, they have no place in the immediate area.)

Interpersonal and communication skills

Residents must be able to demonstrate interpersonal and communication skills that result in effective information exchange and teaming with patients, their patients' families, and professional associates.

> Create and sustain a therapeutic and ethically sound relationship with patients.

"I am going to put you to sleep so they can take the knife out of your spine and the giant vessel coming out of your heart" establishes a relationship pretty damn fast. In reality, though, it's the role of the anesthesiologist to be a reassuring and calming presence in what has the potential to be pandemonium.

> Use effective listening skills and elicit and provide information using effective nonverbal, explanatory, questioning, and writing skills.

A case like this invariably has a great deal of information flying around, and therefore the potential exists for any number of mistakes. Properly checking blood products and medications helps prevent potentially devastating errors. While in the heat of a trauma paper work seems tertiary at best, the OR record is a valuable tool for patient care. Trending vitals and noting times and types of blood products, medications and fluids given, and lab results like arterial blood gases (ABGs) can help guide patient care intraoperatively. Also, should the case be reviewed at a later date, anything written (or not written) in the chart can have huge medical and legal implications.

> Work effectively with others as a member or leader of a health care team or other professional group.

Communication with all members of the health care team cannot be overemphasized. Roles may change during the course of care, and the smooth transition of power and communication are paramount.

49

Initially, EMS will come in with the patient and hand off responsibility to the trauma team. A team leader should be recognized, and each member's role should be well defined. As the case progresses, the anesthesia team will likely assume leadership as the patient is anesthetized in the OR. When the patient is stable, the trauma surgeon assumes control of the patient. While this is an oversimplification, constant and clear communication is important. In a trauma such as this, things should be structured but fluid enough to accommodate any changes that occur. Coordination with resources out of the OR (blood bank, chemistry lab, ICU) is also the role of the team leaders.

Systems-based practice

Residents must demonstrate an awareness of and responsiveness to the larger context and system of health care and the ability to effectively call on system resources to provide care that is of optimal value.

> Understand how their patient care and other professional practices affect other health care professionals, the health care organization, and the larger society and how these elements of the system affect their own practice.

This patient definitely had a significant, life-changing event. Goals for this patient should not focus only on his physical well-being. Not only do we want to see him reach a state of optimal function, but we also want to see him return to a productive role in society. Support is going to be necessary after his hospital stay, and access to those resources should be provided as soon as possible.

> Practice cost-effective health care and resource allocation that does not compromise quality of care.

If asked what they find most rewarding about their job, most physicians would rank taking care of patients far above efficiently utilizing resources in an economically sound manner. That being said, it's a grim reality that even medicine is subject to the limits of the bottom line. There are a number of things the anesthesiologist can do to operate in a more cost-effective manner. Using less expensive agents, not opening up equipment or drawing up drugs unless they are going to be used, and disposing of only sharps in sharps containers save significant amounts of money over time. Judicious use of blood products saves not only money, but also a very limited resource. The smooth transfer of patient care not only improves safety, but also more efficiently utilizes manpower and time.

> Advocate for quality patient care and assist patients in dealing with system complexities.

After his surgery is complete, this poor guy still has a world of obstacles ahead of him. Assuming no major complications from the surgery itself, this person with Brown-Sequard syndrome will have to learn to cope with his new neurological impairment. For a 32-year-old, this means not only loss of function, but possibly also loss of employment and social and psychological issues (let's not forget that a good piece of his support structure just planted a knife in him like she was raising a flag on Everest). Getting him in touch with social work as early as possible will help him gain access to the resources necessary to help him regain and redefine a meaningful existence.

Additional reading

1. Jonker Frederik HW, Schlösser Felix JV, Moll Frans L, Muhs Bart E. Dissection of the abdominal aorta: current evidence and implications for treatment strategies: a review and meta-analysis of 92 patients. J Endovasc Ther 2009;16:71–80.

2. Harris P. Stab wound of the back causing an acute subdural haematoma and a Brown-Sequard neurological syndrome. Spinal Cord 2005;43:678–679.

3. Simsek O, Kilincer C, Sunar H, et al. Surgical management of combined stab injury of the spinal cord and the aorta – case report. Neurol Med Chir (Tokyo) 2004;44:263–265.

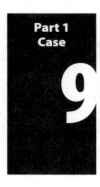

Contributions from Stony Brook University under Christopher J. Gallagher

9 *When* were those stents placed?

Christopher J. Gallagher and Matthew Neal

The case

A 65-year-old man has leukoplakia on his vocal cords. One of your hospital's top referral bases (this ear-nose-throat [ENT] doctor brings bazillions into the hospital, and people come from far and wide for her expertise) schedules him for a vocal cord biopsy tomorrow.

You get the nod because you're a heart guy, and this guy has "a little heart problem."

"Yes?" you ask, ever curious.

"He had two eluting stents placed two days ago, but the cardiologist says his vessels are fine now. They're stented open, after all!" The ENT surgeon, who doesn't like to hear no for an answer, says, "I gave the cardiologist your cell phone number to talk to you, in case you get the heeby-jeebies. Have a nice day."

Patient care

Residents must be able to provide patient care that is compassionate, appropriate, and effective for the treatment of health problems and the promotion of health.

Communicate effectively and demonstrate caring and respectful behaviors when interacting with patients and their families.

In this case, the patient needs to be brought into the loop. Even if the patient doesn't connect the dots between anticoagulation (i.e., aspirin and Plavix) and electively cutting on the airway, you, as a responsible health care provider, are obligated to connect the dots for him. Effective communication with the patient includes explaining the benefits as well as the risks of the proposed procedure. That being said, the situation needs to be handled tactfully; don't open with something like "Sir, I've met a lot of jackasses in my day, but that surgeon of yours sure takes the cake." You need to find a way to explain the situation to the patient without alarming him and without throwing the surgeon underneath the bus. A better opening line might be "Sir, I understand that you recently had a procedure

on your heart, and we need to discuss the implications of this on your surgery today."

Gather essential and accurate information about their patients.

When a case is taking longer than you planned and the surgeon looks up and says, "I should be done in about 30 minutes," it is usually safe to assume that you aren't going anywhere for at least an hour, probably more like an hour and a half. No anesthesiologist I know takes a surgeon at his word on something as benign as op time, so why would we take them at their words on something as important as the patency (or lack thereof) of a coronary or two? Patient care dictates that you gather a little more information. You should get the patient's records from cardiology, for instance, a cath report. Sure, the coronaries are stented open now, but oops … the ejection fraction is only 15%. It is amazing how many fun surprises you can uncover by digging into the patient's chart, instead of just reading "medically cleared for surgery" off a prescription pad and calling it a day.

The other important piece of information that is missing is why the patient went for cath 2 days ago. Was it a routine follow-up, was it a failed stress test, or is the patient now 2 days out from an acute myocardial infarction (MI)? These are all things you may want to find out about. If the patient had an MI in the last few days, he is at risk for having another MI in the perioperative period.

Make informed decisions about diagnostic and therapeutic interventions based on patient information and preferences, up-to-date scientific evidence, and clinical judgment.

Elective surgery should be postponed for a minimum of 12 months after placement of drug-eluting stents, though exact guidelines for eluting stents are tough to nail down. Even if the patient had a bare metal stent, the procedure should be postponed for a least 6 weeks – not 2 days [2]. Even if the surgeon is willing to operate on a patient who remains on antiplatelet therapy, the perioperative period induces a hypercoagulable state, which makes the risk of stent thrombosis unacceptable. You should be prepared to integrate these facts into your decision-making process when determining whether to go forward with the case.

Counsel and educate patients and their families.

This goes back to knowing the risks and benefits. To properly counsel the patient, you need to know this stuff like the back of your hand. Maybe the reason the surgeon is so gung ho to go ahead is because she doesn't really understand the risks either. This could present a golden opportunity not only to educate your patient, but also to educate one of your surgical colleagues.

Work with health care professionals, including those from other disciplines, to provide patient-focused care.

A phone call and/or face-to-face chat with the surgeon is in order here. It is better to discuss the risks of going ahead with the surgery beforehand than it is to discuss what the hell just happened after you had to shock the patient back to life and send him back to the cath lab for the second time in 3 days. It should also be noted that timing is pretty important here. You should have this conversation in the holding area, not in the operating room (OR), after the patient is strapped to the table or, God forbid, already asleep.

Medical knowledge

Residents must demonstrate knowledge about established and evolving biomedical, clinical, and cognate (e.g., epidemiological and social-behavioral) sciences and the application of this knowledge to patient care.

Demonstrate an investigatory and analytic thinking approach to clinical situations.

Investigate further. Look at the cath report; call the cardiologist. After you have gathered some information, analyze it. What are the benefits of this procedure, and what are the potential risks? With this information, you can decide on the best approach going forward.

Know and apply the basic and clinically supportive sciences that are appropriate to their discipline.

The key issue here is the drug-eluting stents. You need to know that a minimum of 1 year of antiplatelet therapy is recommended after placement of a drug-eluting stent [2]. You also need to know the risks of bleeding if this procedure is performed with the patient 2 days out from his Plavix load.

Practice-based learning and improvement

Residents must be able to investigate and evaluate their patient care practices, appraise and assimilate scientific evidence, and improve their patient care practices.

Locate, appraise, and assimilate evidence from scientific studies related to their patients' health problems.

If you want the surgeon to change her plans, it will probably help if you back up your request with something more substantial than your own opinion. A 5-minute PubMed search for the terms "eluting stent" and "elective surgery" will probably yield the evidence you need. You could also consult a textbook or a more highly regarded colleague – every department has a couple of those.

Professionalism

Residents must demonstrate a commitment to carrying out professional responsibilities, adherence to ethical principles, and sensitivity to a diverse patient population.

Demonstrate respect, compassion, and integrity; a responsiveness to the needs of patients and society that supersedes self-interest; accountability to patients, society, and the profession; and a commitment to excellence and ongoing professional development.

Throw out your own ego and remember that your responsibility is to the patient, not to yourself. If you are having a disagreement with a surgeon, don't take it personally; you should simply think about the implications for the patient. This will help you keep a cool head while dealing with your colleague on the other side of the ether screen.

Demonstrate a commitment to ethical principles pertaining to provision or withholding of clinical care, confidentiality of patient information, informed consent, and business practice.

This is the time to bring the patient into the loop. With the cooperation of surgery, you should explain all the risks and benefits of the procedure in terms the patient can easily understand. If the patient has family members at the bedside, you should always ask permission before discussing sensitive medical issues in front of them.

By involving the patient and his family in the decision-making process, you can ensure that everyone has the patient's best interests at heart. Even if you risk angering a surgeon who brings in a lot of business, the professional thing to do is to involve the patient in the process.

Interpersonal and communication skills

Residents must be able to demonstrate interpersonal and communication skills that result in effective information exchange and teaming with patients, their patients' families, and professional associates.

Use effective listening skills and elicit and provide information using effective nonverbal, explanatory, questioning, and writing skills.

After you speak your peace to the patient, take time to listen to the patient's questions and concerns. Communication does not begin and end with you. If the patient wants references, give him references. If he thinks he will have trouble remembering, then write it down for him. By taking just a few minutes to focus on the patient and his concerns, you can drastically improve your relationship with him.

Systems-based practice

Residents must demonstrate an awareness of and responsiveness to the larger context and system of health care and the ability to effectively call on system resources to provide care that is of optimal value.

Understand how their patient care and other professional practices affect other health care professionals, the health care organization, and the larger society and how these elements of the system affect their own practice.

This is where you must consider the implications of a disagreement with the surgeon. Ticking off a major source of revenue for your hospital could have negative consequences for you and your department. It really comes back to professionalism. You have to gather your evidence and figure out a way to approach the conflict in a professional manner so that nobody's feelings get hurt and the OR can remain a happy and productive workplace. Remember that without the surgeons, you don't have a job; nobody comes into the hospital to get anesthesia just to catch up on his or her sleep.

Practice cost-effective health care and resource allocation that does not compromise quality of care.

Cost-effective health care includes avoidance of unnecessary tests and procedures. In this case, you already have all the information you need to determine the patient's cardiac status, and there is no need for further testing. In other words, if you have a 2-day-old cath report, don't send the patient for an echo. It is amazing how often we order a test without really stopping to think about whether we really need it. A prime example of this is the daily complete blood count and electrolyte panel. If it has been normal 6 days in a row, why order it every day?

An easy way out of the situation for you would be to postpone the case for further testing – maybe you can even postpone it until you are postcall and it becomes someone else's problem. This will probably add costs, and nothing else, to the patient's care. If you have the information you need to make a decision, then make a decision. Don't just pass the buck.

Additional reading

1. Rabbitts JA, Nuttall G, Brown M, et al. Cardiac risk of noncardiac surgery after percutaneous coronary intervention with drug-eluting stents. Anesthesiology 2008;109:596–604.

2. Nuttall GA, Brown M, Stombaugh J, et al. Time and cardiac risk of surgery after bare-metal stent percutaneous coronary intervention. Anesthesiology 2008;109:588–595.

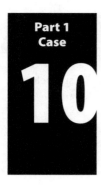

Contributions from Stony Brook University under Christopher J. Gallagher

10 Flame on!

Christopher J. Gallagher and Matthew Neal

The case

A smell like barbeque fills the entire emergency room. "Funny," you think, "no one told me there was a picnic." You note that the smell is coming from the trauma bay, and you go there as a code T (trauma) is called overhead.

Inside, a man is stripped completely bare of his skin and hair. An industrial accident has left him burned over 100% of his body, yet he is talking, coherent, complains only of feeling cool, and has no pain.

"Give him morphine," the resident tells you. "We got an IV in him so just keep giving him morphine."

You ask if you're going to intubate or what exactly the plan is.

"Morphine," the resident tells you again. "That's the plan, you follow me? He's a goner."

Patient care

Residents must be able to provide patient care that is compassionate, appropriate, and effective for the treatment of health problems and the promotion of health.

Communicate effectively and demonstrate caring and respectful behaviors when interacting with patients and their families.

This is based on a real case, believe it or not. No one could find any family members for this patient, and he was eerily and creepily awake and alert for about the first half hour I was with him. Given the extent of his injuries, it was downright *Twilight Zone*–esque that he was so with it, so I had to give it to him straight.

This event is among my most memorable experiences of a lifetime, and I will take this one with me until it's time for *me* to get some morphine. (Now to go from the sublime to the ridiculous.) And this is where you can see the various Core Clinical Competencies tripping over each other because the main thing here is communicating with the patient. If you can figure out where providing patient care that is compassion-

ate ends and interpersonal and communication skills begin, send me an e-mail. They sound awfully close to me!

Bottom line – the patient care that is most compassionate for a truly hopeless case (this patient had third-degree burns over every square inch of his body; the fact that he was even alive at this point was some kind of celestial miracle) is comfort care. He got as much morphine as I could inject through the one IV we were able to get through the burned skin. I warmed the room up, too (he felt cool, which patients sometimes do if all the nerve endings are singed off).

Gather essential and accurate information about their patients.

I did a physical exam to confirm that, indeed, everything was burned off on this man. There were no eyebrows, no eyelashes, and his surface appeared white and meaty, for lack of a better term.

Usually, in such a case, when you are in resuscitation mode, you would be scrambling for a host of laboratory data, as well:

- arterial blood gas, including carbon monoxide level
- hematocrit
- electrocardiogram
- chest X-ray

But in this curious world of "provide comfort only," the approach was different. Why get a bunch of labs that you're not going to act on anyway?

Make informed decisions about diagnostic and therapeutic interventions based on patient information and preferences, up-to-date scientific evidence, and clinical judgment.

I confirmed with the resident, and asked that we confirm with the attending, that this was truly a hopeless case and that we weren't writing someone off who stood a chance. That was the consensus, and the burn people came down and gave us their blessing on this, too.

Develop and carry out patient management plans.

This is where I really hate the Core Clinical Competencies. "Carry out patient management plans." God, what a bloodless and administrato-gobbledygook way of saying "be a doctor and treat the patient."

Counsel and educate patients and their families.

Back to Core Clinical Competency overlap land. This is interpersonal and communications skills as well as professionalism all wrapped into one. I'll get into what I told the guy in the latter section.

Use information technology to support patient care decisions and patient education.

To hell with information technology at this point; it's all hands on and physical exam.

Perform competently all medical and invasive procedures considered essential for the area of practice.

As long as I didn't stick the morphine syringe into the mattress by mistake, I was performing competently. The main thing here was to keep misguided rescuers from running in the room and coding or intubating this guy.

Provide health care services aimed at preventing health problems or maintaining health.

Day late and a dime short here.

Work with health care professionals, including those from other disciplines, to provide patient-focused care.

The most important element here is hooking up with the burn people and making sure that I'm doing the right thing for this poor patient.

Medical knowledge

Residents must demonstrate knowledge about established and evolving biomedical, clinical, and cognate (e.g., epidemiological and social-behavioral) sciences and the application of this knowledge to patient care.

Demonstrate an investigatory and analytic thinking approach to clinical situations.

Shift into high gear and become the world's leading expert on burns in a hurry in this case. Although the focus in this case is comfort care, that doesn't mean that the next burn patient is going to be as badly off. Following are the main points:

- Watch for signs of an upper airway burn (singed nose hairs, carbonaceous sputum) and secure the airway right away in case of any doubt whatsoever. Once the airway swells up, the patient will become an impossible intubation in no time.
- Volume replacement can be tremendous as the "insulation" is lost and the patient loses vast amounts of fluid.
- Carbon monoxide inhalation is as stealthy as it is deadly. A patient can appear perfectly lucid and still have high levels of carbon monoxide, then, later on, suffer severe neurologic damage.

Investigatory and analytic with a burn patient? Snoop around for the hidden problems of a burned airway, lost volume, and "stealth" carbon monoxide.

Know and apply the basic and clinically supportive sciences that are appropriate to their discipline.

For anesthesia, this means the ABCs writ large because this is our stock in trade.

Practice-based learning and improvement

Residents must be able to investigate and evaluate their patient care practices, appraise and assimilate scientific evidence, and improve their patient care practices.

Analyze practice experience and perform practice-based improvement activities using a systematic methodology.

The most practical approach to this Core Clinical Competency is simply this: review the literature pertinent to burn patients and make sure that you are up on the latest.

Locate, appraise, and assimilate evidence from scientific studies related to their patients' health problems.

A modern twist on all this? Google "burns," or do a Medline search to see what the latest thinking is regarding treatment of the burn patient.

> Obtain and use information about their own population of patients and the larger population from which their patients are drawn.

I paged the burn team right away. They deal with this stuff all the time and know the ins and outs of the burn unit, so they were the people to contact regarding this unfortunate patient.

> Apply knowledge of study designs and statistical methods to the appraisal of clinical studies and other information on diagnostic and therapeutic effectiveness.

Much as we hate statistics (most doctors glaze over when biostatistics are mentioned), we still have to know this deadly dull field. If we don't know statistics, we cannot really weigh the validity of a study. Suggestions for the reading public? Here's what I did; you can run with it however you want. Aviva Petrie and Caroline Sabin [1] broke up the forbidding areas of statistics into digestible parts. Give this book a try if you're lost in statistics.

> Use information technology to manage information, access online medical information, and support their own education.

At the time of this case, the year was all of 1984, so the Internet was not yet even a glimmer in Bill Gates's eye. But today, of course, you'd Google anything you didn't know.

Professionalism

Residents must demonstrate a commitment to carrying out professional responsibilities, adherence to ethical principles, and sensitivity to a diverse patient population.

> Demonstrate respect, compassion, and integrity; a responsiveness to the needs of patients and society that supersedes self-interest; accountability to patients, society, and the profession; and a commitment to excellence and ongoing professional development.

Translation for this case? Stick it out with this guy. He deserves that. I made sure I stayed in the room with him, providing pain medication, waving off the code team, and staying until the end. This opens the whole end-of-life discussion.

> Demonstrate a commitment to ethical principles pertaining to provision or withholding of clinical care, confidentiality of patient information, informed consent, and business practice.

The main thing here is to withhold heroic care that would prolong the patient's misery.

Interpersonal and communication skills

Residents must be able to demonstrate interpersonal and communication skills that result in effective information exchange and teaming with patients, their patients' families, and professional associates.

> Use effective listening skills and elicit and provide information using effective nonverbal, explanatory, questioning, and writing skills.

This is the most important aspect of this case, so I'll linger here a while. Following is the conversation I had with this patient, as nearly as I can reconstruct it. (This was such an emotionally wrenching event that it made a hell of an impression on my memory banks.) You can agree or disagree with my approach and choice of words, but here's what I did. I'll call the patient, for the sake of this reconstruction, "Jim Smith."

"Jim, I'm going to be giving you some morphine to make you a little more comfortable."

"It's bad, huh?" (As mentioned earlier, he was surprisingly lucid.)

"Jim, you're burned over all your body, and it's all third degree, that's the worst kind."

"It's cold in here."

I put a blanket over him; his nerve endings were charred, so that didn't hurt him. I turned up the thermostat in the room.

"Jim, this burn is pretty bad. I mean really bad. But I'm going to make sure you're nice and comfortable."

"Will they be doing any operations or anything?"

"No, Jim, we're mainly going to make sure you don't hurt. Do you follow what I'm saying? This is not the kind of burn you can recover from, Jim."

The morphine started kicking in (I was being pretty generous), and he started getting sedated.

"Yeah, yeah, I know what you're saying, Doc."

"Want me to call anyone, Jim? Jim?"

It was probably volume loss and hypotension that finished him. I was hoping that it would go that way and not end up with an obstructed airway.

Work effectively with others as a member or leader of a health care team or other professional group.

We divided up the emergency room that night, and I stayed with Jim.

Systems-based practice

Residents must demonstrate an awareness of and responsiveness to the larger context and system of health care and the ability to effectively call on system resources to provide care that is of optimal value.

Understand how their patient care and other professional practices affect other health care professionals, the health care organization, and the larger society and how these elements of the system affect their own practice.

To subject a person with fatal burns to an epic journey of ventilator dependence, a million skin grafts, and a zillion dollars' worth of treatment is a waste of society's resources when the issue has already been decided. But as treatments improve, the day may come when we "go for it" with such a patient. No easy answers here.

Practice cost-effective health care and resource allocation that does not compromise quality of care.

See the preceding comment.

Additional reading

1. Petrie A, Sabin C. Medical statistics at a glance. 2nd ed. Malden, MA: Blackwell; 2005.

2. Chai JK, Sheng ZY, Yang HM, et al. Treatment strategies for mass burn casualties. Chin Med J (Engl) 2009;122:525–529.

3. Cochran A. Inhalation injury and endotracheal intubation. J Burn Care Res 2009;30:190–191.

4. Belgian Outcome in Burn Injury Study Group. Development and validation of a model for prediction of mortality in patients with acute burn injury. Br J Surg 2009;96:111–117.

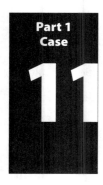

Contributions from Stony Brook University under Christopher J. Gallagher

What date would you like carved in stone?

Christopher J. Gallagher and Anna Kogan

The case

A 73-year-old man is scheduled for a mediastinoscopy. He is emaciated, has positive findings of metastatic disease on his chest X-ray, and is unable to lie down in the least, getting short of breath if he's anything other than bolt upright.

He is to have this mediastinoscopy for a tissue diagnosis of an obviously horrible cancer. He is now on the operating table with the back all the way up, and you're preoxygenating him. It's all you can do to get the saturation up to 92%.

Suddenly, you throw up your hands, call for the surgeon, and say, "This is ridiculous, I'm not doing this case. What the hell are we doing this for?"

The surgeon gets mad as a wet hen and takes you outside. You look him in the eyes and say, "What date do you want carved in this guy's stone? You might as well carve today's if I go ahead."

Patient care

Residents must be able to provide patient care that is compassionate, appropriate, and effective for the treatment of health problems and the promotion of health.

Communicate effectively and demonstrate caring and respectful behaviors when interacting with patients and their families.

OK, so maybe saying "what the hell are we doing this for" was not, precisely, *caring and respectful*, but it sure was *effective*! The main thing here was to take a step back and look at the whole picture, not just this one procedure.

Gather essential and accurate information about their patients.

A review of the chart and a physical exam confirmed everything I needed to know about this man. The severe degree of disability and advanced state of emaciation could only confirm the obvious – no matter what they found on this patient, he was not going to be able to endure chemo, radiation, or surgical therapy.

Make informed decisions about diagnostic and therapeutic interventions based on patient information and preferences, up-to-date scientific evidence, and clinical judgment.

The main point about this case and this write-up is that you have to be a perioperative physician, not just an anesthetic accessory to a surgical procedure.

Develop and carry out patient management plans.

Cancel the stupid case!

Counsel and educate patients and their families.

Believe it or not, it often falls to us, the anesthesiologists, to go out, sit down with the family, and spell out the entire picture. When I went out and talked with the patient's family, I asked what they pictured us doing, and they all agreed that he was far too sick to be subjected to some monstrous cure. Better to let him be. (After the burn case discussed in Case 10, you're going to think I'm some sort of angel of death, stalking the hallways of the hospitals with my scythe and robe!)

Use information technology to support patient care decisions and patient education.

A complete review of the computed tomography scans confirmed that this guy's entire mediastinum was involved and that nothing was going to save the day here.

Perform competently all medical and invasive procedures considered essential for the area of practice.

I *could* have done the anesthetic, taking into account the considerations of mediastinal mass. But that was not the point; rather, the point was to *decide what's best*, not just *dish up an anesthetic*.

Provide health care services aimed at preventing health problems or maintaining health.

It's a little late to tell the patient to stop smoking.

Work with health care professionals, including those from other disciplines, to provide patient-focused care.

I didn't have to slap the surgeon around to see my point of view. I just had to threaten to slap him around to get him to see my point.

Medical knowledge

Residents must demonstrate knowledge about established and evolving biomedical, clinical, and cognate (e.g., epidemiological and social-behavioral) sciences and the application of this knowledge to patient care.

Demonstrate an investigatory and analytic thinking approach to clinical situations.

The biggest analysis that needed doing here was *seeing the forest for the trees*. Don't think "do anesthesia for this one procedure"; rather, think "do what's best for the patient given his overall situation."

Practice-based learning and improvement

Residents must be able to investigate and evaluate their patient care practices, appraise and assimilate scientific evidence, and improve their patient care practices.

Analyze practice experience and perform practice-based improvement activities using a systematic methodology.

This is where being clinically and scientifically precise can be very tough. Where, oh, where, in the world is there a well-controlled, large study that looked at this exact situation – an emaciated patient with advanced everything, and you wonder whether you should proceed with a mediastinoscopy. This is where medicine is more art than science, all due apologies to practice-based learning and improvement.

Locate, appraise, and assimilate evidence from scientific studies related to their patients' health problems.

By all means, know about the implications of a mediastinal mass on the airways and vascular structures. The biggest concern is sedating, anesthetizing, and giving muscle relaxants and ending up with the patient getting cardiorespiratory collapse from the mass.

Apply knowledge of study designs and statistical methods to the appraisal of clinical studies and other information on diagnostic and therapeutic effectiveness.

Oy! Statistics again. There's no avoiding it – sort of like death and taxes.

Professionalism

Residents must demonstrate a commitment to carrying out professional responsibilities, adherence to ethical principles, and sensitivity to a diverse patient population.

Demonstrate respect, compassion, and integrity; a responsiveness to the needs of patients and society that supersedes self-interest; accountability to patients, society, and the profession; and a commitment to excellence and ongoing professional development.

To beat the same drum here, the best way to express respect for this man is to spare him a useless procedure that won't help him or alter his treatment anyway.

Demonstrate a commitment to ethical principles pertaining to provision or withholding of clinical care, confidentiality of patient information, informed consent, and business practice.

When I went out in the hall to talk with his family, I made sure I followed HIPAA and commonsense guidelines. We went to a private room and discussed all this far from prying ears.

Interpersonal and communication skills

Residents must be able to demonstrate interpersonal and communication skills that result in effective information exchange and teaming with patients, their patients' families, and professional associates.

> Use effective listening skills and elicit and provide information using effective nonverbal, explanatory, questioning, and writing skills.

Most of the listening came in that private room, as I dealt with the family's concerns. A major point is to let them have their say and not try to steer the conversation so much.

> Work effectively with others as a member or leader of a health care team or other professional group.

Of course, the surgeon got fussy, but what can you do? They're always mad. Maybe we should sneak Prozac into their cornflakes?

Systems-based practice

Residents must demonstrate an awareness of and responsiveness to the larger context and system of health care and the ability to effectively call on system resources to provide care that is of optimal value.

> Understand how their patient care and other professional practices affect other health care professionals, the health care organization, and the larger society and how these elements of the system affect their own practice.

The main thing in this case was "think what we'll do with this information." That's what made me throw up my hands and say, "Enough!" So we find out it's this or that cancer. Are we going to treat it anyway? If the answer is no, then don't do the case in the first place.

Additional reading

1. Slinger P, Kursli C. Management of the patient with a large anterior mediastinal mass: recurring myths. Curr Opin Anaesthesiol 2007;20:1–3.

2. Marik PE, Callahan A, Paganelli G, Reville B, Parks SM, Delgado EM. Multidisciplinary family meetings in the ICU facilitate end-of-life decision making. Am J Hosp Palliat Care 2009.

3. Pantilat S. Communicating with seriously ill patients: better words to say. JAMA 2009;301: 1279–1281.

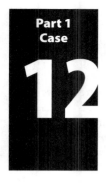

Contributions from Stony Brook University under Christopher J. Gallagher

Spasm, spasm, how do I treat thee?
Bronchospasm in a stage IV breast cancer patient

Bharathi Scott and Shiena Sharma

The case

A 54-year-old black female presented with a lung nodule of unknown origin for thoracosopy and partial resection of the right lower lobe. The patient had a history of breast cancer, reactive airway disease, and high anxiety. The patient was sedated in the holding room, brought back to the operating room, and induced and intubated with a right-sided double lumen tube. The patient subsequently went into bronchospasm, which was ultimately broken by our superb efforts.

The patient was extubated on termination of the case and was completely unaware of our quick and stoic measures to battle the beast of anesthesia, the spasm, a wild and unruly creature whose insidious and sudden onset can throw off even the most experienced of the people under the drapes (OK, so we are behind the drapes, but this phrase reminded me of *People under the Stairs* ... anyone see that movie?).

Patient care

Residents must be able to provide patient care that is compassionate, appropriate, and effective for the treatment of health problems and the promotion of health.

Communicate effectively and demonstrate caring and respectful behaviors when interacting with patients and their families.

On arrival, Mrs. Z had high anxiety, but not the "Oh, my God, am I gonna die?" type. She was quiet and reserved – a true picture of composure. However, a careful, real look into those big, round eyes, and I was reminded of Bambi facing a semi on Interstate 495. We reassured her and her daughter and told them that we would take care of her to the best of our ability and make her as comfortable as possible. I maintained good eye contact, answered the patient's questions, and smiled ... then *versed incoming*!

Gather essential and accurate information about their patients.

It is essential to recognize, acknowledge, and address anxiety preoperatively. This is the compassion component of being a physician, as applied to anesthesia, in particular. A reassuring smile or squeeze of the hand can do wonders in alleviating preop jitters and utilizes the one competency seldom taught in textbooks: the power of human touch.

Make informed decisions about diagnostic and therapeutic interventions based on patient information and preferences, up-to-date scientific evidence, and clinical judgment.

We spoke to the patient after careful review of the chart and confirmed her history, allergies, and all the good stuff that goes into a thorough preoperative evaluation. We identified that her history of reactive airway disease had no relation to smoking and was related to anxiety and weather. We decided that having an inhaler intraop would be a good idea, hence the Proventil.

Develop and carry out patient management plans.

The master plan was induction, intubation (smooth as butter, of course), ALine, surgical procedure, extubation ... lunch!

Use information technology to support patient care decisions and patient education.

General anesthesia was explained, followed by an explanation of standard monitors and invasive monitors.

Perform competently all medical and invasive procedures considered essential for the area of practice.

Because this case involved isolating a lung for surgical procedure, it was important to have read about the surgical requirements of the procedure in the preop period. Effective placement of the double lumen tube, including confirmation of placement with a fiber-optic scope, should be reviewed.

Provide health care services aimed at preventing health problems or maintaining health.

The patient took albuterol on the morning of the procedure.

Work with health care professionals, including those from other disciplines, to provide patient-focused care.

Surgical considerations and requirements for this type of case are of utmost importance. One must be in sync with the ventilating and dropping of the surgically marked lung per the surgeons' request.

Medical knowledge

Residents must demonstrate knowledge about established and evolving biomedical, clinical, and cognate (e.g., epidemiological and social-behavioral) sciences and the application of this knowledge to patient care.

Demonstrate an investigatory and analytic thinking approach to clinical situations.

When performing a one-lung ventilation case, one must anticipate complications and roadblocks to maintaining adequate ventilation. A physician's job is to consistently adapt and apply his or her fund of knowledge to challenging situations and unforeseen complications in a timely manner. Hence all critical situations require

- investigation
- formulation of a hypothesis
- correction of supposed underlying problems (aided by hours of training, journal clubs, QA, lectures, experience, and mistakes)
- prevention of future occurrences

In our case, shortly after induction with the "regulars," a 35-mm left-sided double lumen tube was placed on the first attempt. Anesthesia's friends were all in attendance to confirm proper placement, including Mr. EtCO$_2$, Mrs. Equal B/L B.S, and, of course, Señor fiber optic.

During this time, it was quickly noted how difficult it was to hand ventilate the patient. Peak airway pressures were in the 50s, and auscultation of squeaky, high-pitched, distant breath sounds were appreciated.

Know and apply the basic and clinically supportive sciences that are appropriate to their discipline.

Rather than collapse in a heap of panic and frenzy and radio every airway specialist overhead, a systematic and structured approach was utilized to identify the problem. The fiber-optic scope was quickly placed to determine if the tube was in an appropriate position, which it was. The patient was maintained on 100% oxygen, and sevoflurane was turned on to highest minimum alveolar concentration. Muscle relaxant was administered, corticosteroids were given intravenously, and Proventil was administered via an endotracheal tube.

Professionalism

Residents must demonstrate a commitment to carrying out professional responsibilities, adherence to ethical principles, and sensitivity to a diverse patient population.

Demonstrate respect, compassion, and integrity; a responsiveness to the needs of patients and society that supersedes self-interest; accountability to patients, society, and the profession; and a commitment to excellence and ongoing professional development.

Sometimes under the legality of medicine, we compromise our most basic instincts of nurturing. We fear touching our patients because it can be interpreted the wrong way. In this case, I felt compassion that superseded any legal guidelines involving physical contact with patients that I had received in those mega (boring) all-resident conferences.

Here was a lady who had been through a lot. She was scared. I felt her fear. So I went with my instinct and stroked her head and verbally consoled her to the best of my ability, as her tired eyelids closed slowly and the milky white snaked its way up her veins. My attending stood by me, one hand in the patient's hand, the other gently on her neck. It was an act of compassion, and it was more than any textbook could ever teach me.

> Demonstrate sensitivity and responsiveness to patients' culture, age, gender, and disabilities.

With the patient being a victim of breast cancer and radiation, my attending and I were very aware of the guarded nature of patients who have been in the health care system. They are often weary of medical professionals and, in general, approach procedures with a sense of impending doom. It is our job not only to treat medical ailments, but also to be sensitive of patients' fragility and fears.

Interpersonal and communication skills

Residents must be able to demonstrate interpersonal and communication skills that result in effective information exchange and teaming with patients, their patients' families, and professional associates.

> Create and sustain a therapeutic and ethically sound relationship with patients.

My attending consistently reminded me that if I treated all patients as my own family, I could never go wrong – good advice!

> Use effective listening skills and elicit and provide information using effective nonverbal, explanatory, questioning, and writing skills.

We all know that at times, anesthesia gets the stigma of being "impersonal and isolated" in terms of establishing good patient relationships due to the mere fact that, hey, we put people to sleep for a living. How can we talk to them – *they're asleep*!

In this case, however, it was demonstrated that effective communication has no time constraint and no indication for verbalization. Simply *listening* attentively and patiently to your patient can give you clues to deliver an above average standard of care.

> Work effectively with others as a member or leader of a health care team or other professional group.

The cardiothoracic (CT) surgeon approached me and said, "You know, I just wanted to thank you for your care with that patient the other day. I saw her today, and she mentioned that the anesthesiologist was so kind and caring and appreciated the gentle stroking of her head as she fell asleep. Thank you for making it a pleasurable experience. Nice touch." *Wow…* yeah, I was grinning ear to ear, no lie! But after all, we are a team!

Surgeons, anesthesiologists, nurses, techs – we are the well-oiled machine that delivers optimal care. Although a patient is considered to be CT-surgery or an ortho patient, they are all *our* patients. This is all the more reason to work with our peers as one big unit, rather than as a subdivision of specialties.

Additional reading

1. Nadaud J, Landy C, Steiner T, Pernod G, Favier JC. Helium-sevoflurane association: a rescue treatment in case of acute severe asthma (in French). Ann Fr Anesth Reanim 2009;28:82–85.

2. Mayne IP, Bagaoisan C. Social support during anesthesia induction in an adult surgical population. AORN J 2009;89:307–310, 313–315, 318–320.

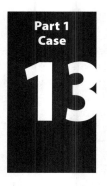
13 Why don't you join the HIT parade?

Contributions from Stony Brook University under
Christopher J. Gallagher

HIT in a cardiac surgery patient

Bharathi Scott and Jason Daras

The case

A 70-year-old male is scheduled for coronary artery bypass graft (CABG) on pump. He has the usual history of unstable angina, diabetes, and hypertension. The cardiac catheterization report shows triple vessel disease with normal left ventricular ejection fraction. You are thrilled that finally, you have a routine CABG this week. No big deal, been there and done that. Just as you are walking down the floor to see the patient, the friendly cardiologist says, "The patient has recently dropped his platelet count and we are waiting for the antibody test. I think the patient has HIT [heparin-induced thrombocytopenia]. We stopped heparin yesterday and started him on argatroban." What the...?

Patient care

Residents must be able to provide patient care that is compassionate, appropriate, and effective for the treatment of health problems and the promotion of health.

Communicate effectively and demonstrate caring and respectful behaviors when interacting with patients and their families.

The anesthesia team must be able to communicate the special issues involved in the anticoagulation management with the patient, surgeon, and other members of the operating room (OR) team, especially the perfusionists.

Gather essential and accurate information about their patients.

The anesthesia team should make sure the appropriate steps are taken to provide alternative anticoagulation for surgery. This includes special attention to platelet count and response to cessation of heparin.

Check the platelet factor 4 antibodies in vitro to confirm the diagnosis of HIT (type II). In addition, it is important to recognize that diagnosis of HIT is made on a clinical basis and is supported with the previously mentioned tests and therapy.

Develop and carry out patient management plans.

Communicate the issues with all members of the surgical team. Choices of alternate method of anticoagulation therapy are argatroban, bivalirudin, and lepirudin. Bivalirudin (Angiomax) is the most commonly used antithrombin agent in cardiac surgical patients. Dosing involves an initial loading dose (1 mg/kg) followed by a maintenance infusion of 2.5 mg/kg/hour. Activated clotting times are monitored and the dosage is adjusted accordingly. Dosage is reduced in patients with renal insufficiency and failure. Argatroban is more commonly used in patients undergoing percutaneous coronary intervention.

Perform competently all medical and invasive procedures considered essential for the area of practice.

Stick to the basics of bypass surgery! Secure your airway, invasive monitors, and, if needed, transesophageal echocardiography (TEE). Be sure to minimize traumatic tube and line placement – the less of the red stuff, the better. Appropriate blood and blood products should be readily available.

Work with health care professionals, including those from other disciplines, to provide patient-focused care.

Whether it is in or out of the OR, health care professionals must understand that they are working toward the same goal. All health care providers must be included.

Medical knowledge

Residents must demonstrate knowledge about established and evolving biomedical, clinical, and cognate (e.g., epidemiological and social-behavioral) sciences and the application of this knowledge to patient care.

> Demonstrate an investigatory and analytic thinking approach to clinical situations.

When you find yourself staring down the belly of HIT, you must think of a differential for the drop in platelets before confirming the HIT diagnosis. Could this patient have leukemia? Could he or she have been exposed to a virus or some other drug that may have caused this?

What does this mean for your intraop management? Alternate anticoagulation and excessive bleeding that may lead to the use of blood and blood products? Managing the hemodynamic response to hypovolemia versus the hemodynamic response to a failing heart – TEE would show all in this case! Get it out and start imaging the heart.

Practice-based learning and improvement

Residents must be able to investigate and evaluate their patient care practices, appraise and assimilate scientific evidence, and improve their patient care practices.

> Analyze practice experience and perform practice-based improvement activities using a systematic methodology.

It is important to learn from your own practice of these cases or your colleagues' cases and discuss the improvements that could be made. Asking questions and following up literature is an important way to improve your practice-based learning.

> Assimilating evidence from your own practice with the literature.

Ultimately, this is a very hard task, and one that separates the experts from the amateurs. Can you look at studies on HIT and, from those studies, create a better method of facilitating diagnosis and/or treatment? It is hard to find a double blind, randomized study on such a not-so-common reaction to heparin.

Professionalism

Residents must demonstrate a commitment to carrying out professional responsibilities, adherence to ethical principles, and sensitivity to a diverse patient population.

> Demonstrate respect, compassion, and integrity; a responsiveness to the needs of patients and society that supersedes self-interest; accountability to patients, society, and the profession; and a commitment to excellence and ongoing professional development.

So this patient with this possibly devastating condition is thrown your way. No sweat . . . or at least, never let them see you sweat. True to life, if you break down and start screaming at others in the OR, they will start screaming back; the patient, if awake, will start to panic, and then you will start to panic – can you see a vicious circle? Think about your own attendings – who are the most composed, professional, and level-headed? I'll bet you the best anesthesiologists are the ones who can calm down a thoracic surgeon who just dissected an aorta. These are the anesthesiologists who command the most respect and communicate best in the OR. So if a patient with HIT comes into your OR, be prepared and make sure the patient and surgeon are prepared for what potential disasters may develop.

> Demonstrate sensitivity and responsiveness to patients' culture, age, gender, and disabilities.

Always remember, you have a life to take care of, which is a unique position for a person to be in. Patients are all different. Some may have more education and may understand a condition and its consequences better than others. They may have the means to research their own medical problems. In a condition so unique as HIT, some patients may need more explanation. Culture can play a huge roll, especially when a Jehovah's Witness appears with the declaration that you may not use blood products – your hands are completely tied, right? Well, maybe to some degree, but there is always autologous blood salvage or transfusions. Assure the patient that you will do your best with the given restrictions, instead of getting upset with the situation or the patient. There is a very important psychosocial aspect to every case you deal with as a physician, so you may as well embrace it.

Interpersonal and communication skills

Residents must be able to demonstrate interpersonal and communication skills that result in effective information exchange and teaming with patients, their patients' families, and professional associates.

Create and sustain a therapeutic and ethically sound relationship with patients.

Many might say that of all physicians, anesthesiologists have more of a problem forming relationships with patients because the majority of our interaction is under anesthesia. However, through our preoperative visit bedside and postoperative visit, we can communicate all our concerns, and the patients can communicate theirs. Devising a plan and allowing the patient to be educated about his or her medical issue will ensure less anxiety pre- and postop.

Work effectively with others as a member or leader of a health care team or other professional group.

A very important aspect is communication of all staff, especially when dealing with a patient who has a unique medical condition. Many people working on the case may not know the extent or ramifications of the illness. Perhaps you may not be comfortable dealing with this patient – it happens. Don't be a cowboy; read and communicate. Don't be afraid to talk to the surgeons because we are all in this together.

Systems-based practice

Residents must demonstrate an awareness of and responsiveness to the larger context and system of health care and the ability to effectively call on system resources to provide care that is of optimal value.

Understand how their patient care and other professional practices affect other health care professionals, the health care organization, and the larger society and how these elements of the system affect their own practice.

We must all understand our role in the health care system and our limitations. Sometimes we go above and beyond what we may have to do to save a patient's life. In the process of treating HIT in a patient undergoing CABG, we act as the cardiologist, hematologist, and anesthesiologist, all the while keeping in mind our own limitations and asking for assistance, if needed.

Practice cost-effective health care and resource allocation that does not compromise quality of care.

The key here is the fact that practicing cost-effective medicine should not compromise patient care. How in HIT can we practice cost-effective medicine? Well, we can take into account that these patients bleed more intraop, and patients will be receiving various blood products. Keeping a mindful watch on the amount of product you are using, placing packed red blood cells in the refrigerator that are not being used, and keeping good communication between the blood bank and OR will contribute toward this. Other cost-effective methods during your anesthetic management can go a long way, so stop cranking up those O_2 flows!

Additional reading

1. Warkentin TE, Greinacher A. Heparin induced
    thrombocytopenia: recognition, treatment and
    prevention. Chest 2004;126:311S–337S.

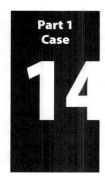

Part 1 Case 14

Contributions from Stony Brook University under Christopher J. Gallagher

Bad lungs in the ICU

Shaji Poovathor and Rany Makaryus

The case

A full-term, 24-year-old, pregnant African American woman was rushed to the operating room (OR) for emergency cesarean section secondary to fetal distress. Post cesarean section, she started to bleed profusely in the abdomen. She was taken back to the OR and ended up having a hysterectomy under general anesthesia. However, she uncontrollably lost around 1.5 L of blood. She received 10 units of packed red blood cells, 10 units of fresh frozen plasmas, 2 units of cryoprecipitate, and multiple boluses of crystalloids. She was left intubated and was admitted to the surgical intensive care unit (SICU). While she was connected to the ventilator, the respiratory therapist noted a copious amount of pink, frothy fluid in her endotracheal (ET) tube.

Patient care

Residents must be able to provide patient care that is compassionate, appropriate, and effective for the treatment of health problems and the promotion of health.

Communicate effectively and demonstrate caring and respectful behaviors when interacting with patients and their families.

After initially attending to the patient and making sure that the patient is stable enough (how stable is enough is a clinical judgment; if the patient is not stable enough, the family members still need to understand the unfortunate outcome), the resident needs to communicate effectively with the primary service who operated on her. Make sure that the family members and next of kin are fully aware. It is the joint responsibility of the primary service and the SICU to keep the family members updated. What can we do? What are the unfortunate outcomes? Could there be any other alternative? Does the patient have a living will?

Gather essential and accurate information about their patients.

Look at the patient. Examine her. Look at the monitor. How bad is her lung (remember the pink, frothy stuff from her ET tube?)? How high is the airway pressure? Order appropriate labs.

Make informed decisions about diagnostic and therapeutic interventions based on patient information and preferences, up-to-date scientific evidence, and clinical judgment.

Can this patient develop disseminated intravascular coagulation? Can this patient develop transfusion-related lung injury (TRALI)? Can she develop acute respiratory distress syndrome (ARDS)? Can she develop pulmonary embolism (PE)? Can she develop sepsis? The answer is yes, she could develop any one of these. Again, clinical judgment warrants looking for these and acting on them.

Develop and carry out patient management plans.

Supportive measures for the lung are important. Remember the ARDS net trial: low tidal volume, low airway pressure to avoid blowing off her lung, and chest X-ray every day to evaluate her lung condition.

An echocardiogram (EKG) to reveal her heart status is needed. What if the EKG had shown a right ventricular dilation (which this patient had)?

Does she need any prophylactic antibiotics? Evidence-based study shows no primary role for antibiotics in terms of prophylaxis, unless and until there is solid evidence of "wrong bugs in the wrong place at the wrong time."

Administer proper sedation and pain killers so that she doesn't yank off her tube. Also give vasopressors, if needed, to support hemodynamics, and get labs to ensure that she is not bleeding, not going into,

73

and not going into kidney failure and to check lytes and repleting lytes, as needed, arterial blood gases, and so on.

Counsel and educate patients and their families.

Now it is time to jump in and evaluate the overall situation. What if things don't work? Think about the living will. Should we involve the organ donation task force?

Use information technology to support patient care decisions and patient education.

Again, look at chest X-rays, labs, ventilator parameters, spirometry, neurological examinations, abdominal examinations, and so on. If an EKG has shown a right ventricular dilation, what are you thinking? Could this be an extra strain on the heart from a PE? How is the patient's hemodynamics? Does she have an alveolar arterial O_2 gradient? (Look at the ABG and the FiO_2. Does she need an increasing O_2 requirement to keep that PaO_2 up?) Should we order a computed tomography (CT) angiogram?

If your instinct says maybe, then don't waste time considering her hemodynamics and other clinical judgments. Go for it. If PE is positive, we need to find out if anticoagulation using heparin is called for, after appropriately discussing this with the primary service.

Perform competently all medical and invasive procedures considered essential for the area of practice.

Make sure that the patient has a central line for access and central venous pressure monitoring and an arterial line for continuous beat-to-beat analysis of blood pressure and frequent ABGs.

Provide health care services aimed at preventing health problems or maintaining health.

Priorities are supportive ventilatory management using extremely low tidal volumes, as per the ARDS net trial, to prevent severe barotrauma. Also important are early diagnosis of PE to prevent catastrophes, and labs, including blood cultures, to discover the hiding bugs, if any, and to treat them appropriately with antibiotics.

Work with health care professionals, including those from other disciplines, to provide patient-focused care.

Work in close association with the primary service, cardiologist (if one was involved for the EKG evaluation), SICU nursing staff, patient relation team (for closer relationships with the next of kin and family members), and organ donation task force (now may be the time to think of a living will, organ donation, etc.).

Medical knowledge

Residents must demonstrate knowledge about established and evolving biomedical, clinical, and cognate (e.g., epidemiological and social-behavioral) sciences and the application of this knowledge to patient care.

Demonstrate an investigatory and analytic thinking approach to clinical situations.

Several situations arise in this particular patient:

1. Multiple blood products – think of transfusion-related lung injury versus adult respiratory distress versus acute lung injury. Look for those bilateral, fluffy, homogenous chest X-rays and increasing FiO_2 requirements.
2. A right ventricular strain on EKG (evidence of right ventricular dilation) may prompt you to think of a PE in combination with severe hemodynamic fluctuations (vasopressor-dependent).
3. With an increasing temperature and white blood cells think of sepsis. Order and look for the blood culture results.
4. Rising creatinine and abnormal lytes will prompt you toward ongoing kidney damage.
5. Avoid the stress gastric ulcer. Have proton pump inhibitors going.
6. Oozing from IV sites, hematuria, bloody sputum – think of DIC? Look for the platelets and fibrinogen.

Know and apply the basic and clinically supportive sciences that are appropriate to their discipline.

Make sure you understand all the physiology that applies to these complex cases: lung parenchymal damage from blood transfusion, physiology of plateau pressure, pathophysiology of ARDS, PE causes and consequences, response of the body to PE and ARDS/TRALI. Following is the sequence:

1. massive blood loss
2. massive transfusion

3. hit to the lungs: TRALI
4. hit to the legs or circulatory system, causing thrombus-embolic phenomena
5. difficulty with oxygenation and ventilation
6. bad, bad, bad lungs!

Practice-based learning and improvement

Residents must be able to investigate and evaluate their patient care practices, appraise and assimilate scientific evidence, and improve their patient care practices.

Analyze practice experience and perform practice-based improvement activities using a systematic methodology.

Again, all is not lost as far as this Core Clinical Competency is concerned! The hospital, obstetric-gynecological (OB-GYN) service, anesthesiology, and the critical care service team should all have continuous quality improvement committees. As previously mentioned, difficult cases, complications, deaths – all these things demand a systematic analysis afterward.

Were there any other alternatives to doing this case in the OR or any other alternatives in managing this case in the ICU? Should the patient never have been allowed a sedation vacation as she had bad lungs hit with transfusion, ARDS, and PE? Were we late in diagnosing the PE? Did we use the concept of permissive hypercapnia and hypoxemia?

Locate, appraise, and assimilate evidence from scientific studies related to their patients' health problems.

This is when we need to turn to the collective experiences of others who have taken care of patients with this reaction. Anesthesia and medicine are ever changing and expanding fields; as continuous adult learners, and for the benefit of our patients, we need to keep abreast of the current literature. It would be prudent for the team members of this patient's care team to look up the most recent literature on TRALI and transfusion-associated circulatory overload (TACO):

1. What's better – a continuous positive airway pressure (CPAP) machine, or no CPAP?
2. Should the patient be placed on an oscillator?
3. What monitoring devices have been proven to be best in this situation?

Obtain and use information about their own population of patients and the larger population from which their patients are drawn.

A study of posttransfusion patients who develop acute pulmonary edema would be beneficial, but of even more benefit would be a study that looked at the prevention of TRALI in multiparous women.

Apply knowledge of study designs and statistical methods to the appraisal of clinical studies and other information on diagnostic and therapeutic effectiveness.

Here are some of the highlights of which we need to be aware:

1. early use of the gold standard CT angiogram to diagnose PE in high-risk cases or in cases with a high index of suspicion
2. the ARDS net trial study with low plateau pressure and low tidal volume, minimizing lung damage
3. literature on deep venous thrombosis prophylaxis: heparin versus fractionated heparin

Use information technology to manage information, access online medical information, and support their own education.

In this case, it is very simply a matter of knowing how to find information about this topic. Entering a PubMed search with institutionalized full-text links is very useful in finding the most up-to-date information. This would include searching for "TRALI" and "TACO" and combining these terms with "multiparous" or "postpartum." Combining these search terms would improve the relevancy of the results to the patient at hand.

Professionalism

Residents must demonstrate a commitment to carrying out professional responsibilities, adherence to ethical principles, and sensitivity to a diverse patient population.

Demonstrate respect, compassion, and integrity; a responsiveness to the needs of patients and society that supersedes self-interest; accountability to patients, society, and the profession; and a commitment to excellence and ongoing professional development.

This is demonstrated by the team's dedication to the care of this patient during this difficult acute situation and continuing to provide the best possible care. Using background medical knowledge, building on this with a review of the current literature, and applying this to the patient show ongoing professional development.

> Demonstrate a commitment to ethical principles pertaining to provision or withholding of clinical care, confidentiality of patient information, informed consent, and business practice.

In these situations, we have to be very careful to keep the patient's wishes in mind. Many times, advanced directives may restrict care that we may be able to give as anesthesiologists. We may sometimes want to do more for the patient, but such directives may limit care; at other times, it is the opposite. The key factor is that the treatments we provide must be consistent with what the patient's wishes are or would have been. Saying that is the easy part, but figuring it out is where it gets a little tough!

> Demonstrate sensitivity and responsiveness to patients' culture, age, gender, and disabilities.

In a nutshell, show respect and compassion to the patient and family members irrespective of age, religion, culture, gender, or race.

Interpersonal and communication skills

Residents must be able to demonstrate interpersonal and communication skills that result in effective information exchange and teaming with patients, their patients' families, and professional associates.

> Create and sustain a therapeutic and ethically sound relationship with patients.

Wash your hands before you go in to examine the patient and after examining the patient. Of course, look professional and give the patient's family your dynamic attention. (Don't be texting while you're talking with them, for example.)

> Use effective listening skills and elicit and provide information using effective nonverbal, explanatory, questioning, and writing skills.

As an ICU physician, your job is to get the information you need with a complete accounting of what happened in the OR, presurgical comorbidities, and a directed history and physical.

Your critical care note will demonstrate your writing skills. Examination of the patient will demonstrate your nonverbal finding skills. History taking from the patient's family members will demonstrate your questioning skills.

> Work effectively with others as a member or leader of a health care team or other professional group.

This involves the following:

- Notify the family of the seriousness of the issue.
- Notify risk management.
- Study the living will and discuss it with family members.
- Involve the organ donation task force.
- Notify the pastor.
- Work in close association with nursing staff and the OB-GYN service.

All should join in the process with appropriate coordination and cooperation.

Systems-based practice

Residents must demonstrate an awareness of and responsiveness to the larger context and system of health care and the ability to effectively call on system resources to provide care that is of optimal value.

> Understand how their patient care and other professional practices affect other health care professionals, the health care organization, and the larger society and how these elements of the system affect their own practice.

This patient has suffered a life-ending hemorrhage, but this could be useful for the general public. Involvement of the organ donation task force early on will help. We have to take the best possible care of this patient to ensure that her organs are best preserved. Maintain hemodynamics and avoid barotrauma/volutrauma to the lungs and heparinization to avoid further embolic phenomena and further damage.

> Practice cost-effective health care and resource allocation that does not compromise quality of care.

The primary concern here is to avoid further damage to the other organs as the lungs are already bad and crunched. Be aware of the hospital's policy on notifying the organ procurement team, how much lead time they need (including, of course, the all-important discussion with family), and also their protocol. Remember that the other organs could be jeopardized as the lungs are already bad. Also keep in mind that careful and professional discussion is warranted as the idea of organ donation for the immediate family members could be extremely painful.

Again, responsible care of the patient at this point mandates standard cost-effective maneuvers. Maintain low nitric oxide ppm (remember that NO is very expensive); avoid frequent and unnecessary labs; and to the best of your ability, shift gears to the least expensive regimen, while always maintaining the optimal physiologic environment for the patient's physiologic status.

Advocate for quality patient care and assist patients in dealing with system complexities.

The main group of people dealing with system complexities at this point are the family members, wrestling with the consequences of the operation. Your advocacy for quality patient care will manifest as you continue to take good care of all physiologic variables (which can be tough, as the brain-dead patient can develop all kinds of instability).

Your assistance with the family will be required:

1. Get everyone in a private room.
2. As usual, turn your beeper and cell phone off; this is no time for interruptions.
3. Allow time for family members to vent their emotions.
4. Repeat information as necessary.

Know how to partner with health care managers and health care providers to assess, coordinate, and improve health care and know how these activities can affect system performance.

Make sure that you keep in touch with hospital administration. The whole team in the SICU and OR should maintain that link with the team outside the OR and ICU that was involved in this patient's care.

Additional reading

1. Terragni PP, Rosboch G, Tealdi A, et al. Tidal hyperinflation during low tidal volume ventilation in acute respiratory distress syndrome. Am J Respir Crit Care Med 2007;175:160–166.

2. Parsons PE, Eisner MD, Thompson BT, et al. Lower tidal volume ventilation and plasma cytokine markers of inflammation in patients with acute lung injury. Crit Care Med 2005;33:1–6.

2. Acute Respiratory Distress Syndrome Network. Ventilation with lower tidal volumes as compared with traditional tidal volumes for acute lung injury and the acute respiratory distress syndrome. N Engl J Med 2000;342:1301–1308.

4. Petersen B, Deja M, Bartholdy R, et al. Inhalation of the ETA receptor antagonist LU-135252 selectively attenuates hypoxic pulmonary vasoconstriction. Am J Physiol Regul Integr Comp Physiol 2008;294:R601–R605.

5. Bloch KD, Ichinose F, Roberts JD Jr, Zapol WM. Inhaled NO as a therapeutic agent. Cardiovasc Res 2007;75:339–348.

6. Pelage J-P, Le Dref O, Jacob D, Soyer P, Herbreteau D, Rymer R. Selective arterial embolization of the uterine arteries in the management of intractable post-partum hemorrhage. Obstet Gynecol Surv 2000;55:204–205.

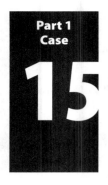

15

Contributions from Stony Brook University under Christopher J. Gallagher

A simple breast biopsy

Neera Tewari and Ramtin Cohanim

The case

A 61-year-old woman is scheduled for a breast biopsy. Her past medical history includes mental retardation and gastroesophageal reflux disease. She lives in a home because she is unable to care for herself. She is nonverbal. Her sister understands her nonverbal cues and is able to communicate with her and calm her.

It is 7:00 A.M. on Monday, and it's nice to be back at work after a relaxing weekend. You've had your first cup of coffee, the drugs are drawn up, the machine is checked, the operating room (OR) is almost ready to go – and the nurses tell you that they need 15 more minutes to set up and see the patient. You go out to holding to meet your first patient. As you draw the curtain, a middle-aged woman is sitting in the stretcher, in street clothes, straddling and hugging your patient while humming in her ear. The patient is wearing a hospital gown, a hair cap, and thick mismatching socks. She sees you and shrieks (*loudly*!). The woman in street clothes motions to you to close the curtains. You do as asked, and the humming just gets louder, and now they are rocking in unison, until the patient is again in a "calm trance."

The patient has no known allergies, has a history of nausea and vomiting from prior general anesthetics, weighs about 68 kg, and has poor dentition and a MP class I airway (you couldn't help but notice as she shrieked on your arrival). You explain to the sister that you need to obtain intravenous (IV) access to anesthetize the patient. After a lengthy discussion considering PO (per oris) sedation, IM (intramuscular) darts, EMLA (eutectic mixture of local anesthetic), mask induction, and IV induction, the sister explains that the patient will allow you to start an IV if you do it in the holding area, while she is present and the curtains are drawn. She explains that the patient has had several successful blood draws. Remembering your rather loud welcome, you quickly locate your resident, present the patient, and observe while she smoothly obtains IV access. *Excellent!*

The patient refused to take PO Bicitra. After 2 mg of IV midazolam, the patient is calm, and you think, "This wasn't that bad." In the OR, the rapid sequence IV induction and intubation [1] are smooth, and the surgery is completed without complications. The patient is given postoperative nausea/vomiting prophylaxis and a propofol infusion was maintained intraoperatively to decrease the amount of volatile agents used. The patient is extubated, comfortable, and taken to recovery. Her sister soon joins her to keep her calm as the anesthetic wears off.

Patient care

Residents must be able to provide patient care that is compassionate, appropriate, and effective for the treatment of health problems and the promotion of health.

Communicate effectively and demonstrate caring and respectful behaviors when interacting with patients and their families.

In this case, it is very important to discuss the details of the anesthetic with the patient's sister. You must also understand how the patient and her sister communicate with each other and how you can make it as comfortable of an experience for both the patient and the family as possible. Including the family in the discussion actually helped our anesthetic plan. The sister was able to comfort and distract the patient while the IV was inserted. Without this smooth IV insertion, the start of the case could have been quite involved. The patient refused PO Bicitra, so attempting PO sedation [2] would have been difficult. A mask induction or an IM injection are possible but would be hard to do in a noncompliant, anxious, combative patient. Remember how she reacted when you drew the curtains in holding. It is obvious that the sister is really in tune with the patient and is able to manage her well. It is to our advantage and the patient's benefit to incorporate the family in her care.

Gather essential and accurate information about their patients.

Again, more of what was said earlier. In this case, it is important to obtain all the information possible from the family because we cannot communicate with the patient. She has gastroesophageal reflux disease (GERD), mental retardation, and a prior history of nausea and vomiting (NV) after general anesthesia.

Make informed decisions about diagnostic and therapeutic interventions based on patient information and preferences, up-to-date scientific evidence, and clinical judgment.

We need to devise an acceptable plan for the care of this patient. She has a history of GERD and is nonverbal – is she a candidate for IV sedation? IV sedation could be a difficult option as she will not be able to express pain or discomfort; likewise, it can be frightening to lie under surgical drapes, and she may become uninhibited or combative under a propofol infusion. With her history, it may be best to proceed with general anesthesia. There are several methods of induction (IV, IM, mask) – which one is best for her? Is a mask induction safe with her history of GERD? A thorough discussion with the family and an understating of the patient's history allows you to make informed decisions about the care of this patient. As discussed earlier, IV induction looks like our best option.

Develop and carry out patient management plans.

Once a sound anesthetic plan is devised and agreeable to all, you must proceed as discussed and always be prepared for emergencies.

Counsel and educate patients and their families.

In our case, the patient may not understand much of what is going on, based on her history. It is our responsibility to educate the family with an open discussion about the risks and benefits of our plans and what will happen in the perioperative period. The patient has a unique medical history that poses certain challenges to her care, and the family must understand this [3].

Use information technology to support patient care decisions and patient education.

You will want to look at prior electrocardiograms and chest X-rays.

Perform competently all medical and invasive procedures considered essential for the area of practice.

All procedures – starting IVs, intubating, maintaining the anesthetic, and waking up the patient – must be done according to standards of care.

Provide health care services aimed at preventing health problems or maintaining health.

The patient can be given a nonparticulate antacid to prevent aspiration pneumonia. To prevent infection, you must make sure that antibiotics are given 1 hour prior to incision.

Work with health care professionals, including those from other disciplines, to provide patient-focused care.

You must discuss your plan with the surgeon and all OR personnel. This patient may be calm at the start of the case (thanks to some IV midazolam), but the wake-up may be a different story. Everyone must be on board to have a quiet and calm OR when the patient is waking up. Manpower should be available if she wakes up thrashing and combative.

Medical knowledge

Residents must demonstrate knowledge about established and evolving biomedical, clinical, and cognate (e.g., epidemiological and social-behavioral) sciences and the application of this knowledge to patient care.

Demonstrate an investigatory and analytic thinking approach to clinical situations.

When you first examine the patient and obtain her history, you realize that good old "propofol, succinylcholine, tube" may not work here. This clinical scenario demands that you tailor your anesthetic plan. Can you do this with some IV sedation, even though the patient has GERD and is nonverbal? If not, how will you proceed with general anesthesia? How can you avoid PONV (postoperative nausea and vomiting)?

Know and apply the basic and clinically supportive sciences that are appropriate to their discipline.

The past medical history includes GERD – you must know how to do a rapid sequence induction. You must also know how to proceed with the different types of induction. What are the drugs and doses for an IM injection? Can you proceed with a mask induction in a patient with GERD [1]?

Professionalism

Residents must demonstrate a commitment to carrying out professional responsibilities, adherence to ethical principles, and sensitivity to a diverse patient population.

Demonstrate respect, compassion, and integrity; a responsiveness to the needs of patients and society that supersedes self-interest; accountability to patients, society, and the profession; and a commitment to excellence and ongoing professional development.

Did you come in on time this morning? Did you set up the room appropriately? Did you get a good night of rest? Did you show compassion to the patient and family, even if she did greet you with a deafening shriek when you first met her? This is not the time to turn around and run, but rather, to be calm and respectful. Your patient is here for an important (maybe even life-saving) procedure, and you must give her the best care you can.

Demonstrate a commitment to ethical principles pertaining to provision or withholding of clinical care, confidentiality of patient information, informed consent, and business practice.

When you are interviewing in the holding area, review the consent with the sister, confirm the site of surgery, and observe all HIPAA rules. It is inappropriate to reveal confidential information and discuss the details of the case while riding the elevator!

Demonstrate sensitivity and responsiveness to patients' culture, age, gender, and disabilities.

This patient is a 61-year-old woman with a history of mental retardation. You must be sensitive to her disabilities. It is inappropriate to make fun of her condition! Be respectful.

Interpersonal and communication skills

Residents must be able to demonstrate interpersonal and communication skills that result in effective information exchange and teaming with patients, their patients' families, and professional associates.

Create and sustain a therapeutic and ethically sound relationship with patients.

In this case, you have a double challenge: you must gain the trust of the patient and her sister. With her sister, you can communicate verbally and develop a relationship, but it is equally important to try to gain the trust of the patient with your nonverbal language. Include her in the discussion as much as possible (don't ignore her). If her sister is able to communicate with her, ask for tips – they may be helpful in the OR!

Use effective listening skills and elicit and provide information using effective nonverbal, explanatory, questioning, and writing skills.

Again, listen carefully to what the family tells you. In our case, that is the only option we will have. Make appropriate eye contact when talking to the patient and the family. Be aware of your body language. Answer all questions appropriately and in simple, lay terms. Defer surgical questions to the surgeon if you are not sure of their answers – it is best not to guess. If you don't know an answer, be *honest* and ask your attending.

Work effectively with others as a member or leader of a health care team or other professional group.

Discuss the plan with the OR team. If the OR is delayed, discuss this with the holding area. Postoperatively, discuss the patient's needs with the recovery room staff and make yourself available for problems or questions.

Additional reading

1. Ng A, Smith G. Gastroesophageal reflux and aspiration of gastric contents in anesthetic practice. Anesth Analg 2001;93:494–513.

2. Petros AJ. Oral ketamine: its use for mentally retarded adults requiring day care dental treatment. Anesthesiology 1991;46:646–647.

3. Butler M, Hayes B, Hathaway M, Begleiter M. Specific genetic disease at risk for sedation/anesthesia complications. Anesth Analg 2000;91:837–855.

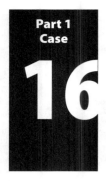

Contributions from Stony Brook University under
Christopher J. Gallagher

16 Fast-track perioperative management of patients having a laparoscopic colectomy for colon cancer

The case

Brian Durkin and Sofie Hussain

Your institution is interested in getting on board the fast-track surgery train that has been traveling across the civilized world, as surgeons and engineers create increasingly innovative ways to take things out of people without them knowing about it. Operations that used to leave incisions measured in feet are now being measured in millimeters, and the resulting postoperative morbidity is shrinking, along with the reimbursement.

You are in charge of your hospital's acute pain service and are responsible for placing and managing all the epidurals used to control postoperative pain. The new colorectal surgeon would like you to help take care of his patients and get them out of the hospital sooner. He says that where he's from in Europe, there is this guy named Dr. Kehlet, and he's always talking about multimodal analgesia and fast-track protocols. You see, the longer you stay in the hospital, the more bad things can happen to you. How are you going to help get this project on track and be successful?

Patient care

Residents must be able to provide patient care that is compassionate, appropriate, and effective for the treatment of health problems and the promotion of health.

Counsel and educate patients and their families.

When seen preoperatively, the patient as well as his or her family should be counseled on the risks and benefits of epidural anesthesia, particularly as it pertains to colorectal surgery. One could explain, for example, that although there is a risk of a postdural puncture headache, it is far less than the chance for postoperative incisional pain, which would compromise early ambulation, which has its own consequences. If patients are taking blood thinners, the risks and benefits of stopping these medications need to be

thoroughly addressed. In so doing, patients and their families are integral members of the decision-making team and, as such, have reported increased satisfaction with their perioperative care. Ideally, the importance of epidural anesthesia for colorectal surgery will be conveyed to the patients by a representative from each interdisciplinary department (i.e., surgery, anesthesia, nursing), and literature further explaining the risks and benefits of the procedure can be distributed.

Medical knowledge

Residents must demonstrate knowledge about established and evolving biomedical, clinical, and cognate (e.g., epidemiological and social-behavioral) sciences and the application of this knowledge to patient care.

Know and apply the basic and clinically supportive sciences that are appropriate to their discipline.

Be able to understand and articulate the risks and benefits of epidural anesthesia. Furthermore, specific to this case, the resident should be able to discuss the pathophysiology of the postoperative patient. For example, to support the use of neuraxial blockade in this setting, one must know the relationship between opiates and paralytic ileus and length of hospital stay. Additionally, fluid management must be understood and applied, multimodal analgesia must be appreciated, and preoperative predictors of postoperative morbidity must be identified and addressed.

Practice-based learning and improvement

Residents must be able to investigate and evaluate their patient care practices, appraise and assimilate scientific evidence, and improve their patient care practices.

Locate, appraise, and assimilate evidence from scientific studies related to their patients' health problems.

Be up to date with the recent literature regarding specific cases. Pertinent to this case are many recent articles exploring the morbidity and mortality of patients undergoing so-called traditional colorectal surgery as compared to those undergoing fast-track colorectal surgery. It is important that the resident be familiar with these studies and guidelines as well as those specifically targeting epidural analgesia and multimodal anesthesia. If the resident is unaware of current literature, he or she must have the tools to access online journals and other sources of current literature.

Professionalism

Residents must demonstrate a commitment to carrying out professional responsibilities, adherence to ethical principles, and sensitivity to a diverse patient population.

Demonstrate respect, compassion, and integrity; a responsiveness to the needs of patients and society that supersedes self-interest; accountability to patients, society, and the profession; and a commitment to excellence and ongoing professional development.

Despite whatever the resident may feel is the best course of action for anesthetic care, if the patient refuses, for example, the resident must not show disappointment or judgment.

Interpersonal and communication skills

Residents must be able to demonstrate interpersonal and communication skills that result in effective information exchange and teaming with patients, their patients' families, and professional associates.

Use effective listening skills and elicit and provide information using effective nonverbal, explanatory, questioning, and writing skills.

Spend some time with the patient and his or her family, discussing treatment options. For instance, when addressing the issue of postoperative pain and the role of epidural anesthesia, it may help to have a surgical colleague present to further the conversation. In so doing, the patient and family are met with a cohesive medical team. It may also behoove one to discuss the likelihood of a shorter hospital course with a fast-track approach. This could help the patient to consider economic factors as well as allow the resident to consider cost-effective health care (without any foreseeable detriment to the patient). Reassurance is also of utmost importance with respect to patient satisfaction, so be certain to listen to the patient and provide contact information should further questions arise.

Additional reading

1. Chase D, Lopez S, Nguyen C, et al. A clinical pathway for postoperative management and early patient discharge: does it work in gynecologic surgery. Am J Ob Gyn 2008;199:541.

2. Ender J, Borger M, Scholz M, et al. Cardiac surgery fast-track treatment in a postanesthetic care unit: six-month results of the Leipzig fast-track concept. Anesthesiology 2008;109:61–66.

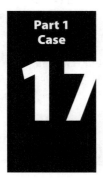

Contributions from Stony Brook University under Christopher J. Gallagher

Treatment of complex regional pain syndrome when the payer doesn't know anything about what you are treating

The case

Marco Palmieri and Brian Durkin

Your patient is a 23-year-old woman who suffered a severe right ankle sprain while exercising her client's dog in the park. She stepped on a rock, twisted her ankle, and ended up in the emergency room, where X-rays showed no fracture – just soft tissue swelling. This happened 6 months ago, and finally, she is sent to your pain clinic for evaluation of possible reflex sympathetic dystrophy (now called complex regional pain syndrome) and medication management. Because this was an on-the-job injury, worker's compensation will be paying her medical bills. She lets you know that her job doesn't provide insurance because she is only part-time. This is one of three part-time jobs that she works while trying to get into graduate school.

Your evaluation leads you to believe that she has complex regional pain syndrome (CRPS) type I – she has allodynia, excessive nail and hair growth, swelling, and color changes, and she is very depressed about the whole thing. She tells you that the hydrocodone/APAP (N-acetyl-p-aminophenol) that her primary care physician is giving her "doesn't even touch the pain." She's taking four to five acetaminophen and seven to eight ibuprofen tablets per day. She tells you that since she has the appointment to see pain management, that she expects you to refill her medications.

Patient care

Residents must be able to provide patient care that is compassionate, appropriate, and effective for the treatment of health problems and the promotion of health.

Communicate effectively and demonstrate caring and respectful behaviors when interacting with patients and their families.

This is very critical for all patients, but especially for a patient who has been told by every health care professional thus far that every test and exam has been essentially normal. Her family and friends may be growing inpatient with her, so it's important that you talk to her and validate her concerns. Assure her that you will not just brush off her symptoms as her being overly dramatic.

Gather essential and accurate information about their patients.

Luckily for your and the patient's sanity, all the lab work and radiology exams were done at your institution and are on the new computer system. You are able to review the plain films, computed tomography scan, magnetic resonance image, and three-phase bone scan done recently as part of the workup completed by the previous physicians who were caring for her. No one has been able to pinpoint a diagnosis, and all the exams were "essentially normal."

Develop and carry out patient management plans.

Your treatment plan will focus on three things: (1) physical therapy, (2) pain control with medications and nerve blocks, and (3) psychological counseling. The patient went to physical therapy after the injury but stopped going because it made the pain worse. You must assure her that with adequate pain control, she should be able to get back to therapy and regain function in her leg. Typically, a diagnostic and, possibly, therapeutic lumbar sympathetic block is done and then followed with a physical therapy session or two. Your office staff reminds you that you have to get authorization before scheduling her for any blocks, and they say that they'll get right on it.

Medication options should focus first on neuropathic pain medications and then anti-inflammatory medications and opioids, if needed to perform adequate physical therapy. You decide to start with pregabalin 75 mg twice per day and titrate up to 150 mg twice per day over a week's time. You also start amitriptyline 25 mg at night and instruct the patient to increase her dose to 75 mg over the next 2 weeks.

Finally, you start her on lidocaine 5% patches and tell her to place three over her right lower leg and foot. You give her some hydrocodone/APAP so she doesn't go into withdrawal and tell her to limit her acetaminophen to less than 3–4 g/day (assuming normal liver function).

From the psychological perspective, you let her know that you are trying to find a psychologist who specializes in pain control, but the closest one available is about an hour away. The pain psychiatrist at your institution is too busy and is not taking any new patients, and the institution is not hiring anyone, ever (I know – it doesn't make sense). So you must now wear the hat of a psychologist and counsel her appropriately. You may even try to find some cognitive-behavioral exercises or desensitization techniques that may be helpful.

That's the plan – start medications, get authorization for lumbar sympathetic blocks, and get her spirits up.

Use information technology to support patient care decisions and patient education.

Perhaps you can direct her and her family members to some useful Web sites to become more informed on her diagnosis and possible treatment options.

Perform competently all medical and invasive procedures considered essential for the area of practice.

Like we said before, part of the treatment for CRPS is pain control with medications and various nerve blocks. Two such blocks are stellate ganglion blocks (upper extremity) and lumbar sympathetic blocks (lower extremity). These blocks are used to see if there is a sympathetic component to the pain. It is hoped, for you and your patient, that the block can be both diagnostic and therapeutic, and *whamo*, you can nail your diagnosis. There is little evidence-based information regarding the proper timing, number, or appropriateness of these nerve blocks for the treatment of CRPS; however, these blocks are used to reduce pain and to enable patients to resume functional rehabilitation, which is our ultimate goal.

Work with health care professionals, including those from other disciplines, to provide patient-focused care.

Your office staff lets you know a couple days after your initial consultation that worker's compensation wants an independent medical examiner (IME) to evaluate the patient. The following week, you find out that the IME has diagnosed "chronic regional pain syndrome" and has recommended a series of three stellate ganglion blocks. You reread this report and can't believe what you see. Did this doctor see the same patient? Did I miss something? Wasn't this an ankle injury? You call the worker's compensation office, and they tell you that they have to stand by what the IME says, and maybe you should call him yourself.

Having been a big fan of the Hardy Boys when you were a kid, you decide to do some investigating. Let's get him on the phone and work this out. You Google him and find several phone numbers scattered around different locations. You also find a Web page that gives a little biography and learn that he is a retired orthopedic surgeon who graduated from medical school in 1958. He was on the faculty at your institution more than 20 years ago, and now he has a little business in retirement, in which he does independent medical exams. Coincidentally, he has a son who is a physician in New Orleans and who is an interventional pain specialist. After Googling yourself and finding nothing but a B movie star who shares your name, you give one of his office numbers a call and leave a message explaining what must be an honest mistake. After all, he has spawned a son who ought to know the right thing to do.

Two days later, a note is on your desk from the IME. "I am returning your phone call to let you know that it is illegal for me to talk to you about this case." Great. You wonder about the choice you made going into medicine and then decide to call New Orleans. You call the IME's son and leave a message with his staff and listen to the uncomfortable silence afterward. "We'll forward this to our doctor. Ya'll from New York, huh?"

Medical knowledge

Residents must demonstrate knowledge about established and evolving biomedical, clinical, and cognate (e.g., epidemiological and social-behavioral) sciences and the application of this knowledge to patient care.

Know and apply the basic and clinically supportive sciences that are appropriate to their discipline.

Before you step into the room and see this patient, you are assured that you know all the critical elements to make the appropriate diagnosis of CRPS. First off, the person has to have pain, *duh*! But seriously, according to the International Association for the Study of Pain, at least one *symptom* in each of the following categories should be present:

1. sensory (i.e., hyperesthesia)
2. vasomotor (temperature or skin color abnormalities)
3. sudomotor-fluid balance (edema or sweating abnormalities)
4. motor (decreased range of motion or weakness, tremor, or neglect)

Also, at least one *sign* in two or more of the following categories should be present:

1. sensory (allodynia or hyperalgesia)
2. vasomotor (objective temperature or skin color abnormalities)
3. sudomotor-fluid balance (objective edema or sweating abnormalities)
4. motor (objective decreased range of motion or weakness, tremor, or neglect)

The diagnosis of CRPS can be difficult, and other diagnoses should be excluded such as diabetic and other peripheral neuropathies, thoracic outlet syndrome, entrapment neuropathies, discogenic disease, deep venous thrombosis, cellulitis, vascular insufficiency, and lymphedema.

Interpersonal and communication skills

Residents must be able to demonstrate interpersonal and communication skills that result in effective information exchange and teaming with patients, their patients' families, and professional associates.

> Advocate for quality patient care and assist patients in dealing with system complexities.

Many patients, like ours in this case, who develop CRPS have to prove their diagnosis to justify treatment. You, the pain physician, must aggressively seek out and document those objective findings on physical exam. Perhaps these findings are not present at all office visits; you must be diligent and help your patient navigate through the endless obstacles she may face as she seeks out treatment for her disease.

> Know how to partner with health care managers and health care providers to assess, coordinate, and improve health care and know how these activities can affect system performance.

As the old saying goes, "if at first you don't succeed, try, try again." Make another phone call to that pain specialist in New Orleans, and perhaps he can provide some insight to the IME as to the proper treatment of CRPS. Of course, when you do so, you are sure to keep all the patient's personal information to yourself, in keeping with HIPAA policy.

Additional reading

1.   Meier P, Zurakowski D, Berde C, Sethna N. Lumbar
     sympathetic blockade in children with complex
     regional pain syndromes: a double blind
     placebo-controlled crossover trial. Anesthesiology
     2009;111:372–380.

2.   Cepeda M, Lau J, Carr DB. Defining the therapeutic
     role of local anesthetic sympathetic blockade in
     complex regional pain syndrome: a narrative and
     systematic review. Clin J Pain 2002;18:216–233.

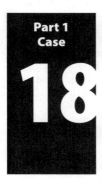

Part 1
Case

18

Contributions from Stony Brook University under Christopher J. Gallagher

OB case with cancer and hypercoagulable state

Joy Schabel and Andrew Rozbruch

The case

A gravida 1 para 0 (G1P0) parturient presented at 38 weeks' gestation with a past medical history significant for breast cancer status post (s/p) bilateral mastectomy, chemotherapy and extensive flap reconstruction, superior vena cava syndrome, expanding brachial plexus mass, chronic pain syndrome, hypercoaguable disorder with bilateral internal jugular (IJ) vein clots, superior vena cava (SVC) clots, and clots in the venous system of bilateral upper extremities. This patient had become pregnant via in vitro fertilization (IVF). On admission to our institution, prior to planned induction of labor, the patient was seen by the obstetrical anesthesia staff for consultation. The main issues of concern regarding the care of this patient were adequate intravenous (IV) access, hypercoagulable status, early epidural placement, surgical backup should cesarean section be necessary, effective pain management, and logistical coordination of necessary resources and personnel.

After interdepartmental discussion with anesthesia, obstetrics, surgery, interventional radiology, pain management, labor and delivery (L&D) personnel, and main operating room (OR) staff, a plan for the care of this patient was established. IV access was particularly challenging in this patient. We were unable to use either upper extremity secondary to lymph node dissection from her mastectomy or extensive venous sclerosing from the chemotherapy; additionally, the patient had bilateral IJ clots, further limiting upper body access. We also wanted to avoid femoral access due to the high risk of clot formation and the need for hip flexion for vaginal delivery. Prior to induction of labor, the patient was sent for placement of a peripherally inserted central (PIC) line with ultrasound guidance to ensure safe and secure access.

Coordination with general surgery and their availability for backup was also arranged in the event of a cesarean because the patient had extensive mesh reconstruction in her abdomen secondary to flap reconstruction after her mastectomy. With the aforementioned contingencies arranged, the patient then received dinoprostone for induction of labor. On arrival to L&D, the patient received an epidural to manage her labor pain and provide a safe mode of anesthesia care in the event of a stat cesarean section. The patient was also placed on a hydromorphone patient-controlled analgesia and fentanyl transdermal patch, as prescribed by the acute pain service, to manage her chronic axilla pain and opioid requirements. Over the course of the next 32 hours, the patient's labor progressed without complications, and the patient delivered vaginally.

Patient care

Residents must be able to provide patient care that is compassionate, appropriate, and effective for the treatment of health problems and the promotion of health.

Communicate effectively and demonstrate caring and respectful behaviors when interacting with patients and their families.

When speaking of bedside manner, either you have it or you don't, right? Wrong – well, sort of. Some of us are better than others at communication, listening, and showing patients that we care. If you have it built in, great; if you don't, you need to learn. Our job as anesthesiologists in establishing trust and building rapport with a patient is a tad more difficult than for the patient's primary care physician or obstetrician-gynecologist because we are often meeting the patient for the first time right before she hands her life over to us. The patient hasn't done any research about us, she hasn't had the opportunity to speak with us before – you catch my drift. So game face on! Approaching a patient with respect and instilling a sense of caring and trust with that patient requires homework. That's right, as old as you get, you still have to do your homework. What do I mean? First, know something about your patient before you meet her. Pick up her chart, review her medical history, speak to other physicians caring for the patient, and have a sense of who the patient is both medically and as a person before you barge into her room and start speaking at her. Which brings me to my next point: don't speak *at* your patients; rather, speak *to* them. Most of our patients have not gone through medical school like we have. Dumb it down a little. Introduce yourself, extend your hand, get down to the patient's eye level, sit down next to her if you can. We are not in a hurry, right? We have nothing else to do, right? Wrong, but the patient does not need to know that. She should feel as though she is your number one priority.

Gather essential and accurate information about their patients.

Know as much about your patient as you can before you meet her. Your history and physical should be an opportunity to confirm what you already know about the patient and clarify some loose ends. This will instantly set the patient at ease and win you many brownie points. If the patient senses that you are learning about her for the first time, as you are speaking to her, she may begin to have doubts, especially if the patient is a nurse, like our patient was. Don't get caught with your pants down – if you always do the right thing, you won't get caught in a compromising situation.

Work with health care professionals, including those from other disciplines, to provide patient-focused care.

Since we are doctors and we know everything, we should dictate to our patients what the plan for them will be. Wrong. While we are highly educated, trained professionals, we don't know everything. If you don't already know that, you need help. Listen to your patient's concerns. For example, with this patient, IV access proved to be a very challenging task, yet of utmost importance. We suggested to the patient the placement of a PIC line. The patient was concerned because of the clots she had in her superior vena cava. Good point; did I think of that? Well, sort of, but I'll just let the interventional radiology people deal with it, right? No, I listened to the patient, acknowledged her concerns, and consulted with the interventional radiologists. I then shared the facts of my conversation with the patient, explained that she need not be

concerned about the clots because the catheter would be placed proximal to her SVC clots, and explained that this intervention would be the safest, most practical plan for her. In this manner, I gained the patient's respect and trust and used good clinical judgment in knowing my limitation of knowledge with respect to PIC lines, and I went to the appropriate resources to get the patient sound, truthful information. Part of good patient care is knowing your limitations and when to ask for help.

Provide health care services aimed at preventing health problems or maintaining health.

So with the PIC line in place, we can go ahead and have the obstetricians induce the patient, right? What if she needs that stat cesarean? All that mesh in her belly from previous surgery, that shouldn't be a problem, we'll deal with it when the time comes. Don't think so! Part of good patient care is always staying one step ahead. Making sure that general surgery would be available for backup prior to induction of this patient was mandatory, not optional. Remember, let's not get caught with our pants down.

Counsel and educate patients and their families.

Although many of our patients homeschool themselves with the Internet and seem to know a good deal about what will happen to them, oftentimes, they are misunderstood or misinformed. Don't believe everything you read. Educating your patients not only enables them to work with you in their care, but it also gives you an opportunity to show how smart you are, which only serves to instill more trust and confidence with the patient.

Medical knowledge

Residents must demonstrate knowledge about established and evolving biomedical, clinical, and cognate (e.g., epidemiological and social-behavioral) sciences and the application of this knowledge to patient care.

Demonstrate an investigatory and analytic thinking approach to clinical situations.

Come to your cases with a plan in mind. Don't leave it to your attending to dictate what you are going to do with your patient. You'll never learn anything that way. Use your cases as a vehicle to draw out important topics and learning issues. Take this case, for example; it's chock full of juicy points. Take some time, identify the important elements, and run with it. Read, talk to others, and be prepared for your sake and the sake of your patient. The more you know, the better it is for all parties involved.

Practice-based learning and improvement

Residents must be able to investigate and evaluate their patient care practices, appraise and assimilate scientific evidence, and improve their patient care practices.

> Analyze practice experience and perform practice-based improvement activities using a systematic methodology.

As we say in the business, some of your worst mistakes can end up being your greatest lessons; it is hoped that you did not harm your patient. During medical school and residency is the time to make your mistakes, but remember not to make the same mistake twice. That's the whole idea behind practice-based learning and improvement. Take the time to discuss both what went wrong and what went right, and always build on your experiences for future practice.

> Use information technology to manage information, access online medical information, and support their own education.

If you don't know, ask; better yet, look it up. Evidence-based medicine, kids – it's the wave of the future. Know your patient and her medical problems, and know them *well*. With the advent of online resources such as PubMed and Google, it has never been easier to look something up and actually have scientific support for what you are saying.

> Obtain and use information about their own population of patients and the larger population from which their patients are drawn.

Talk to your friends and colleagues at other places – HIPAA, of course – and share war stories. Different institutions and different geographical areas see different pathology and do things a little differently. Go to conferences; see what's out there. Suck it all up and incorporate it into your practice as you see fit.

> Apply knowledge of study designs and statistical methods to the appraisal of clinical studies and other information on diagnostic and therapeutic effectiveness.

Think for yourself. "But I read it in a paper." Anyone can get something published. Do your homework, dig deep back to your knowledge of statistical methods and study design, and see if what you're reading is worth reading. If not, move on and find a better article.

Professionalism

Residents must demonstrate a commitment to carrying out professional responsibilities, adherence to ethical principles, and sensitivity to a diverse patient population.

> Demonstrate a commitment to ethical principles pertaining to provision or withholding of clinical care, confidentiality of patient information, informed consent, and business practice.

This complicated patient became pregnant via IVF with donor sperm by an IVF specialist. There was no father of the baby in the picture. One may question the ethics involved in IVF practice for a patient so critically ill. The obstetricians involved in the care of this patient felt that this patient would be denied the ability to adopt a child because of her illnesses, but there are fewer rules and regulations for IVF. Who is going to care for this child in the event of likely health deterioration?

As anesthesiologists, we deal with life-and-death issues more so than social issues. IVF is typically considered more of a social patient issue. However, the IVF of this patient created a life-and-death issue for her. She was already hypercoagulable, which was worsened with getting pregnant. IV access could only be obtained with radiologic assistance. What if she threw a clot to her lungs, heart, or brain? What if she started to hemorrhage after delivery and additional IV access would be necessary to transfuse blood and fluids rapidly? We had to be ready for potential life-threatening disaster created by IVF. I doubt that "life-threatening" appeared anywhere on the IVF consent form. It should have been listed there for this case.

> Demonstrate sensitivity and responsiveness to patients' culture, age, gender, and disabilities.

Though it is difficult to understand and support the incomprehensible decision to impregnate this patient via IVF, what was done was done. We could only be respectful to the patient and her decision making as we anticipated the potential complexities involved in her management. Her medical diseases and limitations challenged our ability to care for her, but we did so with compassion and sensitivity to her many needs.

Interpersonal and communication skills

Residents must be able to demonstrate interpersonal and communication skills that result in effective information exchange and teaming with patients, their patients' families, and professional associates.

> Work effectively with others as a member or leader of a health care team or other professional group.

Taking the necessary time to obtain a thorough history was crucial in this case to understand all the complicated medical and surgical issues, establish the safest management plan, and establish trust. Recent review of closed claim analyses has shown poor communication among health care providers to be a growing and alarming trend among obstetric anesthesia malpractice claims [1]. We need to communicate openly and honestly with patients and other health care teams to maximize patient safety.

Systems-based practice

Residents must demonstrate an awareness of and responsiveness to the larger context and system of health care and the ability to effectively call on system resources to provide care that is of optimal value.

> Understand how their patient care and other professional practices affect other health care professionals, the health care organization, and the larger society and how these elements of the system affect their own practice.

The IVF specialist in this case should have been available to observe the extensive medical and surgical planning necessary to keep this patient out of harm's way. I do not think the IVF specialist was aware of the larger context of health care involved with making this patient pregnant. Lifelong learning in systems-based practice is critical to the practice of medicine, no matter the specialty. Discussion and planning with surgery, obstetrics, anesthesiology, radiology, main OR and L&D staff, and the acute pain team were essential to be prepared for anything from a vaginal delivery to a stat cesarean section in this case.

> Advocate for quality patient care and assist patients in dealing with system complexities.

The multidisciplinary care team worked together to advocate for the best quality care for this patient and her unborn child, given multiple different scenarios. Being prepared was essential to maximizing patient safety and minimizing patient harm.

> Know how to partner with health care managers and health care providers to assess, coordinate, and improve health care and know how these activities can affect system performance.

The coordination of this patient's care maximized patient safety for this patient and her unborn child. What is missing in the coordination of health care in this case is the involvement of the IVF specialist once fertilization had taken place. One would wonder if the IVF specialist would have changed his or her future practice after being part of the delivery end of this patient's care scenario!

Reference

1. Davies JM, Posner KL, Lee L, Cheney FW, Domino KB. Liability associated with obstetric anesthesia: a closed claim analysis. Anesthesiology 2008;109:131–139.

Contributions from Stony Brook University under
Christopher J. Gallagher

19 Extubated and jaws wired shut

Peggy Seidman and Ramon Abola

The case

A 16-year-old male patient is under the care of the pediatric intensive care unit (PICU). He was a pedestrian struck by a motor vehicle and has suffered a traumatic brain injury (TBI) and mandible fracture. He has been stabilized over the past week after endotracheal intubation, intracranial pressure (ICP) monitor placement, ventriculostomy, and decompressive craniectomy. He has required high levels of sedation and paralytics for ICP control.

He undergoes open reduction and internal fixation of the mandible with the oral-maxillary facial surgery (OMFS) service. Preoperative, his oral-tracheal tube is exchanged to a nasal-tracheal tube. The operation proceeds uneventfully. His jaws are wired at the end of the procedure. He returns to the PICU nasally intubated. Overnight, the patient's pulmonary status is favorable. He has maintained normal oxygen saturation with a fractional inspired oxygen (FiO$_2$) of 35% and is spontaneously breathing with 5 mm of pressure support and 5 mm of PEEP.

The patient is following some, but not all, commands. He is evaluated by the PICU staff and the decision is made to extubate. After extubation, he quickly becomes hypoxic, with a SpO$_2$ in the 80s. Chest auscultation reveals clear lungs with course upper airway sounds. The PICU staff is unable to properly suction the oropharynx because of the jaw wires. Anesthesia is called to the bedside. He continues to be hypoxic and in respiratory distress.

As the anesthesia resident on call, you look at the PICU staff, who are searching for answers. The patient's jaws are wired shut, and he's not doing well. You wonder what to do with this handy MAC 3 laryngoscope that you're holding in your left hand.

Patient care

Residents must be able to provide patient care that is compassionate, appropriate, and effective for the treatment of health problems and the promotion of health.

Communicate effectively and demonstrate caring and respectful behaviors when interacting with patients and their families.

There are no family members in the room. Thankfully, the PICU staff made the wise decision to ask Mom and Dad to leave the room during extubation. However, should the family be allowed to stay in the room?

Family members have reported various satisfaction levels when they have been allowed to be present for their loved ones in an emergency resuscitation setting [1]. However this scenario is quite different from an emergency resuscitation in an emergency room. In this situation, the patient would not benefit from family being present, and it is not clear if the family would benefit from being at the bedside.

We often bring parents into the operating room for the induction of anesthesia for the benefit of both the parent and the child. However, the data do not clearly support the benefit to the child of having a parent in the operating room. Apparently, around the world, people are also bringing clowns into the operating room with their pediatric patients [2, 3]. A recent article in the *Canadian Journal of Anesthesia* states, "Contrary to popular belief, in most cases parental presence does not appear to alleviate parents' or children's anxiety. In the rare instances when it does seem to diminish parents' or children's anxiety, premedicating children with midazolam has shown to be a viable alternative. Other anxiety-reducing solutions, such as distracting children with video games, should also be considered" [4, p. 57].

Gather essential and accurate information about their patients.

Consider the following:

1. A quick glance at the patient reveals that he is in respiratory distress. His breathing is labored and noisy.
2. The monitors support this diagnosis – the patient's pulse ox is reading 80% with 100% oxygen administered through a non-rebreathing mask.
3. The PICU resident gives you a quick and brief summary of the patient's history and the events this morning that have led to the present situation.

Make informed decisions about diagnostic and therapeutic interventions based on patient information and preferences, up-to-date scientific evidence, and clinical judgment.

Let's see. The patient was breathing fine with a breathing tube. We have now removed the breathing tube, and patient is no longer doing fine. You try to remember the anesthesia attending who asked you how long the brain can tolerate not receiving oxygen. Four minutes? Maybe it was 5 minutes? (For those who like mnemonics, remember Seidman's rule of 7s: 70 days to starve to death, 7 days to dehydrate to death, 7 minutes of no O_2 until death.) Is that time less because the patient suffered a traumatic brain injury? Wait! Why are you wasting your time? You need to reestablish an airway quickly!

An anesthesiologist needs to be able to assess and manage the emergency airway, which includes determining important equipment and personnel that need to be readily available.

Develop and carry out patient management plans.

Your plan: oral intubation. We'll need to cut those jaw wires to get the tube in there. Thankfully, the OMFS service have placed wire cutters at the head of the patient's bed, as is standard for care for this type of patient for exactly this reason. It's always useful when things are where they are supposed to be. The OMFS service showed the PICU staff how and where to clip the wires during evening rounds last night, and no one actually thought that this information may be needed. You move toward the head of the bed and prepare for direct laryngoscopy.

Counsel and educate patients and their families.

No time to educate the patient and his family during this emergency. However, you hope that the PICU staff has discussed with the family the possibility that the patient may not tolerate extubation. There is the very real possibility of reintubation and, ultimately, the patient may need a tracheostomy.

Use information technology to support patient care decisions and patient education.

Perhaps the use of information technology and online resources is not so useful in the emergency situation. After this episode, a review of the pertinent literature regarding anesthesia management for oral-maxofacial surgery is most useful. "Perioperative Anesthetic Management of Maxillofacial Trauma Including Ophthalmic Injuries" [5] sounds like a good place to start.

Perform competently all medical and invasive procedures considered essential for the area of practice.

A competent anesthesiologist will be able to perform direct laryngoscopy and oral intubation in the presence of a difficult airway. He or she would also be skillful in performing nasal intubation for the original surgery. An anesthesiologist must also assess and determine a proper time for extubation. The anesthesiologist must be prepared for failed extubation and have ready a plan should this occur.

Work with health care professionals, including those from other disciplines, to provide patient-focused care.

The coordination of anesthesia, PICU nursing and physician staff, and oral-maxo-facial surgery is essential to providing the optimal care for this patient, especially in the emergency situation. Future consultation with the pediatric surgery or otolaryngology service to evaluate for placement of a tracheostomy may be warranted.

Medical knowledge

Residents must demonstrate knowledge about established and evolving biomedical, clinical, and cognate (e.g., epidemiological and social-behavioral) sciences and the application of this knowledge to patient care.

Demonstrate an investigatory and analytic thinking approach to clinical situations.

Respiratory distress after extubation occurs. You need to quickly consider a differential diagnosis as to the current situation. Postoperatively, failed extubation could be related to several factors:

1. drugs: too many sedative/hypnotics on board to adequately maintain an airway, inadequate reversal of muscle relaxation
2. pulmonary: pulmonary edema, pneumothorax (hey, we weren't operating anywhere near the lungs, buddy), asthma/bronchospasm, cardiac problems (right ventricular failure, pulmonary edema from congestive heart failure?)
3. airway obstruction from posterior pharyngeal problems or laryngospasm, upper airway secretions unable to clear

This list is obviously not nearly as exhaustive as it should be. The anesthesiologist must also be knowledgeable about determining the appropriateness of extubation. Extubation criteria in the operating room may have some difference to criteria in the ICU setting. However, some basic (and not so basic) principles follow:

1. Is the patient awake or alert enough to protect his own airway?
2. Is the patient hemodynamically stable?
3. Has the initial reason for intubation been resolved?
4. Does the patient demonstrate adequate oxygenation and ventilation during a spontaneous breathing trial or during a T piece trial?
5. Is the patient strong enough to remove ventilator support – does he demonstrate an adequate negative inspiratory force or an adequate vital capacity? Will he be able to maintain effort of respiration in face of nutrional status? Will he fatigue after time?
6. Does the patient demonstrate a favorable rapid, shallow breathing index?

Know and apply the basic and clinically supportive sciences that are appropriate to their discipline.

The medical knowledge that is needed in providing adequate care for this patient is extensive:

1. ICU care
2. approach to the trauma patient
3. approach to the patient with TBI
4. management of ICPs in the head trauma patient
5. ventilator management for the ICU patient

Practice-based learning and improvement

Residents must be able to investigate and evaluate their patient care practices, appraise and assimilate scientific evidence, and improve their patient care practices.

Analyze practice experience and perform practice-based improvement activities using a systematic methodology.

Debriefing and discussion sessions about critical events are important to promote learning and education. Debriefing sessions can come in a variety of different forms: a formal meeting between departments, a discussion between the attending and residents, or even a discussion between physicians and nursing staff. There are a variety of different perspectives about the events, the critical decisions, the implications of those decisions, and lessons for future patient care.

Locate, appraise, and assimilate evidence from scientific studies related to their patients' health problems.

Our PICU has developed an algorithm for the surgical and medical treatment of TBI patients and the management of intracranial pressure. This algorithm was designed after reviewing the pertinent literature and clinical trials that relate to this topic [6]. Algorithms, if designed well, should allow for the implementation of so-called best practices. Critical evaluation of the data from which these algorithms are designed is important to determine the validity of these recommendations and management steps [6].

Our guidelines for the management of TBI patients include some of the following:

PICU Management of High ICP/Low Cerebral Perfusion Pressure (CPP)
First-Tier Therapies

1. administer appropriate sedation/analgesia in patients with secured airways
2. elevate head of bed 30° and in midline
3. manage patient's temperature aggressively to avoid hyperthermia and increased cerebral metabolic rate
4. provide seizure prophylaxis

5. maintain normal glucose levels
6. treat acute increase in ICP or decrease in CPP with sedation, mannitol, or 3% saline
7. treat acute increases in ICP with mild hyperventilation ($PACO_2$ or $ETCO_2$ between 30 and 35) while obtaining one of the preceding therapies

Second-Tier Therapies

1. surgical: neurosurgery to consider placement of an extraventricular drain
2. medical: hyperventilation with goal pCO_2 of 30–35 if ICPs have been unsuccessfully managed with sedation, osmotherapy, and ventricular drainage
3. medical: if these measures do not control ICPs, patient will be placed in a pentobarbital coma with continuous electroencephalography until burst suppression is achieved

Third-Tier Therapies

1. surgical: if continued elevated ICPs, neurosurgery to evaluate for possible decompressive craniectomy
2. medical: consideration of use of 3% saline infusion

Although these recommendations are guidelines that the PICU staff uses to manage head trauma patients, essential to the idea of practice-based learning is to (1) understand the clinical foundation on which these guidelines were made and (2) critically evaluate these recommendations for areas in which change may improve patient outcome. One such idea is considering the use of decompressive craniectomy as an early surgical therapy for these patients. Another example is that hyperventilation was a routine practice in the past for these patients; however, this practice has fallen out of favor. Decreased ICPs secondary to hyperventilation only last 6–12 hours, and there are concerns about decreasing cerebral blood flow to an injured brain with vasoconstriction.

Apply knowledge of study designs and statistical methods to the appraisal of clinical studies and other information on diagnostic and therapeutic effectiveness.

Critical evaluation of clinical studies is important:

1. Does the study group adequately represent the characteristics of my current patient?

2. Do the therapeutic recommendations show a significant improvement to change patient management?
3. Have our own practice experiences been in agreement with clinical studies?

Professionalism

Residents must demonstrate a commitment to carrying out professional responsibilities, adherence to ethical principles, and sensitivity to a diverse patient population.

Demonstrate respect, compassion, and integrity; a responsiveness to the needs of patients and society that supersedes self-interest; accountability to patients, society, and the profession; and a commitment to excellence and ongoing professional development.

Physician A is a participant in this clinical scenario. Physician A begins asking who's to blame for this situation. Who is the responsible party who caused further harm to this patient? Physician A sneers at the accused, stating that the case should have been handled differently and that Physician A should have been called sooner. Physician A stammers that it has always been the policy that these extubations should be handled in this manner to a resident and an attending who are both unaware of any such policy. In a condescending tone, Physician A says, "I hope that you've learned your lesson."

Physician B is a participant in this clinical scenario. He or she gathers information from the various groups involved to obtain a clear picture of what happened. He or she discusses with the various medical services their opinion of the situation, what decisions were made, and how those decisions influenced the results. Physician B tries to identify reasons for why an unintended outcome occurred, not who is the responsible party. Physician B seeks to identify ways to improve both his or her own clinical practice and the clinical practice of the health care unit.

Demonstrate sensitivity and responsiveness to patients' culture, age, gender, and disabilities.

Children are not little adults. This is a phrase recited time and time again by our pediatric colleagues.

Ultimately, our patient failed extubation secondary to his TBI. His pulmonary status appeared to be optimized, but his TBI is the reason for being unable to properly protect his airway and clear his secretions. This is supported by the clinical observation that the patient was not following commands prior to extubation.

In the adult patient, our hospital will routinely place tracheostomy tubes early in a patient's hospital course if it appears that the patient will need prolonged mechanical ventilation. This allows for a decrease in sedation and mobilization of the patient out of bed, if possible. The question is, why not place a tracheostomy in our 16-year-old PICU patient during this first week, when he has demonstrated that he will likely require prolonged ICU care?

Although practices differ between hospitals, our PICU will typically try to avoid placing a tracheostomy tube unless it is absolutely necessary because trachs in children can be very difficult for the families to deal with. This has been the observation of our PICU staff, and it represents an example of how the practice of medicine requires the clinician to be sensitive to the patient's age and also the family members, who become patients themselves, in a way.

Interpersonal and communication skills

Residents must be able to demonstrate interpersonal and communication skills that result in effective information exchange and teaming with patients, their patients' families, and professional associates.

> Create and sustain a therapeutic and ethically sound relationship with patients.

One of the most difficult aspects of the medical practice is providing patients and families with bad news. Similar to history taking or physical exam, giving bad news requires practice.

In this current case, our patient did poorly after extubation. His wires, which were cut, were then noted to be located in both his stomach and pharynx, as they were not accounted for during the airway emergency after extubation. The patient needed to be brought back to the operating room and placed under general anesthesia for endoscopy and direct laryngoscopy to extract these jaw wires and remove them as an infection risk and to prevent them from getting buried into mucosa or other tissues.

Essential to medical practice is being able to provide families with unpleasant information and to be honest about events that occurred during their medical care. Who is the unfortunate resident or physician who has to tell this patient's family that (1) he did not do well after we tried to take out the breathing tube, (2) we have to bring him back to the operating room, and (3) we had to reintubate the patient – essentially everything being a step in the wrong direction? Because you are the emergency consultant without a relationship with the family, the ICU team will need to do this, and they are the most appropriate medical service to inform the family. Often, it is best for the physician who has developed a relationship with the family to meet with the family to discuss bad news. As an anesthesiologist, meeting with a family postoperatively is enhanced by the presence and support of the surgeon, who has developed a patient-physician relationship prior to the day of surgery.

Communication is key to a healthy and working relationship between the medical staff, the patient, and the family. Discussion with patients and families ahead of time about what to expect, plus the possible complications, is essential to help guide patients through medical care. Looking at things from a medicolegal perspective, communication may be beneficial in preventing medical malpractice litigation [7].

> Work effectively with others as a member or leader of a health care team or other professional group.

Essential in any emergency situation is the development of a team leader and team players. The team leader provides the guidance and plan for care, and the team members are just as essential to complete the tasks and provide feedback to the team leader about the situation. Team building is essential for a group of people to respond in an organized fashion to an emergency situation. Think of code blues and cardiac arrests for which there was complete chaos, with no order and people running around like chickens without heads. This is a place where simulation can help by allowing teams to work together in the safety of simulation.

Systems-based practice

Residents must demonstrate an awareness of and responsiveness to the larger context and system of health care and the ability to effectively call on system resources to provide care that is of optimal value.

> Know how types of medical practice and delivery systems differ from one another, including methods of controlling health care costs and allocating resources.

One aspect of ICU care that is relatively new is the ICU checklist. The checklist is a systems-based list that ensures important goals and objectives of the ICU patient on a daily basis such as number of antibiotic days, days since central lines have been placed, or nutritional and feeding management. Checklists allow for important aspects of patient care not to be missed on a daily basis. ICU checklists may also evaluate a patient's need for continued ICU, which may significantly impact the cost of the patient's care.

In addition to the ICU checklist are interdisciplinary rounds, which facilitate communication between the various medical services of ICU patients – the medical staff, nursing staff, nutrition, respiratory therapy, and pharmacy – allowing for optimization of care and keeping all services in agreement.

> Know how to partner with health care managers and health care providers to assess, coordinate, and improve health care and know how these activities can affect system performance.

Important after any critical event is communication between members of the health care team in a professional manner to provide optimal care for future situations. The purpose of these meetings and discussions is to identify systems-based mistakes. Typically, no error in medicine occurs in isolation. Pointing fingers and trying to find who is to blame are typically not very productive means of improving future care.

After this case, it was decided that similar cases should coordinate PICU staff, OMFS, and anesthesia, who are to be readily available at bedside for quick and efficient airway management in the event of a failed trial of extubation.

References

1. Myers TA, Eichhorn DJ, Dezra J, et al. Family presence during invasive procedures and resuscitation. Top Emerg Med 2004;26:61–73.

2. Vagnoli L, Caprilli S, Robiglio A, et al. Clown doctors as a treatment for preoperative anxiety in children: a randomized, prospective study. Pediatrics 2005;116:e563–e567.

3. Golan G, Tighe P, Dobija N, et al. Clowns for the prevention of preoperative anxiety in children: a randomized controlled trial. Paediatr Anaesth 2009;19:262–266.

4. Chundamala J, Wright JG, Kemp SM. An evidence-based review of parental presence during anesthesia induction and parent/child anxiety. Can J Anaesth 2009;56:57–70.

5. Shearer VE, Gardner J, Murphy MT. Perioperative anesthetic management of maxillofacial trauma including ophthalmic injuries. Anesth Clin North Am 1999;17:141–153.

6. Carney NA, Chestnut R, Kochanek PM. Guidelines for the acute medical management of severe traumatic brain injury in infants, children and adolescents. Pediatr Crit Care Med 2003;4(Suppl):S1.

7. Sack K. Doctors say "I'm sorry" before "see you in court." The New York Times 2008 May 18;A1.

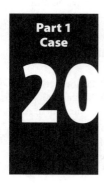
Contributions from Stony Brook University under Christopher J. Gallagher

Code Noelle
A tale of postpartum hemorrhage

Rishimani Adsumelli and Ramon Abola

The case

A 45-year-old woman, gravida 4 para 3, presents at 38 weeks' gestation for cesarean section. The patient has had three previous cesarean sections. Obstetrical colleagues inform you that she has placenta previa and strong possibility for placenta accreta. The patient is originally from Pakistan and speaks only Punjabi and had general anesthesia without complications for her previous three cesarean sections, which were performed in Pakistan. Nursing staff has had a difficult time placing an appropriately sized peripheral IV. The patient's airway examination is unremarkable and her body mass index is within normal limits.

After discussion with colleagues about the risks and benefits of regional versus general anesthesia for this case, a decision is made to recommend regional anesthesia with spinal anesthesia. The patient is reluctant about having a spinal and inquires about general anesthesia. Fortunately, one of the obstetrician residents also speaks Punjabi and facilitates communication. Discussion takes places, informing the patient about the reasons for preferring regional anesthesia, and the patient agrees to this anesthetic plan. Arrangements are made for blood salvage equipment for use in the operating room.

The patient is brought to the operating room and spinal anesthesia is administered successfully. There is routine delivery of a healthy infant. However, after delivery of the placenta, a peek over the field reveals a uterus sitting in a large pool of blood that is steadily growing faster than anyone would like. The patient becomes tachycardic and hypotensive as she's losing quite a bit of blood (up to 700 cc/min, to be exact). The obstetricians inform you that they suspect that the patient does in fact have an accreta and plan for an emergency hysterectomy. "Code Noelle" is called – hospital mobilization for postpartum hemorrhage – which coordinates anesthesia, obstetrics, and the blood bank. Medical therapy is attempted to slow the hemorrhage, with minimal improvement.

Anesthesia colleagues join the operating room to assist in volume resuscitation. The patient becomes anxious and inconsolable secondary to the emergency situation or secondary to the acute loss of blood. The father is escorted from the operating room. The patient is induced with ketamine and succinylcholine and is intubated for general anesthesia.

Patient care

Residents must be able to provide patient care that is compassionate, appropriate, and effective for the treatment of health problems and the promotion of health.

Communicate effectively and demonstrate caring and respectful behaviors when interacting with patients and their families.

When the patient expresses her shock that, when general anesthesia was successfully performed without any complications in her home country of Pakistan, why the sophisticated American anesthesiologists are so concerned about dangerous complications, it is important not to ignore her very pertinent observation. It was important to convey that even we can do GA safely if we need to, but we prefer the regional because it is at least a tad safer [1,2]. Communicating the various nuances via appropriate communicators is very important. Here, having the obstetric resident as an interpreter was very helpful.

Gather essential and accurate information about their patients.

Medical information is important, such as previous uncomplicated GA, other comorbid conditions, blood product availability, and not-so-easy IV access (nurses couldn't get IV, even though the patient was not obese).

Make informed decisions about diagnostic and therapeutic interventions based on patient information and preferences, up-to-date scientific evidence, and clinical judgment.

Prepare for a possible need for interventional radiological procedures such as uterine artery embolization [3] and cell saver use. (The worry that a cell saver might produce amniotic fluid embolism has been unfounded. Moreover, if you salvage the blood after the placenta is removed, there is no worry at all [4,5].)

If you feel that the patient is extremely nervous and that GA can be done safely, you could even choose general anesthesia instead of regional. It all depends on your judgment after careful consideration of risks and benefits.

Develop and carry out patient management plans.

A regional anesthesia with GA backup is planned. Prepare for major blood loss with good IV access, blood products, a cell saver, an arterial line, and central venous access, if needed.

Counsel and educate patients and their families.

The following considerations should be made:

- discussion regarding the possible need for blood transfusion and hysterectomy
- honest discussion about the possible need for interventional radiology help and even intensive care unit (ICU) admission
- discussion of the possible need for postop ventilation

Use information technology to support patient care decisions and patient education.

The pertinent issues in this case are as follows:

- the advantages of regional versus GA
- the useful role of interventional radiology procedures
- recent pharmacological modalities for uterine atony
- the use of a cell saver

Perform competently all medical and invasive procedures considered essential for the area of practice.

The following should be considered:

- competency in performing and conducting regional anesthesia
- competency in administering general anesthesia in a pregnant woman; GA was given when she was hypotensive
- competency in obtaining IV access, both peripheral and central
- competency in placing an arterial line
- competency in using the pharmacotherapy

Provide health care services aimed at preventing health problems or maintaining health.

Pertinent points include the following:

- preparation for counteracting massive blood loss and maintaining hemodynamic stability
- measures to prevent aspiration such as naught per oris status, use of H2 blockers and Bicitra, and rapid sequence induction
- timely antibiotic administration

Work with health care professionals, including those from other disciplines, to provide patient-focused care.

This case is a true reflection of a multidisciplinary approach:

- dialogue with obstetrics
- discussion with the blood bank, labor and delivery nurses, and other support staff
- discussion with the interventional radiology team and surgical ICU team

Medical knowledge

Residents must demonstrate knowledge about established and evolving biomedical, clinical, and cognate (e.g., epidemiological and social-behavioral) sciences and the application of this knowledge to patient care.

Demonstrate an investigatory and analytic thinking approach to clinical situations.

The pertinent points in our case are as follows:

- Is a well-conducted GA really so harmful? What is the current thinking?
- Is it better to do preemptive radiological procedures?
- Am I really prepared for possible blood loss of 700 cc/min?

Know and apply the basic and clinically supportive sciences that are appropriate to their discipline.

The following should be considered:

- thorough knowledge of blood therapy and complications such as transfusion-related acute lung injury
- appropriate use of products
- knowledge of pharmacotherapy of uterotonics
- role of recombinant factor VII

Practice-based learning and improvement

Residents must be able to investigate and evaluate their patient care practices, appraise and assimilate scientific evidence, and improve their patient care practices.

Analyze practice experience and perform practice-based improvement activities using a systematic methodology.

This is based on the following:

- your own experience of exposure to such cases in the past
- your own reflection of how to improve care
- departmental quality control reviews of these cases and debriefings that follow
- knowledge of the departmental protocols that were formulated based on the debriefings

Locate, appraise, and assimilate evidence from scientific studies related to their patients' health problems.

This is based on the following:

- lectures on this topic that you attended
- literature searches
- departmental online resources

Obtain and use information about their own population of patients and the larger population from which their patients are drawn.

Consider the following:

- having knowledge of newer modalities of airway management in case of difficult intubation

- in general, having good exposure to blood product therapy
- application of the knowledge gained from other areas of anesthesia in her situation (at times, knowledge from other areas takes time to trickle down to obstetric anesthesia)
- additionally, debriefing and discussion between anesthesia residents and attendings about case management, critical events, and lessons from the case aid in generating new information
- resident self-reflection on the role of their individual management of the patient, self-reflection on learning and prediction of their performance in this situation if they had been the attending, and aid in continuing practice-based learning

Apply knowledge of study designs and statistical methods to the appraisal of clinical studies and other information on diagnostic and therapeutic effectiveness.

This involves the following:

- knowledge of the statistics needed to evaluate the power of the studies
- ability to analyze statistical significance

Use information technology to manage information, access online medical information, and support their own education.

This involves the following:

- ability to use search engines to get information
- knowledge of departmental online resources

Professionalism

Residents must demonstrate a commitment to carrying out professional responsibilities, adherence to ethical principles, and sensitivity to a diverse patient population.

Demonstrate respect, compassion, and integrity; a responsiveness to the needs of patients and society that supersedes self-interest; accountability to patients, society, and the profession; and a commitment to excellence and ongoing professional development.

This involves the following:

- respectful communication regarding the pros and cons of GA
- respectful communication about the need for an arterial line and large-bore IV when still awake
- overcoming language barriers to connect with the patient
- preparing with necessary skills such as advanced cardiac life support and neonatal advanced life support
- attending departmental grand rounds and continuing use of medical education resources

---

Demonstrate a commitment to ethical principles pertaining to provision or withholding of clinical care, confidentiality of patient information, informed consent, and business practice.

This involves the following:

- ethicality of refusing the care [6] if the patient is adamant about GA
- misplaced worry about additional cost because of the cell saver and all the hotline sets because there is a possibility that she may not need them

---

Demonstrate sensitivity and responsiveness to patients' culture, age, gender, and disabilities.

This involves the following:

- understanding that because of her background, she may be extremely uncomfortable if not covered
- might be more comfortable with women
- care not to be condescending of the medical care in her country

Interpersonal and communication skills

Residents must be able to demonstrate interpersonal and communication skills that result in effective information exchange and teaming with patients, their patients' families, and professional associates.

Create and sustain a therapeutic and ethically sound relationship with patients.

This involves the following:

- honest informed consent and explanation of the rationale behind the use of invasive monitoring

- overcoming language barriers
- effective communication with Dad when he needs to leave the room and continuing the communication about patient status and new developments

---

Use effective listening skills and elicit and provide information using effective nonverbal, explanatory, questioning, and writing skills.

This involves the following:

- judging that there is a severe uterine atony and massive hemorrhage by the expression on the obstetrician's face
- knowing that there is significant hypotension when the patient looks spaced out

---

Work effectively with others as a member or leader of a health care team or other professional group.

This involves the following:

- effective communication about the patient's status, need for GA and blood products, and need for more personnel
- calling code Noelle when extra help is needed

Systems-based practice

Residents must demonstrate an awareness of and responsiveness to the larger context and system of health care and the ability to effectively call on system resources to provide care that is of optimal value.

Understand how their patient care and other professional practices affect other health care professionals, the health care organization, and the larger society and how these elements of the system affect their own practice.

This involves the following:

- understanding of the hospital rules and regulations for narcotic use
- thorough understanding of the impact of a skeleton staff of nurses and other support personnel after 3:00 P.M. [7]
- availability of help from other physicians such as interventional radiologists and gynecologists

Practice cost-effective health care and resource allocation that does not compromise quality of care.

This involves the following:
- having a rapid infuser available but not ready
- cost differences between bupivacaine and ropivacaine
- cost comparison of various inhalational anesthetics

Advocate for quality patient care and assist patients in dealing with system complexities.

The pertinent issue in our case is finding the right person to translate for the patient.

Know how to partner with health care managers and health care providers to assess, coordinate, and improve health care and know how these activities can affect system performance.

The pertinent issue in our case is that in our hospital, systems-based multidisciplinary protocols have been developed for risk stratification, effective treatment, and rapid mobilization of resources by calling code Noelle. Knowledge of the resources that will be mobilized by the code and when to activate this code is important.

References

1. Gulur P, Nishimori M, Ballantyne J. Regional anaesthesia versus general anaesthesia, morbidity and mortality. Best Pract Res Clin Anaesthesiol 2006;20:249–263.

2. Afolabi BB, Lesi F, Merah N. Regional versus general anaesthesia for caesarean section. Cochrane Database Syst Rev 2006;18:CD004350.

3. Hong TM, Tseng H, Lee R, et al. Uterine artery embolization: an effective treatment for intractable obstetric haemorrhage. Clin Radiol 2004;59:96–101.

4. Catling S, William S, Fielding A. Cell salvage in obstetrics: an evaluation of the ability of cell salvage combined with leucocyte depletion filtration to remove amniotic fluid from operative blood loss at caesarean section. Int J Obstet Anesth 1999;8:79–88.

5. King M, Wrench I, Galimberti A, et al. Introduction of cell salvage to a large obstetric unit: the first six months. Int J Obstet Anesth 2009;18:111–117.

6. Chervenak F, McCullough L, Birnbach D. Ethics: an essential dimension of clinical obstetric anesthesia. Anesth Analg 2003;96:1480–1485.

7. Bendavid E, Kaganova Y, Needleman J, et al. Complication rates on weekends and weekdays in US hospitals. Am J Med 2007;120:422–428.

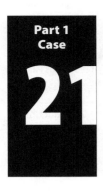
Are you sure there's a baby there?
A tale of the morbidly obese parturient

Ellen Steinberg and Ramon Abola

The case

A 32-year-old gravida 1 para 0 (G1P0) presents to labor and delivery for induction of labor for a large-for-gestational-age fetus. The patient is at 39 weeks' gestation. Past medical history is significant for morbid obesity. She is 5 foot 6 inches but weighs 400 pounds. She presents to the floor for induction in the early evening, a similar practice for most inductions as patients should then be in active labor during the daytime hours. Anesthesia staff is present 24 hours, however, with less help available during the evening hours. During your evening huddle – a meeting between obstetrics (OB), nursing, and anesthesia services – this patient's case is discussed. The patient is also a so-called difficult patient, demanding of the nursing staff, and lacks insight into the severity of her situation. She is unhappy that she is being treated differently than the other expectant mothers on the floor.

Discussion between OB and anesthesia determines that appropriate management will be as follows: (1) placement of an epidural (prior to induction) available for use for emergency cesarean section for maternal or fetal distress, (2) induction of labor, and (3) vaginal delivery – a reasonable plan.

The reality:

1. Nursing staff is unable to obtain intravenous (IV) access.
2. Anesthesia requires IV access prior to epidural placement in case of emergency.
3. Central venous access is placed secondary to inadequate peripheral access.
4. Epidural is placed after multiple attempts, with success after a second anesthesia team attempts epidural placement.
5. Induction of labor is initiated.
6. Patient fails induction of labor.
7. OB and anesthesia staff agree that the best approach will be to perform a cesarean section in a controlled fashion; emergency cesarean section may result in fetal or maternal compromise.
8. Cesarean section is performed under epidural anesthesia; emergency and difficult airway equipment is available in the operating room.
9. The cesarean section proceeds uneventfully under regional anesthesia.

Patient care

Residents must be able to provide patient care that is compassionate, appropriate, and effective for the treatment of health problems and the promotion of health.

Communicate effectively and demonstrate caring and respectful behaviors when interacting with patients and their families.

Communication between the staff and patient is of the utmost importance in the medically challenging and difficult patient. As health care practitioners, we have to be able to convey our concerns to the patient. Educating patients about these concerns helps the patient understand the prescribed care plan.

The patient's body habitus, in our case, complicates medical care:

- difficult IV access
- potential difficult airway management if general anesthesia is needed (mask ventilation in a 400-pound, pregnant patient who will rapidly desaturate secondary to decreased functional residual capacity, with increased metabolic demand and an excess of soft tissue in the airway, does not sound pleasant)
- potentially difficult placement of regional anesthesia (Do you know where the midline is?)
- difficulty in accurate monitoring – both fetal and maternal

- increased comorbid conditions during pregnancy (hypertension, diabetes [1]).
- potentially difficult cesarean section
- increased risk of infection after cesarean section [2]

Gather essential and accurate information about their patients.

A quick review of this patient reveals a morbidly obese patient, G1P0, with an intrauterine pregnancy at term. There is no significant past medical history, and there have been no significant problems during this pregnancy. The patient has had no previous surgeries. Medications include prenatal vitamins.

Physical exam reveals a blood pressure of 110/70, P 76, SpO$_2$ 96% on room air. The patient appears to be in no acute distress. Her airway exam reveals a good mouth opening and a Mallampati class II airway, with good neck extension. Thyromental distance appears to be greater than three finger breadths; however, the patient's neck circumference is quite large. You suspect that the patient would easily exhibit airway obstruction with too much sedation. Auscultation of the chest and heart are difficult secondary to the patient's body habitus. You note the multiple attempts that the nurses have made in placing an IV.

Laboratory studies are reviewed, revealing an appropriate hematocrit of 36, a platelet count of 140, and normal coagulation studies. Gathering the essential information is important to developing an appropriate management plan for this patient.

Develop and carry out patient management plans.

A useful tool in medical practice is to predict what will or what could possibly happen during the care of a patient. Planning for all possible outcomes allows one to better prepare for an emergency. The management plan for this patient was as follows:

1. Placement of IV access prior to epidural anesthesia should be performed. During a regional anesthetic procedure, IV access administers essential IV fluids or emergency medications for resuscitation. Complications with neuraxial anesthesia include hypotension from sympathectomy, high spinal block, and local anesthesia toxicity from intravascular injection.
2. As placement of peripheral IV access was unsuccessful, a central line was placed. A right

internal jugular triple lumen catheter was placed under ultrasound guidance. There is current debate about increased safety, success rate, and time to placement [3]. An article from *Interactive and Cardiovascular Thoracic Surgery* concludes that "in patients with a potentially difficult central line insertion, the ultrasound technique reduces complications and time to insertion. However, in those patients where no difficulty is predicted, there is no evidence that the ultrasound technique confers any advantage" [3, p. 527].

3. Placement of epidural anesthesia prior to induction of labor should be completed. Should the patient develop the need for a stat cesarean section (i.e., nonreassuring fetal heart tracing), having epidural anesthesia in place would allow for rapid administration of surgical-level anesthesia, without instrumentation of the patient's airway.
4. Then, induction of labor for a large-for-gestational-age fetus should be performed.
5. Should general anesthesia become necessary, difficult airway equipment, including different laryngoscope blades, a laryngeal mask airway, an intubating laryngeal mask airway, gum elastic bougie, and other airway tools should be readily available.

Perform competently all medical and invasive procedures considered essential for the area of practice.

Invasive procedures performed during this case include (1) establishing IV access in a difficult patient, (2) placement of an epidural catheter, (3) placement of central venous access for a patient with poor peripheral access, and (4) airway management in the obese patient should general anesthesia be needed. Essential for the anesthesiologist is determination of the appropriateness of each invasive procedure.

Work with health care professionals, including those from other disciplines, to provide patient-focused care.

Labor and delivery requires coordinating the services of anesthesia, obstetrics, and nursing staff to provide optimal care. Each area of expertise provides a different perspective about the current problem, and by communication and discussion, the best medical plan should be established.

Medical knowledge

Residents must demonstrate knowledge about established and evolving biomedical, clinical, and cognate (e.g., epidemiological and social-behavioral) sciences and the application of this knowledge to patient care.

Know and apply the basic and clinically supportive sciences that are appropriate to their discipline.

With any parturient, the anesthesiologist needs to be mindful of the physiological changes in pregnancy and how this will affect their management. Knowledge of increased blood volume and increased edema is important as this will result in increased airway edema, fragile mucosa, and more difficult airway management. Lung volumes are decreased secondary to the gravid uterus, with a decreased functional residual capacity. The pregnant patient will become hypoxic faster with apnea than the nonpregnant patient. Additionally, the pregnant patient has an increased risk of aspirating gastric contents because progesterone relaxes the lower esophageal sphincter tone and there is increased pressure on the abdomen by the gravid uterus [4].

Obesity increases the probability of difficult airway management, certainly making ventilation more difficult and possibly making intubation more difficult [5]. Proper patient positioning for intubation is important.

The morbidly obese patient demonstrates (1) a decreased functional residual capacity and (2) a decreased closing capacity, both of which will result in faster oxygen desaturation with apnea. Increased chest wall weight results in increased airway resistance and higher peak airway pressures during positive pressure ventilation. Patients with morbid obesity have a high incidence of sleep apnea, which can be associated with pulmonary hypertension and, ultimately, cor pulmonale.

These patients may have associated medical conditions that complicate both their anesthetic and obstetric management, including hypertension, diabetes, and coronary artery disease. These patients are at an increased risk of developing gestational hypertension, preeclampsia, gestational diabetes, and fetal birth weight greater than 4,000 g [6].

Regional anesthesia provides an attractive anesthetic plan for these patients as it allows for surgery without manipulation of the airway. A postoperative concern for this patient is pain management, and regional anesthesia allows one to minimize systemic analgesics that may depress respiratory function.

The anesthesiologist must be informed about obstetrics to facilitate decisions regarding patient care. Knowledge of the indications for a cesarean section allows the anesthesiologist to be an advocate for good patient care. Questioning a colleague about the indication for this procedure may allow a patient not to have an unnecessary procedure. Knowledge of the procedure itself is important. In the morbidly obese patient, a cesarean section is not a simple procedure: (1) how much tissue is there between the skin and the uterus? (2) Can you find the uterus to apply fundal pressure when extracting the fetus? (3) An operative delivery can have increased complications of poor wound healing and wound infection. This is surgery that would benefit from as much expertise and assistance as is available. A stat cesarean section in this patient may likely have complications. Alternatively, vaginal delivery may not be a better option. These patients have an increased rate of large-for-gestational-age fetuses, and there is a higher risk of shoulder dystocia.

Practice-based learning and improvement

Residents must be able to investigate and evaluate their patient care practices, appraise and assimilate scientific evidence, and improve their patient care practices.

Analyze practice experience and perform practice-based improvement activities using a systematic methodology.

Essential to anesthesia learning is to review the events of this case, the decisions that were made, the patient outcome, and if alternatives to therapy should have been done.

On our obstetric anesthesia service, we perform a daily debriefing with residents and attendings that reviews the day's critical events, teaching points, and lessons for future care. It is a system that reviews clinical experience to help shape learning and future decision making.

Locate, appraise, and assimilate evidence from scientific studies related to their patients' health problems.

Reviewing pertinent literature before and after this case about the obstetric management of the morbidly obese patient allows one to ensure that one is performing evidenced-based medicine and adhering to good practice principles. Reviewing literature may also provide ways to improve patient care, for example, would the use of ultrasound guidance improve success in epidural placement [7]?

Apply knowledge of study designs and statistical methods to the appraisal of clinical studies and other information on diagnostic and therapeutic effectiveness.

Reviewing the medical literature about the complications noted in the morbidly obese parturient as well as performing a critical review of this information for its validity will allow the medical team to prepare patients for what they should expect in their care. The care of the morbidly obese paturient has a high likelihood of complications, both for the mom and for the fetus.

Professionalism

Residents must demonstrate a commitment to carrying out professional responsibilities, adherence to ethical principles, and sensitivity to a diverse patient population.

Demonstrate a commitment to ethical principles pertaining to provision or withholding of clinical care, confidentiality of patient information, informed consent, and business practice.

One of the most difficult aspects of obstetrical care is that we are caring for two patients: both the mom and the fetus. A principle to review is that fetal well-being is dependent on maternal well-being. If maternal health is jeopardized, then the outcome of the fetus is jeopardized. However, this relationship does not necessarily apply in reverse.

Consider the following scenario: our morbidly obese patient is on labor and delivery with continuous fetal monitoring. The fetus demonstrates nonreassuring fetal heart tracing, and the decision is made to perform a stat cesarean section. Performing an ill-prepared general anesthetic in this patient may result

in loss of the airway, hypoxia, cardiac arrest, and loss of both the mother and the fetus. The physician must remain mindful of this problem and perform the ethical principle of nonmaleficence. This is not to say that an urgent cesarean section cannot be performed, but it should not be done in a matter that may jeopardize the life of the mother.

Interpersonal and communication skills

Residents must be able to demonstrate interpersonal and communication skills that result in effective information exchange and teaming with patients, their patients' families, and professional associates.

Create and sustain a therapeutic and ethically sound relationship with patients.

Communication skills were essential in dealing with this difficult patient. The medical staff needed to develop a trusting relationship with this patient in a very short amount of time. Trust is important from this patient, particularly as several invasive procedures needed to be performed – central line access and epidural placement.

Work effectively with others as a member or leader of a health care team or other professional group.

One practice that we have implemented on labor and delivery is the huddle, which is to occur twice a day. The nursing, anesthesia, and obstetric staff meet briefly to discuss the patients on the unit, any potential problems, and planned medical care. This also provides an opportunity for each medical service to express its concerns about individual patients.

Systems-based practice

Residents must demonstrate an awareness of and responsiveness to the larger context and system of health care and the ability to effectively call on system resources to provide care that is of optimal value.

Understand how their patient care and other professional practices affect other health care professionals, the health care organization, and the larger society and how these elements of the system affect their own practice.

This case highlights some of the challenges of care with a morbidly obese pregnant patient during delivery. A task force was formed to evaluate several of the issues surrounding this case. The task force looked at ways to improve system practices for these patients. What quality improvement measures can be done to optimize patient care? Several policies have been implemented.

We have compiled the data from the medical literature that assess the complication rates and outcomes of pregnancy in the morbidly obese patient. This information has been given both to health care providers and to patients. This education highlights the risks, dangers, and outcomes of the morbidly obese patient during pregnancy. Better educating patients should allow them to modify their expectations should they decide to become pregnant.

Assessing a patient prior to presentation at labor and delivery allows for anesthesia providers to (1) evaluate the airway, (2) evaluate possible peripheral IV access, and (3) provide patient education about anesthetic management at the time of delivery. Educating patients about the placement of an epidural catheter early in labor allows them to understand the benefits of the medical plan. The outpatient setting also allows for more time in a lower-stress environment for questions and concerns to be properly addressed. An anesthetic plan can be formulated prior to presentation on labor and delivery.

As noted in this case, given the difficulty of IV access, our staff has become more aggressive at having peripherally inserted central catheter lines placed by interventional radiology before admission to labor and delivery.

Improving the health care system and using a multidisciplinary approach to these patients should improve patient care.

Additional reading

1. Castro LC, Avina R. Maternal obesity and pregnancy outcomes. Curr Opin Obstetr Gynecol 2002;14:601–666.

2. Schneid-Kofman N, Sheiner E, Levy A, Holcberg G. Risk factors for wound infection following cesarean deliveries. Int J Obstetr Gynecol 2005;90: 10–15.

3. Espinet A, Dunning J. Does ultrasound-guided central line insertion reduce complications and time to placement in elective patients undergoing cardiac surgery. Interact Cardiovasc Thorac Surg 2004;3:523–527.

4. Birnbach D, Browne I. Anesthesia for obstetrics. In: Miller R, editor. Miller's anesthesia. 6th ed. Philadelphia: Elsevier Churchill Livingston; 2005: 2307–2344.

5. Popescu WM, Schwartz JJ. Perioperative considerations for the morbidly obese patient. Adv Anesth 2007;25:59–77.

6. Weiss JL. Obesity, obstetric complications and cesarean delivery rate – a population-based screening study. Am J Obstetr Gynecol 2004;190:1091–1097.

7. Ali ME, Laurito C. Ultrasound guidance for epidural catheter placement: a coming of age? J Clin Anesth 2005;17:235–236.

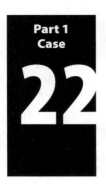

22 Smoking, still smoking, and won't quit

Deborah Richman and Rany Makaryus

The case

"Joe the plumber" is a 44-year-old male who presented to preoperative services with low back pain because of a herniated disc at L5/S1, going for a discectomy. He had been having severe radiating pain, especially down his right leg, and was treating this pain with all the Vicodin he could get his hands on! He did not have any paraesthesias or weakness. As a self-employed contractor, and with no other medical problems besides hypertension (HTN) and gastroesophageal reflux disease, he just wanted to get this surgery done so he could get back to work and pay his bills again. Since he's had surgery before (a laparotomy about 20 years ago, with no problems), of course, he would have no problems with this surgery, right?

On further questioning and a review of systems, it was discovered that he also smokes just a little – only about two packs per day for 30 years! On top of this, he also has a chronic cough, worse in the morning and productive of brown sputum, as well as a wheeze. He denied having frequent urinary tract infections, pneumonia, or bronchitis. He doesn't take any pulmonary medications because he doesn't have insurance. He was also suspect for obstructive sleep apnea, being that he snores, has daytime tiredness, has been observed to stop breathing in his sleep, and has a history of HTN. He can't, however, afford a sleep study because his darned health insurance, which, again, doesn't exist, can't pay!

On the positive side, though, he is a contractor and works hard with great effort and tolerance. He is self-employed; he can't work because he's in too much pain, and he can't afford not to work because he has way too many bills to pay.

His only medication at this time is Vicodin. A physical exam revealed that he is 5 feet 11 inches tall, weighing in at 225 pounds, with a blood pressure of 158/92 and with bilateral wheezes – mainly in the upper airway – that improve with coughing and in an open-mouth sniffing position, but not completely. The rest of the physical exam was noncontributory.

Patient care

Residents must be able to provide patient care that is compassionate, appropriate, and effective for the treatment of health problems and the promotion of health.

Communicate effectively and demonstrate caring and respectful behaviors when interacting with patients and their families.

Joe the plumber is a model U.S. citizen! He definitely deserves respect! This is a difficult situation, in which we must understand the difficult dilemma this patient is in and respect his decision in going forward with surgery, even though his medical condition is not optimized. Part of the problem is that he may not be able to afford the surgery if he puts all his hard-earned money into medical optimization.

Gather essential and accurate information about their patients.

A great deal of time was spent trying to gain information from this patient to establish a working diagnosis and optimize this patient with as little further testing as possible so as not to impart much cost to the patient. Careful assessment of his pulmonary function and stability of his presumed chronic obstructive pulmonary disease (COPD) are mainly done on history and physical exam.

Make informed decisions about diagnostic and therapeutic interventions based on patient information and preferences, up-to-date scientific evidence, and clinical judgment.

This is where being a clinician, and individualizing medical care for each patient, becomes very important. Ideally, this patient should do the following:

- see a pulmonologist for optimization
- be encouraged to quit smoking and have his surgery scheduled for 8 weeks after he quits
- have his sleep apnea evaluated and treated

However, for him, it may be much more beneficial to go ahead with surgery, simply assuming that he won't quit smoking and that he has severe sleep apnea, and to provide anesthesia with these facts and assumptions in mind.

Develop and carry out patient management plans.

The patient's plan includes smoking cessation, incentive spirometry education preoperatively, and beta agonist nebulizer prior to surgery; combined local and general anesthesia; and postoperative monitoring, incentive spirometry, and deep venous thrombosis prophylaxis.

The physician should keep careful documentation of these plans and the reasoning behind them. Communication with the anesthesia and surgical teams who will be providing care for this patient should be maintained to ensure the best possible care for this patient.

Counsel and educate patients and their families.

This patient needs to be educated on multiple health care concerns. First and foremost is education on the negative effects of smoking, especially in such little – oh, sorry, I mean large … oh, sorry, I mean enormous – amounts!

Also important to discuss with this patient is the fact that taking Vicodin for pain should be done in moderation – not only because of the possibility of opioid toxicity, but also because of the adverse hepatic effects of acetaminophen. Sometimes it would be better to provide the patient with opioid medications separately from the acetaminophen.

Finally, if it is decided to go ahead without further optimization, the patient needs to be aware of the extra risks he is taking on – specifically postoperative pulmonary complications, and worse, the risk of being canceled on the day of surgery by the anesthesiologist due to lack of optimization.

Use information technology to support patient care decisions and patient education.

This patient's probable diagnosis of obstructive sleep apnea (OSA) would not have been discovered had the STOP screen questionnaire not been used, which, in the literature, has been proven to be effective in detecting this disease in the preoperative population.

Perform competently all medical and invasive procedures considered essential for the area of practice.

Chest X ray, pulmonary function tests, and blood gases are not proven to change management or outcome in these patients and are not indicated.

Provide health care services aimed at preventing health problems or maintaining health.

Teach the patient preoperatively how to use the incentive spirometer and send him home with one. Offer a prescription for nicotine patches. If sputum is infected (green or yellow), have the patient take an antibiotic for at least 48 hours prior to surgery, with the goal of preventing pulmonary complications postoperatively.

Work with health care professionals, including those from other disciplines, to provide patient-focused care.

Hold discussions with the surgical team, the operating room (OR) anesthesia team, the postanesthesia care unit team, pulmonary experts, and the patient to provide the best possible anesthesia care.

Medical knowledge

Residents must demonstrate knowledge about established and evolving biomedical, clinical, and cognate (e.g., epidemiological and social-behavioral) sciences and the application of this knowledge to patient care.

Demonstrate an investigatory and analytic thinking approach to clinical situations.

Think about how to treat chronic bronchitis/COPD. Think about how to treat OSA.

Know and apply the basic and clinically supportive sciences that are appropriate to their discipline.

Preop use of nebulizers and/or albuterol – to use or not to use? If you gave the patient an inhaler, would his inhaler technique be adequate enough to get the drug delivered, or would most be drifting into the ozone? Also, consider the advantages and disadvantages of preoperative steroids.

How long should the patient stop smoking for? Six hours (CO effects)? Twenty-four hours (sympathetic effects of nicotine withdrawal)? Two weeks (return of ciliary function)? Eight weeks (decreased postoperative pulmonary complications)? Ten years (return to nonsmoking population risk of coronary artery disease and lung cancer)? Or my personal favorite – whenever you stop is good, excellent, and wonderful!

Practice-based learning and improvement

Residents must be able to investigate and evaluate their patient care practices, appraise and assimilate scientific evidence, and improve their patient care practices.

Analyze practice experience and perform practice-based improvement activities using a systematic methodology.

Consider carefully why this patient is different from a 75-year-old with the same history and if that patient could be sent to surgery without further workup – it's all about the risk–benefit ratio. Remember age and closing capacity.

Locate, appraise, and assimilate evidence from scientific studies related to their patients' health problems.

Look up management of COPD, preop optimization for smokers, advantages of quitting tobacco use, and so on. Also look up the usefulness of the STOP screen, what to do with the screen, what is a positive screen, and the importance of identifying patients with OSA.

Obtain and use information about their own population of patients and the larger population from which their patients are drawn.

This patient needs individualized care, and this must be drawn from known information on how to deal with patients with similar disease processes.

Apply knowledge of study designs and statistical methods to the appraisal of clinical studies and other information on diagnostic and therapeutic effectiveness.

Have studies shown that screening for OSA is effective in preventing complications? What about these study designs and/or statistical methods supports that assertion?

Use information technology to manage information, access online medical information, and support their own education.

Much information about COPD, OSA, smoking cessation, local support groups, and so on is available online and in pamphlets that can be handed out to patients.

Professionalism

Residents must demonstrate a commitment to carrying out professional responsibilities, adherence to ethical principles, and sensitivity to a diverse patient population.

Demonstrate respect, compassion, and integrity; a responsiveness to the needs of patients and society that supersedes self-interest; accountability to patients, society, and the profession; and a commitment to excellence and ongoing professional development.

In this case, responding to the needs of the patient is top priority – the need to have surgery to regain the ability to make a living is most important for this patient and thus needs to be most important for the clinician, as well.

Demonstrate a commitment to ethical principles pertaining to provision or withholding of clinical care, confidentiality of patient information, informed consent, and business practice.

Respecting the patient's decision to go ahead with surgery without medical optimization, while he continues to smoke, is important, as is the ethical principle to the patient of "first, do no harm …"

Demonstrate sensitivity and responsiveness to patients' culture, age, gender, and disabilities.

Keeping these factors in mind, making the decision to go with surgery on this patient, while giving the patient all the important information and medical education for surgical optimization, is the result of being sensitive to the patient's disabilities, lack of insurance, and need for employment.

Interpersonal and communication skills

Residents must be able to demonstrate interpersonal and communication skills that result in effective information exchange and teaming with patients, their patients' families, and professional associates.

Create and sustain a therapeutic and ethically sound relationship with patients.

Take care of the patient as a person, not as another subject of medical treatment.

Use effective listening skills and elicit and provide information using effective nonverbal, explanatory, questioning, and writing skills.

Listening to the patient brought out the fact that he lacks insurance, yet needs this surgery. Using inexpensive tests and interventions, for example, the STOP screen and incentive spirometry, to assess and manage this patient provided necessary medical information and allowed the patient to make appropriate medical decisions.

Work effectively with others as a member or leader of a health care team or other professional group.

Communication with the surgical team and the anesthesiologist providing the patient's care is *huge* – the anesthesiologist of the day would not be wrong to cancel our friend Joe the plumber. Find the right guy or gal, give him or her a head's up, and let him or her think it over, bounce it off the boss/spouse/dog, and make an informed decision to anesthetize this patient because of the unique circumstances of 2009.

Systems-based practice

Residents must demonstrate an awareness of and responsiveness to the larger context and system of health care and the ability to effectively call on system resources to provide care that is of optimal value.

Understand how their patient care and other professional practices affect other health care professionals, the health care organization, and the larger society and how these elements of the system affect their own practice.

Deciding that this guy is OK to do might fit your clinical judgment and moral values – you've spoken with a real person, not a cold chart that looks sick or an anxious supine patient without his teeth. But if the surgeon and anesthesiologist of the day do not agree with your opinion – the OR stands, the surgeon fumes, and your colleague thinks you are an idiot (the feeling will probably be mutual) – there is going to be downtime in the OR (mega bucks).

If your judgment is not sound, the patient may suffer postop pneumonia, increased length of stay, tests, consults, and more mega bucks! And the state just cut our budget again.

Practice cost-effective health care and resource allocation that does not compromise quality of care.

Providing this patient with surgery that will empower him to return to work and regain a functional lifestyle is very important – all the while using effective health care, while maintaining the least possible cost to the patient, is key in this case.

Advocate for quality patient care and assist patients in dealing with system complexities.

Helping this patient gain the benefits of surgery, without giving him undue financial stress, is important here.

Know how to partner with health care managers and health care providers to assess, coordinate, and improve health care and know how these activities can affect system performance.

The patient's surgery and recovery period were uneventful. He was discharged home on postop day 1 and has significant improvement in his symptoms, enabling him to return to work ... and smoking.

Additional reading

1. Qaseem A, Snow Q, Fitterman N, et al. Risk assessment for and strategies to reduce perioperative pulmonary complications for patients undergoing noncardiothoracic surgery: a guideline from the American College of Physicians. Ann Intern Med 2006;144:575–580.

2. Pasquina P, Tramèr MR, Granier J, Walder B. Respiratory physiotherapy to prevent pulmonary complications after abdominal surgery: a systematic review. Chest 2006;130:1887–1899.

3. Wong D, Weber E, Schell M, Wong A, Anderson C, Barker S. Factors associated with postoperative pulmonary complications in patients with severe chronic obstructive pulmonary disease. Anesth Analg 1995;80:276–284.

4. Smetana GW, Lawrence VA, Cornell JE. Preoperative pulmonary risk stratification for noncardiothoracic

surgery: systematic review for the American College of Physicians. Ann Intern Med 2006;144: 581–595.

5. Warner DO. Perioperative abstinence from cigarettes: physiological and clinical consequences. Anesthesiology 2006;104:356–367.

6. Egan TD, Wong KC. Perioperative smoking cessation and anesthesia: a review. J Clin Anesth 1992;4: 63–72.

7. Practice guidelines for the perioperative management of patients with obstructive sleep apnea: a report by the American Society of Anesthesiologists Task Force on Perioperative Management of Patients with Obstructive Sleep Apnea. Anesthesiology 2006;104:1081–1093.

8. Chung F, Yegneswaran B, Liao P, et al. STOP questionnaire: a tool to screen obstructive sleep apnea. Anesthesiology 2008;108:812–821.

Contributions from Stony Brook University under Christopher J. Gallagher

Pseudoseizures following office extubation

Ralph Epstein and Andrew Drollinger

The case

This is a case of a 19-year-old female college student presenting to a private dental office for comprehensive dental care under general anesthesia. Her medical history includes depression, panic disorder, "problems with mental health," needle phobia, anemia, latex allergy, and seasonal allergies. She takes sertraline for depression, lorazepam for anxiety, and amoxicillin for dental infection.

At a recent dental appointment under general anesthesia by the same anesthesiologist, blood studies were obtained, including complete blood count (CBC) with platelets and differential and a thyroid panel. All results were found to be within normal limits. Evaluation of her airway classified her as Mallampati class I, with full range of motion of her neck and with adequate thyromental distance.

Owing to the patient's needle phobia, general anesthesia was initiated via mask induction with sevoflurane, nitrous oxide, and oxygen. A 7.0 nasal endotracheal tube was inserted atraumatically through the patient's left naris. Monitoring included electrocardiogram, blood pressure, heart rate, pulse oximetry, pretracheal auscultation, capnography, temperature, and bispectral index (BIS). Anesthesia was maintained by propofol and dexmedetomidine infusion, and her dental work, which included root canal on nine teeth, was completed as expected. The anesthetic course was smooth, with no aberrations. At the completion of treatment, infusions were discontinued, and she was extubated without complications (6:50 P.M.).

At 7:00 P.M., the patient's mother, a physician, was brought into the recovery area with the patient being awake, responsive, and resting comfortably. At 7:20 P.M., the patient's behavior began to change. She started shaking and shuttering and was no longer responsive. Her blood pressure was 113/70, with a pulse of 88 and oxygen saturation at 98%. A BIS monitor was placed, and a reading of greater than 90 was noted. At this point in time, the mother reported that her daughter exhibited this behavior previously in a medical office. Not knowing if the patient was actually having a seizure, intravenous (IV) access was obtained via a 20-gauge catheter and with D5-1/2 as the IV fluid. The patient was administered midazolam 10 mg over 10 minutes with no change in her seizurelike behavior. Diazepam 5 mg was then administered, also with no changes noted. Her BIS was noted to be in the 70s, as expected after the administration of benzodiazepines.

It was noted that this seizurelike behavior would start and stop and increase and decrease in intensity, particularly with her mother's involvement. About 20 minutes into this event, when she was called by the wrong name, she opened her eyes slightly and jokingly became upset that such a mistake was made, and then slipped back into shaking and shuttering.

At 8:20 P.M., emergency medical services (EMS) were called to transport the patient to the local emergency department. This decision was made collectively, including with the mother. The patient was transported to the emergency department via ambulance. All the involved dentists went to the emergency department to provide necessary information to the emergency department physician and to provide support to the patient and her mother.

After about 1 hour in the emergency department, the physician, in hearing the distance of the patient, recommended sedation with propofol and reintubation to take a brain magnetic resonance image (MRI). The mother was opposed to the reintubation and, following the advice of the anesthesiologist, she left the treatment room to call her husband, also a physician. Approximately 3 minutes after the mother left the room, the patient opened her eyes, woke up, and the seizurelike behavior stopped. A brain MRI was taken and the patient was admitted overnight. The brain MRI was read out without any positive findings.

When the IV started by the anesthesiologist in the private office was removed the next morning, the patient exhibited 5 minutes of the seizurelike activity.

The same seizurelike activity occurred later in the afternoon, when the IV started in the emergency department was removed.

Later follow-up indicated that the patient had a video electroencephalogram (EEG) performed. During the video EEG, the patient exhibited four episodes of the seizurelike activity. The official impression from the neurophysiologist conducting the video EEG was as follows:

- four nonepileptic events
- EEG normal
- large beta may be secondary to Ativan

The mother reports that the primary neurologist has made a diagnosis of pseudoseizures.

Patient care

Residents must be able to provide patient care that is compassionate, appropriate, and effective for the treatment of health problems and the promotion of health.

> Communicate effectively and demonstrate caring and respectful behaviors when interacting with patients and their families.

The decision was made early on to involve the patient's mother.

> Gather essential and accurate information about their patients.

Vital signs and BIS were recorded, and seizure activity was highly suspected.

> Make informed decisions about diagnostic and therapeutic interventions based on patient information and preferences, up-to-date scientific evidence, and clinical judgment.

> Suspected seizure activity was treated accordingly.

> Develop and carry out patient management plans.

The patient was treated for seizures and transported to the emergency department via EMS within an appropriate time frame.

> Counsel and educate patients and their families.

The patient's mother was included in the decision-making process.

> Perform competently all medical and invasive procedures considered essential for the area of practice.

General anesthesia was performed as planned and without incident. After pseudoseizures began, IV access was obtained and benzodiazepines were administered.

> Work with health care professionals, including those from other disciplines, to provide patient-focused care.

Everyone who was involved in patient care escorted the patient to the emergency department to provide all necessary information to the emergency department physician.

Medical knowledge

Residents must demonstrate knowledge about established and evolving biomedical, clinical, and cognate (e.g., epidemiological and social-behavioral) sciences and the application of this knowledge to patient care.

> Demonstrate an investigatory and analytic thinking approach to clinical situations.

The patient's behavior was immediately suspected to be seizure and was treated accordingly.

Practice-based learning and improvement

Residents must be able to investigate and evaluate their patient care practices, appraise and assimilate scientific evidence, and improve their patient care practices.

> Locate, appraise, and assimilate evidence from scientific studies related to their patients' health problems.

This patient presented with a psychological history of anxiety and depression.

Professionalism

Residents must demonstrate a commitment to carrying out professional responsibilities, adherence to ethical principles, and sensitivity to a diverse patient population.

Demonstrate respect, compassion, and integrity; a responsiveness to the needs of patients and society that supersedes self-interest; accountability to patients, society, and the profession; and a commitment to excellence and ongoing professional development.

Everyone involved in the patient's care went to the emergency department and stayed until her care was complete.

Additional reading

1. Ng L, Chambers N. Postoperative pseudoepileptic seizures in a known epileptic: complications in recovery. Br J Anaesth 2003;91:598–600.

2. Allen G, Farling P, Ng L, Chambers N. Anaesthesia and pseudoseizures. Br J Anaesth 2004;92:451–452.

3. Parry T, Hirsch N. Psychogenic seizures after general anaesthesia. Anaesthesia 2007;47:534.

4. Taylor DC. Pseudoseizures and the predicament: pseudoseeing is pseudobelieving. Epilepsy Behav 2001;2:78–84.

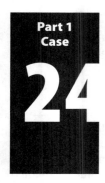

24

Contributions from Stony Brook University under
Christopher J. Gallagher

What happened to the ETT tip?

Ralph Epstein and Tate Montgomery

The case

A 16-kg, 2-year, 6-month-old male presented to the dental office with multiple carious, nonrestorable teeth. His past medical history and family history were noncontributory. On examination, it was determined that he would require a more extensive examination, radiographs, multiple restorations, cleaning, and extractions. It was decided that because of age and behavior, the treatment would be done with the patient under general anesthesia in the dental office. Prior to the date of treatment, the anesthesiologist evaluated the patient and determined that he was a good candidate for office-based general anesthesia.

The child was seen preoperatively by his pediatrician and was found to be healthy, with no contraindications to general anesthesia. Prior to the start of anesthesia, the patient was evaluated by the anesthesiologist and found to be in good condition for office-based general anesthesia on this date. The patient was given 15 mg oral midazolam in the waiting room. Twenty minutes later, he was taken to the treatment room and general anesthesia was induced by sevoflurane and nitrous oxide/oxygen. Intravenous access was obtained with a 22-gauge Jelco catheter in the right anticubital fossa. Standard ASA monitors were placed as well a BIS monitor and a precordial stethoscope.

Both nares were prepared with oxymetazoline drops, and nasal airways 20–26, which were lubricated with 2% lidocaine jelly, were successively placed in the right naris. To decrease the trauma to the naris, an uncuffed Mallinckrodt 4.5 nasal RAE was removed from its package and placed in very hot water. Immediately prior to insertion of the NRAE in the right naris, the tube was lubricated with 2% lidocaine jelly that was on a 4 by 4 inch gauze. The patient was intubated on the first attempt, and it was atraumatic. The tube was secured, eyes were taped, and the head was wrapped in the usual manner for a dental procedure. The dentist placed one throat pack. Maintenance anesthesia was sevoflurane and nitrous oxide/oxygen for

2 hours and 30 minutes. All vital signs, respiratory sounds and $ETCO_2$, SpO_2, temperature, and BIS readings were within normal limits.

When the dentist finished, she removed the throat pack and allowed the anesthesiologist to extubate the patient. It was done atraumatically, although some secretion or something came out with the tube. The tube was placed on a tray to the right, and all attention was returned to the patient. He was recovering very well. On glancing to the right, the anesthesiologist noticed that the tip of the NRAE was abnormal and that part of it was missing. A direct laryngoscopy was performed and there was no sign of a foreign body. The patient continued to have an oxygen saturation of 98%. His lungs were clear to auscultation and he was then transferred to another room to continue recovery and monitoring. The operatory was thoroughly inspected and cleaned in an attempt to find the missing tip from the NRAE, but nothing was found.

The entire situation was explained to the parents. Following consultation with a pediatric radiologist at University Hospital 1 mile away, the patient was transported by the anesthesiologist to the hospital, without discontinuing his IV. A pediatric radiologist reviewed the patient's chest PA and a lateral and found an area of prominent markings in the right upper lobe due to atelectasis or infiltrate, no air trapping, and no opaque foreign body. A pediatric mag study was also done, and there was atelectasis or infiltrate in the right upper lung field; no radiopaque foreign body and no nonopaque foreign body surrounded by air was found. Intravenous access was discontinued, and the patient was transported to the private office of the chief of otolaryngology.

The patient was inspected via anterior rhinoscopy, direct fiber-optic nasal endoscopy, and laryngoscopy with phenylephrine. There was no evidence of a foreign body, abrasion, or any airway compromise. The patient was then sent home, and instructions were given to the parents that if anything abnormal occurred with regard to his breathing, they should inform the anesthesiologist and immediately go to the emergency department. The patient was followed by his pediatrician, radiographs were retaken 3–4 days posttreatment, and he was evaluated in the office 6 days later. The patient did well, and the parents never reported any problems.

Mallinckrodt was informed of the situation via e-mail, and digital photographs of the tube were sent. After several months, by letter, Mallinckrodt explained that the tubes are manufactured in one piece. The Murphy eye is then punched after the tube is formed. They explained that the tube was probably punched twice and not detected by their quality control procedures. This defect was reported to both the quality and manufacturing departments, and they requested that corrective action be implemented to avoid the reoccurrence of this problem.

This was a situation that was challenging to manage because it occurred in a private office, where all means where not immediately available to address the concerns of an incomplete tube discovered on extubation. All information was disclosed to the parents, and they were assisted and informed throughout the entire process. We are reminded by this incidence that we must always be ready to manage unexpected situations in a professional and ethical manner. I currently check not only the cuff on my endotracheal tubes, but the entire tube every time I intubate! Will you now?

Patient care

Residents must be able to provide patient care that is compassionate, appropriate, and effective for the treatment of health problems and the promotion of health.

Communicate effectively and demonstrate caring and respectful behaviors when interacting with patients and their families.

It was necessary for the anesthesiologist to carefully explain, in full detail, in a manner that the parents could understand, what happened and what was going to need to be done.

Gather essential and accurate information about their patients.

As the patient was so young, it was necessary to discuss with the parents the health of the child and to ask appropriate questions.

Make informed decisions about diagnostic and therapeutic interventions based on patient information and preferences, up-to-date scientific evidence, and clinical judgment.

It was decided to first transport the patient to the hospital for further examination, and when satisfactory results were not found, the patient was then transferred to a specialist to further determine what could be done to ensure that the best care was provided.

Develop and carry out patient management plans.

The postoperative management was handled as described previously.

Counsel and educate patients and their families.

Most information was given to the parents because of the patient's age. The parents were informed about everything and were very cooperative.

Use information technology to support patient care decisions and patient education.

It was explained to the parents that everything was done to find the missing piece of the endotracheal tube. In the past, the most that might have been done would have been to take a chest X-ray, but with the aid of the specialist, much more was done to maintain the health of the patient.

Perform competently all medical and invasive procedures considered essential for the area of practice.

The anesthesiologist transferred the patient to two different and independent health care providers to reevaluate and confirm that nothing was abnormal.

Medical knowledge

Residents must demonstrate knowledge about established and evolving biomedical, clinical, and cognate (e.g., epidemiological and social-behavioral) sciences and the application of this knowledge to patient care.

Demonstrate an investigatory and analytic thinking approach to clinical situations.

Before the patient was transferred to the hospital, the room was thoroughly searched to see if the missing piece could be found. After the situation occurred, the manufacturer was contacted to further explain what happened.

Practice-based learning and improvement

Residents must be able to investigate and evaluate their patient care practices, appraise and assimilate scientific evidence, and improve their patient care practices.

Locate, appraise, and assimilate evidence from scientific studies related to their patients' health problems.

The manufacturer was contacted to determine if this has been a problem and to see what would be done to ensure that this did not happen again.

Obtain and use information about their own population of patients and the larger population from which their patients are drawn.

This was an unexpected issue that was not specific to this patient's population; however, it could occur to anyone undergoing intubated general anesthesia.

Professionalism

Residents must demonstrate a commitment to carrying out professional responsibilities, adherence to ethical principles, and sensitivity to a diverse patient population.

Demonstrate respect, compassion, and integrity; a responsiveness to the needs of patients and society that supersedes self-interest; accountability to patients, society, and the profession; and a commitment to excellence and ongoing professional development.

Because this patient required unexpected additional care, other patients had to be rescheduled to another day. Total productivity for the day was decreased, which resulted in a decrease of income for the operating dentist and the anesthesiologist.

Demonstrate a commitment to ethical principles pertaining to provision or withholding of clinical care, confidentiality of patient information, informed consent, and business practice.

Throughout this entire case, the parents were fully informed and involved to make sure they knew that the best health care available was provided to their child.

Interpersonal and communication skills

Residents must be able to demonstrate interpersonal and communication skills that result in effective information exchange and teaming with patients, their patients' families, and professional associates.

Create and sustain a therapeutic and ethically sound relationship with patients.

The family was kept informed of the status of their child during the posttreatment evaluation process. Multiple postoperative phone calls were made to answer questions and to make sure the child had no further complications.

Work effectively with others as a member or leader of a health care team or other professional group.

The entire staff was involved in attempts to find the missing piece and to determine a plausible cause for the issue. Multiple other health care providers were consulted, but the anesthesiologist took the lead, gathered information from all possible resources, and made leadership decisions for the benefit of the patient.

Systems-based practice

Residents must demonstrate an awareness of and responsiveness to the larger context and system of health care and the ability to effectively call on system resources to provide care that is of optimal value.

Understand how their patient care and other professional practices affect other health care professionals, the health care organization, and the larger society and how these elements of the system affect their own practice.

This case demonstrates how office-based general anesthesia care affects multiple health care practitioners and institutions and also how dependent we are on multiple providers to ensure the best care for our patients.

> Practice cost-effective health care and resource allocation that does not compromise quality of care.

This case demonstrates that when providing cost-effective office-based general anesthesia and being presented with the most unexpected of complications, the patient's quality of care was not compromised.

> Advocate for quality patient care and assist patients in dealing with system complexities.

The anesthesiologist was with the patient throughout the multiple visits he received. He was there to explain the results that were obtained from the different specialists. The complexities of accessing specialty consultant care were far from normal. While attending to the recovery of the child, multiple phone consultations outside the treatment facility were required to schedule and organize the best treatment for the patient.

> Know how to partner with health care managers and health care providers to assess, coordinate, and improve health care and know how these activities can affect system performance.

The private office had predetermined where a patient would be transported if it were ever necessary. This way, there was no time wasted when it was actually necessary.

Additional reading

1. Pritt B, Harmon M, Schwartz M, et al. A tale of three aspirations: foreign bodies in the airway. J Clin Pathol 2003;56:791–794.

2. Lampl L. Tracheobronchial injuries: conservative treatment. Interact Cardiovasc Thorac Surg 2004;3:401–405.

3. Wang PC, Tseng GY, Yang HB, et al. Inadvertent tracheobronchial placement of feeding tube in a mechanically ventilated patient. J Chin Med Assoc 2008;71:365–367.

4. Krzanowski TJ, Mazur W. A complication associated with the Murphy eye of an endotracheal tube. Anesth Analg 2005;100:1854–1855.

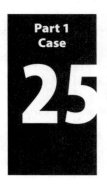

25 Jerry and Terry want one more baby

Rishimani Adsumelli and Vishal Sharma

The case

A 39-year-old gravida 10 para 9 (G10P9) is admitted for treatment and evaluation to the obstetrics floor for abdominal pain. The obstetricians are telling you that the patient probably has placenta accreta and placenta previa on ultrasound. Furthermore, the obstetricians relate to you that the baby has no heart rate and no movement is visualized on ultrasound at 36 weeks' gestation. The patient has no significant past medical history. Her obstetric history is extensive, including five vaginal births and four previous cesarean sections. Her cesarean sections were complicated by uterine atony after each procedure, requiring blood transfusions and an intensive care unit stay for the last one. It is recommended to the patient that she undergo bilateral uterine artery embolization as well as abdominal hysterectomy to remove the dead fetus and to prevent postpartum hemorrhage from previa and accreta. The patient is devastated at the loss of her child and is refusing all medical care. She just wanted to be given some sedation and sleep.

After extensive discussion with the patient and the obstetrician, it is determined that an initial attempt to perform a cesarean section will be made; if, however, the patient begins to have bleeding of any kind, no further attempts will be made to deliver the placenta, and the patient will then undergo abdominal hysterectomy.

The patient is brought to the operating room and an epidural catheter is placed successfully with a T5 thoracic level obtained using 2% lidocaine with 1:200,000 epinephrine, approximately 20 mL. An arterial line and three large-bore IVs are placed. The patient is sedated with versed and incremental doses of ketamine. During the surgery, the obstetricians perform a cesarean section; after opening the uterus, a large amount of brownish amniotic fluid is expelled, and it becomes readily apparent that the cause of IUFD was, in fact, placental abruption. The obstetricians discontinue efforts to remove the placenta after initial attempts reveal brisk bleeding and then successfully

perform abdominal hysterectomy. During the surgery, the patient develops hypotension and bradycardia. The patient is transfused 5 units of packed red blood cells, 2 units of platelets, and 2 units of fresh frozen plasma. Her lowest hemoglobin was 6.7 and her hematocrit was 24. The patient is transported to the recovery room, where she recovers from her surgery. She has no other complications and is eventually discharged after 5 days of hospitalization.

Patient care

Residents must be able to provide patient care that is compassionate, appropriate, and effective for the treatment of health problems and the promotion of health.

Communicate effectively and demonstrate caring and respectful behaviors when interacting with patients and their families.

Although the patient wanted only sedation and wasn't willing to discuss any other medical management, it was not an option for the medical team. We couldn't sedate unless consents were signed for management.

Faced with this situation, the only option was to give her some time for this devastating event to sink in, while continuing discussions with her husband. We showed empathy by having different staff try to get across to her, even a pastor. After 2 hours, one of the labor and delivery nurses managed to convince her that the rest of her children needed her and that she needed to consent to the treatment plan. After the consent was obtained, sedation was given.

It must be said that this mother of nine children has an abundance of progeny, and although the loss of a child may be devastating, the clear course of action in this case would be to prevent postpartum hemorrhage. You must put aside any resentment and difficulties you might have with providing care for a patient not willing to comply with the advice of doctors. The patient is making the best decision for her, and not for you. The role that the physician should play in this situation is to inform the patient of the risks, benefits, and alternatives of surgery and anesthesia and advise a course of action that is both safe and effective in treating this mother. Adapting to the patient is part of being a good anesthesiologist.

Gather essential and accurate information about their patients.

The patient had many risk factors for postpartum hemorrhage. This patient had advanced maternal age. The patient had four previous cesarean sections. The patient had a previous history of uterine atony. The patient had an ultrasound consistent with placenta previa and accreta.

Make informed decisions about diagnostic and therapeutic interventions based on patient information and preferences, up-to-date scientific evidence, and clinical judgment.

Placenta previa is a condition in which the placental tissue covers the cervix. There are both partial and complete varieties, which refer to the degree of previa covering the cervical os. The incidence of previa is 1 in 200 pregnancies and increases with prior cesarean sections, advanced maternal age, and multiparity. Ultrasound remains the most useful diagnostic test used to detect previa.

Placenta accreta is an abnormal adherence of the placenta to the uterine wall. This degree of invasion of the uterine wall can be graded as accreta when the chorionic villi are in contact with myometrium (80% of cases), placenta increta when the chorionic villi invade into myometrium (15% of cases), or the most serious, percreta, when the chorionic villi invade into serosa (5% of cases).

Develop and carry out patient management plans.

Since there was no live baby, hysterectomy without opening the uterus was an option in this situation. That will decrease the bleeding. However, the ultrasound diagnosis of placenta accreta is not specific. Moreover, the patient was adamant that the uterus be preserved. She only consented to hysterectomy as a life-saving measure.

Our initial plan, which was defeated by the patient, included uterine artery embolization. This is a process in which a balloon can be inserted into the uterine artery, or the hypogastric artery, to prevent intra-operative hemorrhage. The option of general anesthesia was offered to the patient in view of her emotional status and high risk of hemodynamic instability. Her airway examination was optimal. However, the patient refused general anesthesia, and the procedure was performed with epidural. Obviously, hemodynamic instability in this case would warrant an arterial line and several large-bore IVs for the administration of fluid, blood products, and vasopressors.

Discussion with interventional radiology about the possible need for intervention subsequent to the surgery was warranted.

Counsel and educate patients and their families.

A discussion with your patient is needed to facilitate understanding and trust between doctor and patient. In this difficult situation, you are trying to provide anesthesia safely, while trying to appease not only the mother, but also the father. It is important not to neglect the father in this situation because the mother may have some degree of trust in you, but not nearly the amount of trust that she has in her husband. Medical decisions are not made by patients; rather, they are made by the patients and their families.

Here, discussing the options of GA versus regional was important. It is also important to discuss possible conversion to GA, if need be.

Use information technology to support patient care decisions and patient education.

The preoperative discussion is when information from the obstetrician and anesthesiologist can be presented to the patient so that she can have an abundance of understanding about the risks that she is undertaking and can make an informed decision about her health care. In this case, the high incidence of bleeding and the useful role of interventional radiology can be discussed.

Perform competently all medical and invasive procedures considered essential for the area of practice.

It is important to remember that this is not an emergency. All proper steps should be undertaken to reduce risk to the patient. Having an epidural with an adequate level is key to providing anesthesia and keeping the patient comfortable throughout the procedure.

There is a need for large-bore IVs, and an ALine must be in place prior to incision. Ensuring an adequate supply of blood and blood products is also critical for this procedure. Having additional means of placing access, that is, an introducer, and devices to give large volumes of fluid or blood products, such as a level 1 rapid transfuser, is also important. Adequate sedation is also needed here to keep the patient calm throughout the procedure – you must remember that this isn't the procedure the patient wanted or expected. Pharmacologic interventions would include oxytocin, methylergonovine, and prostaglandin F2alpha. These drugs are used frequently in the obstetric population to treat uterine atony.

> Provide health care services aimed at preventing health problems or maintaining health.

All the steps mentioned previously are designed to prevent hemorrhage in the operating room and afterward.

> Work with health care professionals, including those from other disciplines, to provide patient-focused care.

Having good communication with an obstetrician is critical to get a sense of when critical events will occur in the operating room and the overall state of their concerns with regard to this patient. Being able to talk to a surgeon alleviates stress and ensures that things are not omitted. In this situation, the decision to perform hysterectomy was made immediately when the uterus was opened. Knowing this, we can plan our anesthesia accordingly.

Also, communication with the interventional radiology in case there is continuing oozing even after hysterectomy is warranted.

Medical knowledge

Residents must demonstrate knowledge about established and evolving biomedical, clinical, and cognate (e.g., epidemiological and social-behavioral) sciences and the application of this knowledge to patient care.

> Demonstrate an investigatory and analytic thinking approach to clinical situations.

The sudden cause of hypotension in this patient should alert the anesthesiologist to the possibility of occult bleeding. No vigorous attempts were made to remove the placenta, the partially abrupted placenta was left relatively intact without significant blood loss when the hysterectomy was initiated. However, the patient became hypotensive. Remember that with a closed uterus, an obstetrician may not readily identify bleeding from a previa. With all the IV access, this did not become an issue, and the patient was given crystalloid solutions and blood products to keep her hemodynamically stable.

> Know and apply the basic and clinically supportive sciences that are appropriate to their discipline.

An appreciation of intraoperative obstetrical hemorrhage is key to being prepared for this situation. The uterine artery at term delivers 700 mL/min of blood to the uterus. With unchecked bleeding, it can become very clear that this patient can exsanguinate in merely 4–5 minutes.

Practice-based learning and improvement

Residents must be able to investigate and evaluate their patient care practices, appraise and assimilate scientific evidence, and improve their patient care practices.

> Analyze practice experience and perform practice-based improvement activities using a systematic methodology.

This is what can never be taught, but rather, must be experienced in the operating room from previous cases. The vigilance that must be provided for this patient is heightened not only by knowledge of the literature, but also by previous cases. Experience teaches us the finer nuances that cannot be learned from a book.

For example, in this case, when the patient looks as if she is spacing out, it probably means that she is losing blood rapidly and in shock. Bleeding in obstetrics is difficult to assess. Alert the surgeon.

Your previous experience tells you that at times, the blood products may not reach you in a timely fashion, so make arrangements so that you have enough support staff to help you.

Locate, appraise, and assimilate evidence from scientific studies related to their patients' health problems.

This is mostly accumulated knowledge. In our case, it is also good to know the newer options to treat bleeding such as recombinant activated factor VII.

Obtain and use information about their own population of patients and the larger population from which their patients are drawn.

This is the knowledge acquired from departmental statistics and also the literature. For example, in this case, how effective is uterine artery embolization? How effective is recombinant factor VII? Understand possible adverse reactions to the blood products and their presentation.

Apply knowledge of study designs and statistical methods to the appraisal of clinical studies and other information on diagnostic and therapeutic effectiveness.

Although randomized controlled studies are the gold standard, in cases like this, we have to consider observational studies and case reports. The knowledge that somebody had a good result with recombinant factor VII is useful, even though it is not a controlled study.

Use information technology to manage information, access online medical information, and support their own education.

The ability to perform a literature search and use your hospital's resources for full text articles and review articles any time of the day is important. Maybe the obstetric anesthesia department has compiled important articles and study materials, which are made available via the resident portal.

Professionalism

Residents must demonstrate a commitment to carrying out professional responsibilities, adherence to ethical principles, and sensitivity to a diverse patient population.

Demonstrate respect, compassion, and integrity; a responsiveness to the needs of patients and society that supersedes self-interest; accountability to

patients, society, and the profession; and a commitment to excellence and ongoing professional development.

In this case, it would have been so much better if the patient had agreed to the management options that were presented to her, instead of refusing medical care and wanting to die with her baby. However busy you might be in labor and delivery during the night, giving her time to come to terms with the situation and letting various health care personnel reach out to her was being respectful of her beliefs.

Demonstrate sensitivity and responsiveness to patients' culture, age, gender, and disabilities.

In this case, her wish to have more children might sound irrational. However, keep in mind that nobody is rational all the time, and engaging in nonjudgmental dialogue is important.

Interpersonal and communication skills

Residents must be able to demonstrate interpersonal and communication skills that result in effective information exchange and teaming with patients, their patients' families, and professional associates.

Create and sustain a therapeutic and ethically sound relationship with patients.

In our case, explaining all the patient's options in a nonjudgmental way, while giving her time to absorb the barrage of information, really helped in communicating with her. Furthermore, using the help of labor and delivery nurses, who might have different communication styles, to help the patient come to terms with the situation before presenting the technical information was also important.

Good communication with obstetrics about all the aspects of planning, including involvement of interventional radiology, is also essential.

Use effective listening skills and elicit and provide information using effective nonverbal, explanatory, questioning, and writing skills.

Here, even though the patient expressed that she wished to die, knowing that she really didn't want to die and making her feel that we empathized with her situation was very important. It is also important to include in the chart all the important elements of the conversation, while waiting for the patient to make a decision.

> Work effectively with others as a member or leader of a health care team or other professional group.

This situation is a true example of a multidisciplinary approach. It would have been inappropriate to give sedation, even though the patient was demanding it, before obtaining consent. Planning and coordination of care involves a team approach.

Systems-based practice

Residents must demonstrate an awareness of and responsiveness to the larger context and system of health care and the ability to effectively call on system resources to provide care that is of optimal value.

> Understand how their patient care and other professional practices affect other health care professionals, the health care organization, and the larger society and how these elements of the system affect their own practice.

In our situation, the following would fall under this category:
- ability of the blood bank to provide much needed products in a timely fashion
- availability of interventional services at odd hours
- availability of experts, such as a trauma team or, even better, a gynecologist, in case the surgical bleeding becomes hard to control
- availability of any help that may be needed down the line, such as a need for intensive care unit care

> Practice cost-effective health care and resource allocation that does not compromise quality of care.

Here, the appropriate examples are as follows:
- keep a level 1 rapid transfuser available but not set up
- ropivacaine versus bupivacaine

> Advocate for quality patient care and assist patients in dealing with system complexities.

The appropriate examples in our case follow:
- help Mom and Dad find the resources to deal with their grief such as bereavement support groups
- help Mom and Dad understand how to navigate the physical facility
- help Mom and Dad understand what to do with the little child who accompanied them to the hospital

> Know how to partner with health care managers and health care providers to assess, coordinate, and improve health care and know how these activities can affect system performance.

This category includes the following:
- take an appropriate time-out
- administer antibiotics
- fill out a QA form if there are any issues that need to be addressed so that care can be improved
- fill in log books for data collection and management

Additional reading

1. Teo TH, Law YM, Tay KH, Tan BS, Cheah FK. Use of magnetic resonance imaging in evaluation of placental invasion. Clin Radiol 2009;64:511–516.

2. Delotte J, Novellas S, Koh C, Bongain A, Chevallier P. Obstetrical prognosis and pregnancy outcome following pelvic arterial embolisation for post-partum hemorrhage. Eur J Obstetr Gynecol Reprod Biol 2009;145:129–132.

3. Breathnach F, Geary M. Uterine atony: definition, prevention, nonsurgical management, and uterine tamponade. Sem Perinatol 2009;33:82–87.

4. O'Brien D, Babiker E, O'Sullivan O, MCauliffe F, Geary M, Bryne B. Causes of massive obstetric haemorrhage and outcomes of medical and surgical management strategies. Am J Obstetr Gynecol 2008;199(Suppl 1):S93.

5. Esakoff T, Sparks T, Poder L, et al. How good are ultrasound and MRI for the diagnosis of placenta accreta? Am J Obstetr Gynecol 2008;199(Suppl 1):S189.

6. Laird R, Carabine U. Recombinant factor VIIa for major obstetric haemorrhage in a Jehovah's Witness. Int J Obstetr Anesth 2008;17:193–194.

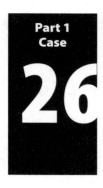

26 Overhextending yourself

Helene Benveniste and Jonida Zeqo

The case

A 68-year-old woman goes to the operating room (OR) for elective resection of a meningioma. She has hypertension (HTN) (reasonably treated!), a history of deep venous thrombosis (DVT), and is obese. After a smooth intravenous (IV) induction, relaxation, and intubation, an arterial line is placed, as are two large-bore IVs. The mean arterial blood pressure (MABP) is approximately 60 mmHg, and a bag of Hextend is started to counteract mild hypotension during the expected long (1-hour) neurosurgical prepping and draping, delaying surgical stimulation. A Foley is also placed. The attending leaves to start another case. Twenty minutes later, the attending returns to check on things and finds the resident bending over the arterial line. "It's not working," he says. The attending notices that there is sinus tachycardia and a no/low end-tidal carbon dioxide ($ETCO_2$) on the respiratory trace monitors and immediately starts resuscitating, while telling the resident that there is no problem with the arterial line – something else is going on, but what? At this point, the patient is oxygenating well, tachycardia is present, but there is not yet any profound hypotension. No antibiotics have yet been given.

The neurosurgical prepping is stopped; the pressure is maintained now with an epinephrine drip. Fluids and Hextend are continued for maintaining MABP, and anesthesia is discontinued as surgery is canceled; a femoral venous catheter is quickly placed for central venous access. Given the history of DVT, it is suggested that the patient might have thrown a pulmonary embolism. We rush to radiology; the computed tomography (CT) scan is negative. The anesthesiologist notices a rash on the chest of the patient and decides to give diphenydramine, ranitidine, and steroids in case of a possible anaphylactic reaction – to what? The MABP stabilizes within 10 minutes, and the epinephrine drip is off in no time. "But the patient did not get anything that could cause this reaction,"

somebody says. "The only thing she has gotten since induction is a bag of…Hextend!" Oh, we better stop that, just to be sure.

Now, back at the farm, the patient is stable; she is not yet fully awake but will soon be ready to be extubated. The next day, the patient is fine. A later workup clarified an allergic reaction to Hextend.

Patient care

Residents must be able to provide patient care that is compassionate, appropriate, and effective for the treatment of health problems and the promotion of health.

Communicate effectively and demonstrate caring and respectful behaviors when interacting with patients and their families.

This patient did not have any relatives at the hospital. The appropriate action is therefore to stay with the patient at all costs during the acute and subacute phases and to explain to the slowly awakening patient what is going on and why she has not yet had any surgery for her primary condition. It will also be appropriate to contact her relatives by phone and to communicate the current state of the patient and the plan for workup and rescheduling of surgery.

Gather essential and accurate information about their patients.

Continue to astutely follow the vital signs from the monitors; alert the surgeon about the situation and maintain resuscitation procedures until the cause of the situation has been established. Call for help to get a plan together. Examine the patient: check breath sounds; get a neurological exam, if possible; and what about temperature? It would also be appropriate to assess urine output and to get an ABG (arterial blood gas).

Make informed decisions about diagnostic and therapeutic interventions based on patient information and preferences, up-to-date scientific evidence, and clinical judgment.

The patient is suddenly hypotensive without apparent reason; go through the list of possibilities: airway, ventilation/oxygenation, circulation, cardiac history (electrocardiogram shows normal sinus, although there is tachycardia). Given the history of DVT, rule out a pulmonary embolism.

Develop and carry out patient management plans.

Make preparations to transport the patient from the OR to the radiology suite, while maintaining patient stability. Call for help transporting and for monitors, and alert radiology that there is an acute situation. Coordinate and communicate.

Counsel and educate patients and their families.

It is essential to stay with the patient through this episode; she has no relatives nearby, and you are her closest "relative" at this time as well as her patient advocate. In parallel, her family should be informed continuously about her status.

Use information technology to support patient care decisions and patient education.

As all most likely possibilities were ruled out (pulmonary embolism, intracerebral hematoma), it is appropriate to go to scientific and clinical databases to seek information on the possibility of Hextend causing an anaphylactic reaction.

Perform competently all medical and invasive procedures considered essential for the area of practice.

An arterial line was placed immediately after induction, which was appropriate for a case involving resection of a large meningioma. Two large-bore IVs were also placed. Resuscitation was continued through a femoral venous catheter – was that really necessary? Probably, given the need to infuse pressor drugs. Can epinephrine safely be given through a peripheral venous catheter? Yes, you can, and people do give epinephrine through peripheral intravenous lines, however in a code situation you would prefer to use a central line. And of course a concern arises that if the peripheral line would infiltrate, you can get skin necrosis at the site.

Provide health care services aimed at preventing health problems or maintaining health.

Aseptic technique when placing all invasive lines is paramount; the femoral line is probably in the worst place, given infection, and should not stay in. Consider antibiotic coverage – given the anaphylactic reaction, can an antibiotic be given safely? During the acute phase, the patient was intubated because she was anesthetized, but the plan after she was stabilized was to extubate as soon as possible. She was admitted to the surgical intensive care unit and placed under a standard of care that included suctioning of the endotracheal tube and turning, including DVT prophylaxis.

Additional reading

1. Mertes PM, Laxenaire MC, Alla F. Anaphylactic and anaphylactoid reactions occurring during anesthesia in France in 1999–2000. Anesthesiology 2003;99:536–545.

2. Sampson HA, Munoz-Furlong A, Bock SA, et al. Symposium on the definition and management of anaphylaxis: summary report. J Allergy Clin Immunol 2005;115:584–591.

3. Smith PL, Kagey-Sobotka A, Bleecker ER, et al. Physiologic manifestations of human anaphylaxis. J Clin Invest 1980;66:1072–1080.

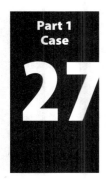

Contributions from Stony Brook University under
Christopher J. Gallagher

Broken catheter after Whipple

Xiaojun Guo and Khoa Nguyen

The case

Bruce was about to undergo a major operation with removal of several internal organs – the "Whipple." He received the standard spiel about the anesthesia and received the pain-destroying epidural catheter prior to entering the operating room (OR). The case went as smoothly as it could have, considering it was a Whipple. As he was being moved over to the stretcher for transport to the recovery room, he hit a snag, or at least, his catheter did. The tip of the catheter became caught up on a rail on the bed and the tension was too much for the small catheter. It gave way after stretching to its fullest. No problem, thought the anesthesiologist, who assumed that the catheter was just pulled out of its snug position in the thoracic spine. On closer inspection, the catheter was missing something peculiar – the *tip*!

Patient care

Residents must be able to provide patient care that is compassionate, appropriate, and effective for the treatment of health problems and the promotion of health.

Communicate effectively and demonstrate caring and respectful behaviors when interacting with patients and their families.

The patient is just waking up after general anesthesia and no family is present now, so the most caring and respectful interaction we can have is making sure that the patient arrives to the recovery room in stable condition and that no other lines or catheters become dislodged or removed.

Gather essential and accurate information about their patients.

As the patient is waking up, make sure a quick neurological exam is done to determine if there is any deficit, considering that there is now a small plastic foreign body floating around the patient's epidural space. Having that exam gives a baseline level of function to compare to, should there be a change later on. Measure the broken catheter to determine how much of the tip may have broken off. Also, examine the insertion site to make sure that no further trauma has been missed on movement.

Make informed decisions about diagnostic and therapeutic interventions based on patient information and preferences, up-to-date scientific evidence, and clinical judgment.

Based on the textbooks that you have read regarding epidural catheters, you decide to leave the broken catheter piece in place, assuming the patient remains asymptomatic. The literature on broken catheters recommends watchful vigilance with asymptomatic patients, imaging to determine exact location of the fragmented catheter, and a possible neurosurgical consult should you need their expertise to remove it.

Develop and carry out patient management plans.

As the patient becomes more awake, you make him aware of the event that has transpired regarding the catheter. You explain to him the risks of having a foreign body in the epidural space (i.e., infection, migration leading to nerve irritation or compression) and the red flags to watch out for symptomatically. You then send him for the appropriate imaging studies to get an exact idea of the catheter's current location, while sending out a consult to your neurosurgical friends so they can get to know the patient should they take him to the OR in the future.

Counsel and educate patients and their families.

The patient and his family should be counseled about the fact that most of the cases like this have no further sequelae related to the broken catheter. Answer all questions regarding the situation as honestly as possible. Make sure the patient understands that he should be aware of red flags such as pain, weakness, or fever in the affected areas. He must be advised to call his surgeon or the anesthesiologists if complications do arise and be ready to return to the emergency room if things worsen quickly. During his recovery at home, his family should also be made aware to watch for the same symptoms and act accordingly.

> Use information technology to support patient care decisions and patient education.

We have done that by looking up the latest recommendations regarding the handling of such situations. We reviewed the case reports and are acting on the current knowledge base to support our decisions about the patient's care.

> Perform competently all medical and invasive procedures considered essential for the area of practice.

All imaging and physical exams should be performed competently so that we have a baseline should anything change with the catheter position or the patient's status.

> Provide health care services aimed at preventing health problems or maintaining health.

Giving the patient a course of antibiotics may not be a bad idea considering that he does have a foreign body in a usually sterile place that may be a nidus for infection. Also, give the patient the appropriate contact information for the anesthesia department and arrange a follow-up appointment in the near future to assess for any changes in the catheter position and any possible related symptoms.

> Work with health care professionals, including those from other disciplines, to provide patient-focused care.

We have already contacted our colleagues in the neurosurgery department, but it is hoped that we will not need their services.

Medical knowledge

Residents must demonstrate knowledge about established and evolving biomedical, clinical, and cognate

(e.g., epidemiological and social-behavioral) sciences and the application of this knowledge to patient care.

> Demonstrate an investigatory and analytic thinking approach to clinical situations.

Removing an epidural catheter is usually uneventful, but not in this case. Your first investigative thought is where exactly the tip is located. To answer that question, you send the patient for a computed tomography or magnetic resonance scan. Your analytical thought leads you to possible outcomes of the broken catheter, including neurological deficits or dysfunction and possible infection. You start antibiotics and do routine neurological exams.

Practice-based learning and improvement

Residents must be able to investigate and evaluate their patient care practices, appraise and assimilate scientific evidence, and improve their patient care practices.

> Analyze practice experience and perform practice-based improvement activities using a systematic methodology.

Using the case reports and review articles you found, you act according to what the experts recommend. After following this patient, writing up your own case reports to add to the information that already exists for situations like this may allow for improvements in catheter manufacturing or appropriate management when catheters are sheared in patients. Also, reeducate all operating personnel about proper patient movement and the dangers that lie within.

> Locate, appraise, and assimilate evidence from scientific studies related to their patients' health problems.

It is known that this situation does not happen very often, and thus there are not many studies regarding its management. What does exist is advice from textbooks, the experience of others in case reports, and a few reviews of the current literature. Currently most literature recommends leaving the catheter in place, assuming that the patient is asymptomatic, and immediate removal should the catheter lead to problems. Sounds simple enough.

Use information technology to manage information, access online medical information, and support their own education.

We know you feel badly enough about the situation, but reliving it through literature searches about the subject is necessary to learn from the mistake and see how others managed the situation.

Professionalism

Residents must demonstrate a commitment to carrying out professional responsibilities, adherence to ethical principles, and sensitivity to a diverse patient population.

Demonstrate respect, compassion, and integrity; a responsiveness to the needs of patients and society that supersedes self-interest; accountability to patients, society, and the profession; and a commitment to excellence and ongoing professional development.

You apologize to the patient and his family, explain exactly what occurred, and offer any resource that the hospital has should they need it to demonstrate respect, compassion, and integrity.

Demonstrate a commitment to ethical principles pertaining to provision or withholding of clinical care, confidentiality of patient information, informed consent, and business practice.

Observe all HIPAA regulations and keep the patient's information confidential when you present this case at the next quality assurance meeting.

Demonstrate sensitivity and responsiveness to patients' culture, age, gender, and disabilities.

Follow the golden rule. Enough said.

Interpersonal and communication skills

Residents must be able to demonstrate interpersonal and communication skills that result in effective information exchange and teaming with patients, their patients' families, and professional associates.

Create and sustain a therapeutic and ethically sound relationship with patients.

Develop a rapport with the patient and his family. Arrange a follow-up appointment for the patient with a neurologist or neurosurgeon and make sure that you are at that follow-up appointment to demonstrate to the patient that you are committed to his care, which should contribute to a sound relationship with him.

Use effective listening skills and elicit and provide information using effective nonverbal, explanatory, questioning, and writing skills.

During the preop visit, a focused history and physical was obtained. You listened to the patient's questions and concerns and addressed them all appropriately using language he could understand. You then documented the history and physical and conversation in the chart and have now become a consultant in interpersonal and communication skills.

Work effectively with others as a member or leader of a health care team or other professional group.

Since you were the one ultimately responsible for the epidural catheter, you arrange the appropriate imaging modalities needed as well as any consults and follow-up appointments. Make sure that all involved are on the same page regarding the management of the situation.

Systems-based practice

Residents must demonstrate an awareness of and responsiveness to the larger context and system of health care and the ability to effectively call on system resources to provide care that is of optimal value.

Understand how their patient care and other professional practices affect other health care professionals, the health care organization, and the larger society and how these elements of the system affect their own practice.

The patient had an unfortunate event occur with the breakage of the catheter. It is now your responsibility to make sure that the patient has appropriate follow-up for the possible complications that may occur. That means further studies and visits to other health professionals to ensure the best outcome of this situation.

> Practice cost-effective health care and resource allocation that does not compromise quality of care.

Cost-effective health care at this point probably involves not ordering every imaging modality known to medicine to find the catheter, but rather, ordering one that will provide adequate visualization so that you only need one test, and also one with the least radiation to the patient to maintain quality of care.

> Advocate for quality patient care and assist patients in dealing with system complexities.

Make sure to remind the patient that you are available to assist the patient with further follow-up should he run into difficulty with scheduling office visits or other appointments.

> Know how to partner with health care managers and health care providers to assess, coordinate, and improve health care and know how these activities can affect system performance.

Writing up this case as a report can aid in the improvement of handling these types of situations. With enough reports and expert opinions, a consensus may be reached about how to systematically deal with such situations.

Additional reading

1.   Mitra R, Fleischmann K. Management of the sheared epidural catheter: is surgical extraction really necessary? J Clin Anesth 2007;19:310–314.

2.   Fragneto RY. The broken epidural catheter: an anesthesiologist's dilemma. J Clin Anesth 2007;19:243–244.

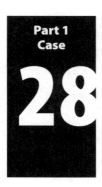

28 Pierre who?

Ron Jasiewicz and Khoa Nguyen

The case

We were having an enjoyable morning in the endoscopy suite, and then we were told that we would have an add-on endoscopy from the neonatal intensive care unit (NICU) by our pediatric gastroenterology colleague. The patient was a 1-month-old with frequent emesis after feeding. And yes, he was premature, but without "apneas and bradycardias" while in the NICU. He had been diagnosed with Pierre Robin malformation. Our friend was 2.5 kg and quite active. Although he could not roll yet, we were convinced that he wanted to run out of the room! He must have suspected what was going to happen to him and didn't want any part of it.

He was brought into our world as an elective cesarean section because his mother's preeclampsia was worsening. Born with Apgar scores of 7 and 8, he appeared to have a murmur on oscillation. He presented to our suite with no other medical history. At the time of delivery, he was 35 weeks postconception. Currently he was a "feed and grow" in the NICU nearing discharge, but had trouble keeping it down.

Patient care

Residents must be able to provide patient care that is compassionate, appropriate, and effective for the treatment of health problems and the promotion of health.

Communicate effectively and demonstrate caring and respectful behaviors when interacting with patients and their families.

Considering that our patient is a neonate, most of our interaction will be with the parents. Speak with the parents about the procedure in a compassionate way, as this must be a difficult time for them. Respect them by making sure that you use language they understand. For truly effective communication, give them a chance to ask questions, while you listen attentively, and answer them as best you can.

Gather essential and accurate information about their patients.

Getting a detailed history of the pregnancy and birth as well as the patient's short medical history is vital in anesthetizing such a unique patient. In addition to speaking with the parents, it is necessary to speak to our NICU colleagues about the patient's medical course so far. Important issues to consider are cardiac and respiratory status as many of these patients often have cardiac abnormalities. Nutritional status is also a concern as children with Pierre Robin syndrome have cleft palates, which can cause respiratory and feeding difficulties. Malnourishment may lead to anemia, causing decreased oxygen delivery for the infant, so the patient's hematocrit may be useful to obtain. Be aware of current medications the infant may be taking which may interact with the anesthetic medications. Naught per oris (NPO) status must be determined as this patient is about to undergo a procedure in which aspiration is a concern.

Make informed decisions about diagnostic and therapeutic interventions based on patient information and preferences, up-to-date scientific evidence, and clinical judgment.

This patient is considered to have a difficult airway, so a plan must be made regarding securing the airway for the procedure. Numerous case reports have led to several review articles with recommendations for securing the airway in Pierre Robin syndrome patients. Infants may be intubated awake and unanesthetized as they usually tolerate the stress well. Maintaining spontaneous respiration is recommended as there is a high risk of airway collapse with induction or muscle relaxation. Intubation may be carried out via fiber-optic scope or with direct visualization with laryngoscopy. Inhalational inductions may be done with an emphasis on keeping the patient spontaneously breathing due to a risk of loss of the airway.

Develop and carry out patient management plans.

After appropriate monitors are placed, the patient is allowed to spontaneously breathe, while an intravenous (IV) is placed. Once the IV is functional, an awake intubation is attempted but is unsuccessful due to the patient's vigorous activity. Inhalational agents are then used to help with sedation for another attempt at intubation, but due to the severity of the patient's airway issues, the intubation attempt is aborted as the patient begins to obstruct. The patient is then emerged. Oral midazolam is agreed on by the team to help with sedation with causing airway obstruction. The midazolam works well, and the airway is obtained, though it did require some serious external airway manipulation.

Counsel and educate patients and their families.

Again, this is mainly directed to the patient's family. Every effort should be made to explain to the parents the severity of the situation. The patient needs an urgent procedure to help with a diagnosis, but there are always risks involved. Airway collapse is the major concern. Counseling the parents must include the possibility that the endotracheal tube may remain in place after the procedure, until it is determined to be absolutely safe to remove it.

Use information technology to support patient care decisions and patient education.

The parents may not fully understand the scope of Pierre Robin syndrome and can be directed to the many Web sites and support groups for parents of children with similar issues.

Perform competently all medical and invasive procedures considered essential for the area of practice.

IV placement should be done quickly and competently to minimize stress to the patient as well as to confirm that a patent IV is available should the patient require rescue medications. The most important procedure in this case was obtaining the airway, which was successful, but only after several attempts due to the abnormal anatomy related to the patient's disease.

Provide health care services aimed at preventing health problems or maintaining health.

This is the whole reason for the case. We were attempting to provide a service to the patient (the endoscopy) with the aim of preventing any further deterioration and maintaining his health!

Work with health care professionals, including those from other disciplines, to provide patient-focused care.

With the help of our NICU and gastrointestinal (GI) colleagues, in this case, we were able to provide a high level of patient-focused care.

Medical knowledge

Residents must demonstrate knowledge about established and evolving biomedical, clinical, and cognate (e.g., epidemiological and social-behavioral) sciences and the application of this knowledge to patient care.

Demonstrate an investigatory and analytic thinking approach to clinical situations.

Hearing the words *Pierre Robin* should automatically generate the three common entities associated with the syndrome. The three include micrognathia, glossoptosis, and cleft palate. Also, we must also be ready for other congenital anomalies the patient may have other than the three just mentioned, especially the cardiac anomalies. Difficult airway is synonymous with Pierre Robin patients, and thus we develop an analytical approach to obtaining the airway, with a backup plan and a backup plan for the backup plan, which was put into action in this case.

Practice-based learning and improvement

Residents must be able to investigate and evaluate their patient care practices, appraise and assimilate scientific evidence, and improve their patient care practices.

Analyze practice experience and perform practice-based improvement activities using a systematic methodology.

At the conclusion of the procedure, it would make sense to sit down with our NICU and GI colleagues to analyze what we did correctly and what we could improve. Attention to what worked well in this patient may serve us well in the future with patients like him or others with difficult airways.

> Locate, appraise, and assimilate evidence from scientific studies related to their patients' health problems.

This is exactly what was done prior to taking this case on. We made sure that we had an idea of what to expect when we looked into the patient's airway. We also tried to read and learn about what worked for our colleagues around the world when dealing with Pierre Robin syndrome patients. Thus we had all our airway equipment ready as well as medications to help allow us to obtain the airway.

> Obtain and use information about their own population of patients and the larger population from which their patients are drawn.

We will be sure to record the experience with this case for future reference, and in time, we should have a sizable database from which to learn.

Professionalism

Residents must demonstrate a commitment to carrying out professional responsibilities, adherence to ethical principles, and sensitivity to a diverse patient population.

> Demonstrate respect, compassion, and integrity; a responsiveness to the needs of patients and society that supersedes self-interest; accountability to patients, society, and the profession; and a commitment to excellence and ongoing professional development.

It is very easy to act responsively to the needs of such a young and unique patient in a way that supersedes our own self-interest. Your commitment to excellence is shown by the extensive preparation done to make sure this case goes off without any complications. Your commitment to ongoing professional development is evidenced by your writing a case report of this case to add to your repertoire of anesthesia experience.

> Demonstrate a commitment to ethical principles pertaining to provision or withholding of clinical

care, confidentiality of patient information, informed consent, and business practice.

When referencing this case in the future, during presentations or case reports, be sure to respect HIPAA policies and do not divulge any confidential patient information.

> Demonstrate sensitivity and responsiveness to patients' culture, age, gender, and disabilities.

You did your best to demonstrate your sensitivity to the patient's disabilities by speaking in depth with the parents and showing compassion when discussing the specifics about the case. Answering all their questions appropriately shows your responsiveness.

Interpersonal and communication skills

Residents must be able to demonstrate interpersonal and communication skills that result in effective information exchange and teaming with patients, their patients' families, and professional associates.

> Create and sustain a therapeutic and ethically sound relationship with patients.

This seems so obvious and redundant, but the rapport that you develop with the parents will help create a level of trust that contributes to a sound relationship with the patient and his family.

> Use effective listening skills and elicit and provide information using effective nonverbal, explanatory, questioning, and writing skills.

Summoning all that you learned in grade school, you use your ears and eyes as much as your hands and mouth to practice effective listening and explanatory skills.

> Work effectively with others as a member or leader of a health care team or other professional group.

Before and after the procedure, you work as a member of the health care team to ensure that the patient and his family are on the same page as the health care team. During the procedure, you become the team leader and manage the patient and team to ensure that the procedure is completed safely so that the appropriate treatment can be determined.

Systems-based practice

Residents must demonstrate an awareness of and responsiveness to the larger context and system of health care and the ability to effectively call on system resources to provide care that is of optimal value.

Understand how their patient care and other professional practices affect other health care professionals, the health care organization, and the larger society and how these elements of the system affect their own practice.

This patient has a constellation of issues that may require further medical intervention in the future. Making sure that this patient gets appropriate diagnosis and treatment early on for his medical issues may help reduce his chances of having more serious medical issues in the future. That alone affects everyone involved in his care, from his parents to his physicians and, finally, the big health care organizations.

Practice cost-effective health care and resource allocation that does not compromise quality of care.

You do your best to be cost-effective by not opening instruments or drugs that you may not need so that their integrity is intact for the next patient, but by no means do you compromise the quality of care for any patient, especially this one, with such unique needs.

Advocate for quality patient care and assist patients in dealing with system complexities.

Provide the parents with documentation of the management of the patient's airway for future reference, if necessary. Make sure that the parents understand that you are always available for consultation from an anesthesia perspective for their child.

Additional reading

1. Shprintzen RJ, Singer L. Upper airway obstruction and the Robin sequence. Int Anesthesiol Clin 1992;30: 109–114.

2. Olasoji HO, Ambe PJ, Adesina OA. Pierre Robin syndrome: an update. Niger Postgrad Med J 2007;14:140–145.

3. Meyer AC, Lidsky ME, Sampson DE, Lander TA, Liu M, Sidman JD. Airway interventions in children with Pierre Robin sequence. Otolaryngol Head Neck Surg 2008;138:782–787.

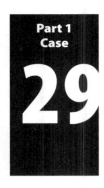

Part 1 Case

29

Contributions from Stony Brook University under Christopher J. Gallagher

Submandibular abscess

Syed Azim and Jane Yi

The case

A 44-year-old male presented for an incision and drainage of a left submandibular abscess. The patient had presented to the emergency department with a chief complaint of pain and swelling for 15 days, limited mouth opening, and difficulty swallowing. Computed tomography (CT) scan of the head and neck revealed moderate displacement of the trachea to the right. Physical exam by oral maxillo-facial surgery (OMFS) revealed trismus and a carious mandibular left third molar, with periapical pathology.

Patient care

Residents must be able to provide patient care that is compassionate, appropriate, and effective for the treatment of health problems and the promotion of health.

Communicate effectively and demonstrate caring and respectful behaviors when interacting with patients and their families.

Always introduce yourself to the patient and family members. Keep in mind that most people are afraid of the unknown. You may have been involved in dozens of surgical procedures, but this might be the patient's first surgery.

Gather essential and accurate information about their patients.

Before administering anesthesia, you want to know the patient's past medical history (PMH), past surgical history (PSH), current medications, allergies, naught per oris (NPO) status, and Mallampati airway assessment. It is also important to get a history of present illness, family history (especially of anesthesia), and social history. Many patients are not completely forthcoming with information. Sometimes they don't remember; sometimes they don't think it's important; and sometimes they lie. I once had a patient deny having had any medical conditions, but when I asked her if she had high blood pressure, she said yes. As I continued with the interview and asked about her past surgical history, she revealed that she had coronary artery disease, with a history of myocardial infarction (MI), and was status post (s/p) coronary artery bypass graft (CABG) × 4!

This is why we should ask pointed questions. For example, one could ask, "Do you have any allergies to any medications, latex, or foods?" rather than asking, "Do you have any allergies?" Speaking of allergies, it is also important to confirm whether a documented allergy is an *actual* allergy. Once I read in a patient's chart that she had an "allergy to general anesthesia." What does that even mean? Did she have a history of malignant hyperthermia? It turned out that she had a history of postoperative nausea and vomiting.

Develop and carry out patient management plans.

Abscesses that invade the fascial spaces can become airway nightmares, especially if it is bilateral-Ludwig's angina. Furthermore, if imaging studies show tracheal deviation, the abscess should be properly drained urgently. So, needless to say, the most important part of this anesthetic plan lay in successfully securing the airway.

The anesthesia plan was general anesthesia (GA) with awake, fiber-optic, nasal intubation. Equipment included a fiber-optic scope; nasal endotracheal tubes, preferably soaked in warm water to soften; and nasal airways, with lubrication. Drugs used included glycopyrrolate (antisialogogue), dexmedetomidine (sedative), 4% lidocaine nebulizer and 5% lidocaine jelly (topical anesthetic), and oxymetazoline spray (topical decongestant).

Counsel and educate patients and their families.

147

Explain the following:

1. nasal versus oral intubation: nasal intubation is preferred because the approach for the I&D was going to be both extraoral and intraoral
2. awake versus asleep intubation: awake is preferred because of the risk of losing the airway

The idea of being awake for the intubation might be frightening to some patients. I explained it as such: "Because of the changes in your airway brought on by the abscess, we need to use a camera to place the breathing tube for you. You will be awake because it is safer if you are breathing on your own, but you will be sedated and your throat will be numb." Remember, the patient is probably already feeling quite anxious – imagine being unable to open your mouth and unable to swallow, and having difficulty breathing.

Use information technology to support patient care decisions and patient education.

Use the CT of the head and neck as an illustration for the patient. For the most part, patients like to be informed and appreciate having an active role in their health care. Showing this patient the deviation of his trachea emphasized the importance of an awake, fiber-optic intubation.

Perform competently all medical and invasive procedures considered essential for the area of practice.

Make sure you have adequate peripheral access, especially when the patient arrives with an IV already in place. If the IV is running poorly but is not infiltrated, do yourself and the patient a favor and use it to induce but start a new one, once the patient is asleep. Also, try to avoid the ante-cubital fossa (ACF) so you don't have to concern yourself with making sure the patient's elbow isn't bent. Most likely, the patient will be continued on IV antibiotics postoperatively, so he will appreciate having an IV elsewhere.

Once the IV is placed, you can start the steps toward a successful awake, fiber-optic, nasal intubation. A little bit of glycopyrrolate goes a long way. It's amazing how much easier it is to make out anatomy when you don't have salivary juices getting in your way. Start the dexmedetomidine $0.5–1$ µg/kg since this loading dose should be infused over a period of 10–15 minutes. During this time, have the patient start puffing on the nebulizer containing 4% lidocaine. Then squeeze some 5% lidocaine on a tongue depressor and

tell the patient to think of it as a lollipop or popsicle, advancing it further, as tolerated.

Provide health care services aimed at preventing health problems or maintaining health.

Make sure antibiotics ordered by surgery are administered appropriately. Ideally, antibiotics should be delivered within 1 hour of surgical incision. Know your patient's allergies and know the antibiotics. Some antibiotics, such as vancomycin, should be administered over a longer period of time, whereas others, such as aminoglycosides, will potentiate the effects of neuromuscular blocking drugs. Usually, the preferred antibiotic for dental infections is penicillin, but because of the patient's allergy to penicillin, clindamycin was ordered. Once you start the antibiotics, watch for signs of an allergic reaction.

Work with health care professionals, including those from other disciplines, to provide patient-focused care.

It is really important to communicate with the surgical team. OMFS explained that they will take an extraoral and intraoral approach as well as extracting the carious tooth. Therefore nasal intubation was preferred so that the tube would not be in the way of the surgical site. It is also a good idea to know that the surgeon is planning on using local anesthesia. In this case, the surgeon used 2% lidocaine with 1:100,000 epinephrine. We should know that the maximum dose is 7 mg/kg and make sure surgeons and nurses are aware.

Medical knowledge

Residents must demonstrate knowledge about established and evolving biomedical, clinical, and cognate (e.g., epidemiological and social-behavioral) sciences and the application of this knowledge to patient care.

Demonstrate an investigatory and analytic thinking approach to clinical situations.

Infection of the submandibular space causes swelling that begins at the inferior border of the mandible and extends medially to the digastric muscle and posteriorly to the hyoid bone. Some clinical signs can include the following: trismus, drooling, dysphagia, and dyspnea. Progression of this swelling can lead to upper airway obstruction. The most common cause of this abscess is a dental infection, usually involving the mandibular third molars.

Knowing this, we should expect that we won't be able to properly assess the airway due to trismus and swelling. We also know that it would be even more beneficial to administer an antisialogogue, to counteract the drooling due to dysphagia. Let's not forget the obvious; this can become a true airway emergency.

Practice-based learning and improvement

Residents must be able to investigate and evaluate their patient care practices, appraise and assimilate scientific evidence, and improve their patient care practices.

> Analyze practice experience and perform practice-based improvement activities using a systematic methodology.

As you proceed in a case like this, you realize how overwhelming things can get, especially when it comes to the airway. It is therefore important to develop a systematic approach to the steps taken, from the moment the patient enters the OR to the point at which he settles down in the recovery room. Institution-specific protocols call for certain types and dosages of antibiotics to be administered, requiring use of multiple lines. Have the difficult airway cart ready and checked. With proper preparation and practice, experience, and practice-based improvement activities, there should be little variation in the way this surgery is handled, even among different clinicians.

> Locate, appraise, and assimilate evidence from scientific studies related to their patients' health problems.

When a patient presents with an abscess that invades fascial spaces, always keep in mind the possibility of an airway complication. Larawin et al. [1] reported upper airway obstruction that required tracheotomies in 8.3% of patients. Other complications included septic shock, asphyxiation and descending mediastinitis, and respiratory failure. Moreover, death was reported in 8.7% of patients.

> Apply knowledge of study designs and statistical methods to the appraisal of clinical studies and other information on diagnostic and therapeutic effectiveness.

Once it is determined that an awake, nasal, fiber-optic intubation is the plan of choice, one has to decide the appropriate steps to follow through with this plan. The literature supports the use of different drugs to provide adequate sedation and analgesia for the patient during what can be a frightening experience (and I'm not just talking about the patient here). The most important thing we need for successful awake fiber-optic intubation is spontaneous respiration. In addition to that, it would be nice to have analgesia, amnesia, and sedation.

Reusche and Egan [2] reported the use of remifentanil as a sedative-analgesic for an awake intubation in a patient with Ludwig's angina. The patient was premedicated with glycopyrrolate 0.2 mg IV, droperidol 0.625 mg IV, and midazolam 2 mg IV over 10 minutes. The airway was topicalized with 4 mL of 4% lidocaine through the use of a nebulizer, and the right naris was swabbed with 4% cocaine. Then a remifentanil infusion at 0.05 μg/kg/min was started before nasal fiber-optic intubation. Spontaneous ventilation was maintained and the vocal cords were sprayed with 2 mL of 4% lidocaine via the suction port located on the fiber-optic scope. Moreover, this article reports the advantages of using remifentanil as the following: short context-sensitive half-time, analgesia, synergistic with sedatives, and the ability to suppress laryngeal reflexes. The disadvantage of using remifentanil is that it is an opioid and has all the side effects that come with that classification of drug. Remifentanil can cause respiratory depression, bradycardia, hypotension, nausea, vomiting, muscle rigidity, and pruritis [2].

Abdelmalak et al. [3] described the use of dexmedetomidine as a sedative for awake intubation in the management of a critical airway. Dexmedetomidine is an α2-agonist that has the desirable properties of analgesia and amnesia and that acts as an antisialogogue. Abdelmalak et al. further describe a case of a patient with a submandibular abscess presenting with progressive respiratory difficulty. A loading dose of dexmedetomidine 1 μg/kg was initiated for 10 minutes, followed by a maintenance dose of 0.6 μg/kg/hour. Additionally, 4% lidocaine via nebulizer and 2% lidocaine gel were used to topicalize the oropharynx. Four percent lidocaine was also administered during bronchoscopy in what the author described as a "spray-as-you-go-technique." Once general anesthesia was induced, the dexmedetomidine infusion was discontinued. The advantage of using dexmedetomidine is that you have the desired effect of sedation with minimal risk of respiratory depression. The disadvantages

149

of dexmedetomidine include possible bradycardia and hypotension [3].

Is there an alternative to an awake fiber-optic intubation? Shteif et al. [4] describe the use of the superficial cervical plexus block to drain a submandibular and submental abscess as an alternative to general anesthesia. The patient is placed in the supine position and draped in a sterile fashion. The landmarks identified are the following: the mastoid process and Chassaignac's tubercle of C6 transverse process. Using a 25-gauge needle, local anesthetic is delivered with the fan technique. The goal is to block all four major branches of the superficial cervical plexus. Supplemental anesthesia may be required in the form of the long buccal for a submandibular abscess and an inferior alveolar block for a submental abscess. Shteif et al. describe advantages of using a block as opposed to general anesthesia as the following: lowered patient cost, decreased recovery time, and decreased surgical time. However, the disadvantages would include complications such as hematoma, local anesthetic toxicity, nerve injury, phrenic nerve block, and possible spinal anesthesia. Furthermore, a contraindication for the use of a superficial cervical plexus block would be patients with significant respiratory disease and highly stressed or anxious patients [4].

Professionalism

Residents must demonstrate a commitment to carrying out professional responsibilities, adherence to ethical principles, and sensitivity to a diverse patient population.

Demonstrate a commitment to ethical principles pertaining to provision or withholding of clinical care, confidentiality of patient information, informed consent, and business practice.

Review informed consent, double-check on surgery site, and be cognizant that there are others around you as you discuss details of your patient's medical record in the holding area. Also, make sure the surgeon has seen the patient prior to taking him to the OR.

Demonstrate sensitivity and responsiveness to patients' culture, age, gender, and disabilities.

What may transcend all cultures, ages, gender, and disabilities is the notion of treating your patients as you would wish to be treated.

Interpersonal and communication skills

Residents must be able to demonstrate interpersonal and communication skills that result in effective information exchange and teaming with patients, their patients' families, and professional associates.

Create and sustain a therapeutic and ethically sound relationship with patients.

Hand washing is an important habit to develop, especially when seeing patients with infectious processes going on in the system, like this particular patient had.

Use effective listening skills and elicit and provide information using effective nonverbal, explanatory, questioning, and writing skills.

The patient will likely have many questions, some of which you may not be able to answer in detail. You may even be asked a question more appropriately answered by the surgeons, in which case, you should respectfully defer to your colleagues.

Work effectively with others as a member or leader of a health care team or other professional group.

The significance of working effectively with other members of the OR staff should be reiterated. In addition, as you transition to the recovery room, your input may be requested not only by the recovery room staff, but also by ENT and OFMS and intensive care unit personnel.

Systems-based practice

Residents must demonstrate an awareness of and responsiveness to the larger context and system of health care and the ability to effectively call on system resources to provide care that is of optimal value.

Understand how their patient care and other professional practices affect other health care professionals, the health care organization, and the larger society and how these elements of the system affect their own practice.

Many levels of coordination are involved in airway cases. It is important to understand the urgency of the case and scarce resources that should be handled with utmost diligence. You have a challenge to contribute to the likelihood of success by being vigilant in the OR and by effectively handling the situation in a controlled fashion.

Practice cost-effective health care and resource allocation that does not compromise quality of care.

For this case, we discontinued the dexmedetomidine after induction of anesthesia. However, you might want to consider continuing the infusion. This would decrease the amount of anesthetic needed and also decrease the amount of waste. Just know the surgery and know when to discontinue the dexmedetomidine. There are some reports of delayed awakening when it is not discontinued at the appropriate time [1].

Advocate for quality patient care and assist patients in dealing with system complexities.

Understand the immediate postoperative concerns for this patient and be prepared to react appropriately in certain situations. For example, what do you do if the patient develops stridors or becomes short of breath? What if he develops high-grade fever and is not responding to antipyretics? Knowing what to do beforehand allows for a smoother postoperative course and a potentially better surgical outcome.

Know how to partner with health care managers and health care providers to assess, coordinate, and improve health care and know how these activities can affect system performance.

The immediate postoperative period is important in terms of laying out the goals, standards, and protocols for the care of the patient. Usually, medication orders will be clearly preprinted. Communication with the ENT and OFMS teams is imperative.

References

1. Larawin V, Naipao J, Dubey SP. Head and neck space infections. Otolaryngol Head Neck Surg 2006;135:889–893.

2. Reusche MD, Egan TD. Remifentanil for conscious sedation and analgesia during awake fiberoptic tracheal intubation: a case report with pharmacokinetic simulations. J Clin Anesth 1999;11:64–68.

3. Abdelmalak B, Makary L, Hoban J, Doyle DJ. Dexmedetomidine as sole sedative for awake intubation in management of the critical airway. J Clin Anesth 2007;19:370–373.

4. Shteif M, Lesmes D, Hartman G, Ruffino S, Laster Z. The use of the superficial cervical plexus block in the drainage of submandibular and submental abscesses – an alternative for general anesthesia. J Oral Maxillofac Surg 2008;66:2642–2645.

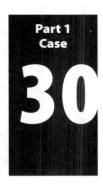

Contributions from Stony Brook University under Christopher J. Gallagher

30 ERCP with sedation
A Big MAC (monitored anesthesia care), supersized!

Tazeen Beg and Michelle DiGuglielmo

The case

A brand-new anesthesia attending, you have just finished a case and the anesthesia coordinator asks you to go get some lunch and then go to the endoscopy unit for an ERCP (endoscopic retrograde cholangiopancreatography). ERCP? You remember learning about it in medical school but never got a chance to observe one being done. While wolfing down a greasy cheeseburger deluxe from the cafeteria, you Google it and find that it is usually done prone and under sedation. "Easy MAC, let me grab a bunch of propofol," you think to yourself.

You reach the endoscopy unit after getting lost a few times on the way there and introduce yourself to the gastroenterologist. He explains that the patient is in-house and "not that sick" and that the gastroenterologist needs to get to office hours, "so can we do this quickly?" Wanting to develop a good rapport in the endoscopy suite as a new attending, you reassure him that you'll get things moving along – it's just a MAC case after all! You then go to the room, draw up your propofol syringes, and, as a final thought, crack open the succinylcholine vial.

The patient arrives. She is a 52-year-old female with a history of hypertension (HTN), 65 kg, and recently diagnosed with gallstone pancreatitis. She looks as if she's in pain. You approach the patient and introduce yourself. The patient looks around and asks, "Are there any real doctors here? You look like my granddaughter!" You reassure her that you've been practicing anesthesia "for years," and she relents by shrugging her shoulders. After a quick airway (class II with upper dentures) and physical exam, you explain the risks and benefits of anesthesia and the prone position. The patient is then moved over to the procedure table and makes herself as comfortable as possible in the prone position. You place the monitors and make sure the IV is secured and flushing well. You put a nasal cannula on her at 2 L/min, see that you're getting adequate end-tidal CO_2, and proceed by pushing 50 mcg of fentanyl ("for the pain") with a 150-mg chaser of propofol. The patient becomes apneic, so you tell the gastrointestinal (GI) doctor to place his endoscope, thinking the stimulation will make her breathe again. His scope is in but the oxygen saturation monitor is reading 80%; you attempt jaw thrust, and he yells, "I cannot have you in my field or the patient moving!" As you point to the monitors, a look of fear comes over his face and he quiets down, whispering, "Do whatever you need to do." The saturation monitor continues to go down, so you grab for your circuit to bag the patient back up with some positive pressure ventilation. Uh-oh, there's no mask on the end of the circuit – in your new surroundings, you forgot to do a machine check! You ask the nurse to bring in the stretcher and put the patient back in the supine position quickly, as the endoscope is removed by the gastroenterologist. You realize that you never looked at her preoperative potassium levels, so you forget the succinylcholine and just do direct laryngoscopy. Luckily, you have a grade 1 view of the vocal cords, so you throw in an entotracheal tube, hook up the circuit, and bag her back to a saturation of 98%. You tape your tube in and calmly say to the GI attending, "Proceed with your ERCP." That cheeseburger you scarfed down at lunch might be making a reappearance soon!

Patient care

Residents must be able to provide patient care that is compassionate, appropriate, and effective for the treatment of health problems and the promotion of health.

Communicate effectively and demonstrate caring and respectful behaviors when interacting with patients and their families.

Preoperatively, the patient seemed concerned about how young you look! Reassurance is crucial; the patient needs to know that you are a trained medical doctor and that you have had years of experience specifically in the field of anesthesia. In addition, it was noted that the patient appeared to be in pain. Emphasize to your patient that pain control is a vital part of anesthesia and that you will do all you can to provide pain relief in a safe manner.

Gather essential and accurate information about their patients.

The patient's history can come from a variety of sources. In this particular instance, we learn from the attending doing the procedure that she was "not that sick." Recognize that other physicians may simplify medical conditions that to an anesthesiologist are critical. Did she vomit prior to reaching the endoscopy suite? Is she a full stomach, or will she aspirate? Are her electrolytes out of whack, and is succinylcholine a possibility if an emergency situation surfaces? A history and physical exam (H&P) with the patient are also crucial – after all, a good H&P is the very heart of medicine! Realize that some patients do not know the extent of their medical conditions, so a chart review is important, particularly for inpatients who may have seen several physicians in consultation and/or have had many diagnostic exams. This patient was known to have HTN – what medications is she on? Was there an electrocardiogram (EKG) done?

Develop and carry out patient management plans.

Let's look at this case retrospectively. You did the Google search over lunch – most review articles report that ERCP is done under MAC in American Society of Anesthesiology (ASA) I–II patients; her HTN was presumed to be under control, she was thin, and she had a good airway with upper dentures. You were pretty certain you could intubate her if you needed to, and sure enough, you ultimately had to! But remember that the ABCs are not always easy as 1-2-3; perhaps general anesthesia with an endotracheal tube should have been instituted from the start, especially given the prone positioning.

Counsel and educate patients and their families.

You informed the patient of the risks and benefits of anesthesia as well as the risks of the prone position – corneal abrasions, facial and upper airway edema, and postoperative vision loss. This is particularly

true for cases under general anesthesia greater than 6 hours.

Perform competently all medical and invasive procedures considered essential for the area of practice.

Remember to always do a machine check! You would have picked up on the fact that there was no mask attached to the circuit had you adequately checked your ventilator. Off-site anesthesia is quickly becoming the norm in many hospitals, and your anesthesia equipment is not always ready and available to you as in your comfort zone of the main operating rooms.

Use information technology to support patient care decisions and patient education.

Preoperatively, the anesthesiologist can review diagnostic studies to determine the number and size of the gallstones for removal – this may give an indication as to the length of time the procedure will take and whether or not the patient will be able to tolerate ERCP under MAC.

Work with health care professionals, including those from other disciplines, to provide patient-focused care.

Preprocedure, the GI and anesthesiology attendings discussed carrying out this case quickly under MAC in an otherwise healthy lady. Remember, with any procedure, it's not about doing it fast, but rather, it's about doing it right! Intraoperatively, as critical events develop, the anesthesiologist must adapt calmly to changes and direct those in the room on what they can do to help in stabilizing the patient. Postoperatively, a debriefing of critical events is beneficial to see what went wrong and how to avoid such situations in the future.

Medical knowledge

Residents must demonstrate knowledge about established and evolving biomedical, clinical, and cognate (e.g., epidemiological and social-behavioral) sciences and the application of this knowledge to patient care.

Know and apply the basic and clinically supportive sciences that are appropriate to their discipline.

Our patient became apneic after a small dose of fentanyl and what can be considered an induction dose of propofol. Although approximately 2 mg/kg of propofol are necessary for tolerating the placement of an upper endoscope in most patients, anesthesiologists should not treat all cases like a chocolate chip cookie recipe (milk of anesthesia and cookies – yum!). Use your knowledge of anesthesia to figure out a quick algorithm for yourself in this situation. You need to maintain the ABCs airway, breathing, circulation; you just took away your A and B with the drugs you pushed, and you know that if you don't do something soon, you'll lose your C as well:

1. You tell the GI doc to place his scope, hoping that that will stimulate ventilation, but alas, it does not, and saturations are dropping.
2. Hmmm, the fentanyl dose was small, Narcan won't help the situation, and why has no one designed an antidote to propofol?
3. Jaw thrust next to open the airway and, it is hoped, provide a painful stimulation to breathe. Negative.
4. On to positive-pressure ventilation – ugh, there's no mask! Hypoxia continues as you hear your saturation alarm drop – don't let it follow with bradycardia and cardiopulmonary resuscitation (CPR).
5. OK, think of the Nike ads – "Just tube it!" Intubate the patient, confirm tube placement, secure the airway, and proceed with ERCP under general anesthesia.

Practice-based learning and improvement

Residents must be able to investigate and evaluate their patient care practices, appraise and assimilate scientific evidence, and improve their patient care practices.

Locate, appraise, and assimilate evidence from scientific studies related to their patients' health problems.

Unsure of what an ERCP entailed, the anesthesiologist utilized time well by doing an online search of the procedure and the usual anesthetic management

of this case during a lunch break! As stated earlier, multiple review articles revealed that ERCP is an off-site procedure performed under MAC in the prone position in most patients with average ASA classifications of 1–3. When administering monitored anesthesia care, one must realize that just as with a general anesthetic, each patient is individualized, and extra care must be taken not to be heavy-handed with medications – your airway is *not* secured. In addition, the airway in the prone position is not readily available to you, and it is being shared with the gastroenterologist! Have a backup plan if apnea ensues, and if the airway was difficult from the beginning or the patient was vomiting perioperatively, then have a low threshold for endotracheal intubation.

Professionalism

Residents must demonstrate a commitment to carrying out professional responsibilities, adherence to ethical principles, and sensitivity to a diverse patient population.

Demonstrate sensitivity and responsiveness to patients' culture, age, gender, and disabilities.

This patient was middle-aged and concerned that you, as a junior attending, looked like her granddaughter. Regardless of your specialty in medicine, introductions and first impressions are key. Dress professionally, whether in a shirt and tie or scrubs. Keep your scrubs clean; if you dirty them, then change – patients do not want to see blood running down your scrub pants or vomit on your scrub top! Wear your white coat when not in a sterile location, and have your ID badge visible at all times in the hospital. If you're fatigued from too many hours on call and it shows on your face, take 5 minutes to wash up and reapply that makeup! In sum, look the part of a doctor, and your age should not matter to the patient. The patient will see that at the core, you are clinically competent (how's that for alliteration?).

Demonstrate a commitment to ethical principles pertaining to provision or withholding of clinical care, confidentiality of patient information, informed consent, and business practice.

The patient was adequately informed of the risks of the procedure by the gastroenterologist as well as the risks for anesthesia. Particularly crucial to this case was

155

explaining to the patient that she would be sedated in the prone position, which can be uncomfortable and intimidating to a patient.

Interpersonal and communication skills

Residents must be able to demonstrate interpersonal and communication skills that result in effective information exchange and teaming with patients, their patients' families, and professional associates.

> Work effectively with others as a member or leader of a health care team or other professional group.

This case is chock full of communication and interpersonal skills! As a new attending, it is important to be cordial to your colleagues, especially in this era of off-site anesthesia. You never know to which corner or crevice of the hospital you will be asked to go to provide your services! The preoperative conversation between the anesthesiologist and the gastroenterologist was necessary to determine how stable the patient was and to agree on monitored anesthesia care in the prone position. The GI doc had office hours to follow, and of course, you want to keep him happy by having things go efficiently and smoothly, but remember that patient safety does not always follow a time line.

When gallstones hit the fan and the patient quickly became hypoxic from sustained apnea, the anesthesiologist in the case maintained composure; the GI doctor began yelling about patient movement, but instead of raising a voice in retaliation, a quick point to the monitors can get your intentions across. In fact, the gastroenterologist quickly humbled after this. When

things are spiraling downward in a crucial situation, it is important to firmly delegate tasks so that all hands are helping. Remember that people panic and freeze in emergencies, and you as an anesthesiologist have only two hands to do many, many tasks. If an anesthesia tech had been in the room, he or she could have been a valuable source for finding a mask to ventilate the patient. You told the GI doctor to remove the endoscope; you told the nurse to get the stretcher; collectively, you turned the patient from prone to supine and were able to secure the airway. At the end, you said with calm composure to the gastroenterologist to continue, even though, on the inside, you were dying!

Systems-based practice

Residents must demonstrate an awareness of and responsiveness to the larger context and system of health care and the ability to effectively call on system resources to provide care that is of optimal value.

> Understand how their patient care and other professional practices affect other health care professionals, the health care organization, and the larger society and how these elements of the system affect their own practice.

When critical events arise, do not underestimate the power of a debriefing session with all those involved – sometimes even the patients themselves – so that a thorough review of the situation can occur. Attempt to answer the question of how this situation can be avoided in the future. Perhaps an ERCP protocol can be developed; perhaps all ERCPs should be done under general anesthesia with endotracheal tube (ETT) from the very beginning.

In sum, don't supersize that Big MAC!

Additional reading

1. Tagaito Y, Isono S, Nishino T. Upper airway reflexes during a combination of propofol and fentanyl anesthesia. Anesthesiology 1998;88:1459–1466.

2. Langley MS, Heel RC. Propofol: a review of its pharmacodynamic and pharmacokinetic properties and use as an intravenous anesthetic. Drugs 1988;35:334–372.

3. Wehrmann T, Kokabpick S, Lembcke B, et al. Efficacy and safety of intravenous propofol sedation during routine ERCP: a prospective controlled study. Gastrointest Endosc 1999;49:677–683.

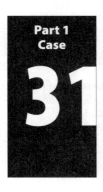

Contributions from Stony Brook University under Christopher J. Gallagher

On call in labor and delivery
The morbidly obese nightmare

Ursula Landman and Kathleen Dubrow

The case

There is a 30-year-old, 450-pound plus, as stated in the chart, gravida 1 para 0 (G1P0) in labor and delivery room 4 who is being induced with no epidural, and there is still no IV. The patient's blood pressure is 120/70, pulse 70, respirations 15, fetal heart rate (FHR) 140s. Past medical history/past surgical history none. Her meds included perinatal vitamins, and she had no known drug allergies. There were multiple IV attempts during the afternoon, without success. The obstetric anesthesiologist states that "the patient wants general anesthesia if she is to have a c-section." The obstetrician states that he does not need anesthesia now. The obstetric anesthesiologist has left. What do you do?

Patient care

Residents must be able to provide patient care that is compassionate, appropriate, and effective for the treatment of health problems and the promotion of health.

> Communicate effectively and demonstrate caring and respectful behaviors when interacting with patients and their families.

A mutually agreed on plan is of the utmost importance. The patient needed to gain the trust of the new team so that a further attempt at an epidural and IV could be done. It was also important to note that the day team had tried multiple times to get an epidural and an IV. The first concern would be to check the patient's airway – just in case she does have a cesarean section. Next, the patient would have to be asked directly about retrying for an epidural, given all the risks that would go along with a general anesthetic. Although multiple attempts for an epidural were made, I felt it necessary to try to get an epidural in this morbidly obese patient, in addition to large-bore IV access. The patient actually agreed to another attempt and, if an epidural was obtained, realized it would be used for cesarean section.

> Gather essential and accurate information about their patients.

The patient was actually much larger than 450 pounds – that was an understatement. One area of the chart stated that her weight was 600 pounds plus. On repeat interview of the patient, she admitted to 600. I always like to recheck history and physical exam for myself. Many times, I will gain additional important information, just by asking the question again.

> Make informed decisions about diagnostic and therapeutic interventions based on patient information and preferences, up-to-date scientific evidence, and clinical judgment.

It doesn't take a genius to see that this is a disaster about to happen. The patient has no IV and no epidural and wants general anesthesia for cesarean section if she needs one. Patient preference here is not an option. The risks had to be clearly spelled out to this patient and her husband. She was also being induced after normal hours.

> Develop and carry out patient management plans.

It was necessary to try to get an epidural in this morbidly obese patient, in addition to large-bore IV access. This was discussed with the obstetric attending. Of course, this obstetric attending then left, and a new obstetrician attending took over. The plan for an epidural was discussed again. Communication is very important between the team, especially so that they understand the possibility of a difficult airway and difficult IV access. Attempts were made again, without success. The difficult airway box was checked, as was availability of the fiber optic and other necessary equipment. You should use what you are most comfortable with and have that available in the operating room. The other attending in-house was also made aware but stated that he was unable to help if there was a need for cesarean section.

Counsel and educate patients and their families.

Here is a patient who was as healthy as a 600-pound plus patient could be up to this point, but there is a genuine worry that things may end up very badly. It is best not to sugarcoat the risks, but just tell it like it is: the risks are *x*, *y*, and *z*, and this could very well happen because you are at increased risk. I explained to the patient the possibility of having a difficult airway. She appeared to understand this and became more willing to have an epidural attempted again.

Use information technology to support patient care decisions and patient education.

If the obstetricians have done a bedside ultrasound, it is great to hear their estimate of the baby's size and how the placenta is lying. This can alert you to further needs, for example, blood availability if the placenta is low lying. This patient did not have a low-lying placenta. Also, the baby was predicted to be of average weight.

Perform competently all medical and invasive procedures considered essential for the area of practice.

A competent anesthesiologist would skillfully place adequate venous access and an arterial line (to monitor blood pressure on a beat-to-beat basis, especially if there is lack of an adequate cuff size).

Provide health care services aimed at preventing health problems or maintaining health.

One preventive measure that we can take in this size of a patient is application of compression stockings to avoid deep venous thrombosis (DVT) later on. Also, if this patient were to have a cesarean section, then during such a case, timing the delivery of prophylactic antibiotics is important. Current standards are for antibiotics to be delivered within an hour of incision.

Work with health care professionals, including those from other disciplines, to provide patient-focused care.

We must work with the obstetricians closely and develop a plan for this type of patient. A huddle to debrief about the patient was done so that we could all be on the same page regarding her care. The problem was the change of shift, so this had to be done multiple times, and each time, we had to convince the new obstetrician taking over that we could not just throw our hands up and hope for the best if she were to be sectioned. We needed to attempt an IV and an epidural again. It is also in the obstetrician's best interests to have an appropriate anesthetic on board – it will make his or her job easier and be the safest for the patient.

Medical knowledge

Residents must demonstrate knowledge about established and evolving biomedical, clinical, and cognate (e.g., epidemiological and social-behavioral) sciences and the application of this knowledge to patient care.

Demonstrate an investigatory and analytic thinking approach to clinical situations.

It was also necessary to have the longer Tuohy needle for the additional attempt at an epidural. We had various sizes available, and the one that was successful was almost "harpoonlike," in the words of the nurse who was assisting me. Persistence truly paid off after about 2.5 hours of attempts for an epidural. A pearl for these obese patients: the excess soft tissue was taped up to help visualize the back better. This was a much needed intervention. Sometimes it is necessary to think outside the box and use other means to maximize the best attempt. It made a world of difference in comparison to just attempting without the tape. Don't underestimate the importance of this taping. A crisscross *V* was made with tape, and the area was prepped with povidone-iodine.

Know and apply the basic and clinically supportive sciences that are appropriate to their discipline.

The FHR was checked multiple times, and it was fine. A Doppler transducer was used at first, and then, because it was taking a while to obtain an anesthetic, a fetal scalp electrode was placed. The fetal scalp electrode is most accurate. The cervix does need to be 1–3 cm dilated for use, and membranes must be ruptured. A cardiotachometer uses the peak or threshold voltage of the fetal *r*-wave to measure the interval between each fetal cardiac cycle. There was good FHR baseline variability (fluctuations in the baseline FHR of

2 cycles per minute). Normal baseline FHR remained 140–150. This gave me the leisure to continue epidural attempts. In actuality, a spinal was purposefully done with the epidural needle because the epidural space could not be located.

Practice-based learning and improvement

Residents must be able to investigate and evaluate their patient care practices, appraise and assimilate scientific evidence, and improve their patient care practices.

Analyze practice experience and perform practice-based improvement activities using a systematic methodology.

It took some time, but after more and more of these morbidly obese patients began to come to deliver, a task force was formed to develop practice guidelines for these patients, who are now frequent in labor and delivery. There was a systematic analysis done with the obstetricians and the anesthesiologists, and now anesthesia is consulted in advance on these patients. They are seen in clinic, and they may now have lines placed preemptively if they are such a difficult stick.

Locate, appraise, and assimilate evidence from scientific studies related to their patients' health problems.

The literature was reviewed and recommendations were made based on it. Early preoperative evaluation by the obstetric anesthesia team is a necessity. The ultimate disaster can be averted here. It was helpful to have the obstetricians hear our needs and us theirs. We are all looking to have the best outcome – a healthy baby and mother.

Obtain and use information about their own population of patients and the larger population from which their patients are drawn.

It is important to revisit this literature in case new developments occur regarding morbidly obese pregnant patients.

Use information technology to manage information, access online medical information; and support their own education.

The Internet can be a great place to keep up to date on the latest knowledge in the field. Also, the American College of Obstetricians and Gynecologists and Society for Obstetric Anesthesia and Perinatology publications can be great to review for information in the field.

Professionalism

Residents must demonstrate a commitment to carrying out professional responsibilities, adherence to ethical principles, and sensitivity to a diverse patient population.

Demonstrate respect, compassion, and integrity; a responsiveness to the needs of patients and society that supersedes self-interest; accountability to patients, society, and the profession; and a commitment to excellence and ongoing professional development.

It is always important to treat the patient and family with respect and compassion, even if they seem to have crazy ideas. This patient wanted general anesthesia, but once her concerns were addressed and all was explained, then she was amenable to another attempt at epidural. As always, even for a regional anesthetic, it is important to set up for a general anesthetic, just in case – this means that you should always check your machine and have medications prepared and ready.

The best way to be responsive to patient needs is to listen – it sounds simple, but many physicians do not, and they can miss information or miss cues regarding the patient's needs. Facial expressions and body language are very important, and this can help the patient if you can pick up on them. Also, patients can pick up on the anesthesiologist's facial expressions and body language, so it's best to be nonjudgmental and not to approach the patient with hands on your hips – many times, the patient will not open up to you about the situation.

Professionalism encompasses a commitment to excellence and your own development. If you have been attending hospital and teaching rounds and going to meetings, this will help you keep up to date in the field. There is always new information in medicine, and we cannot ignore that – you have to be a lifelong learner as a physician.

Demonstrate a commitment to ethical principles pertaining to provision or withholding of clinical care, confidentiality of patient information, informed consent, and business practice.

It is unprofessional to talk about other patients in front of your patient. Many times, we have multiple laboring patients, and it is best to take the discussion outside of labor and delivery so that it can be discussed in privacy. Patient privacy should be respected. I always make it a practice to knock on the door before I enter the labor and delivery room and to wash my hands in front of the patient before and after seeing her. It also seems silly, but a time-out should be held with the patient, nurse, and physician to ensure that the patient is receiving the correct procedure. Many times, patients will comment, "Of course I am having a c-section – don't we all know that? Just look at my belly!"

Demonstrate sensitivity and responsiveness to patients' culture, age, gender, and disabilities.

Many of the female laboring patients come to us from different backgrounds, and although they have to "bare their bottom" to deliver, they still want to preserve modesty. I always tell my residents to place a drape up while the patient is being prepped in the operating room. This is then switched out with the sterile drape afterward. Patients who have modesty and/or cultural issues will then be more at ease. They will only see the anesthesiologists, and although they know very well that they are naked for all in the room, it will now not be so disturbing to them.

Interpersonal and communication skills

Residents must be able to demonstrate interpersonal and communication skills that result in effective information exchange and teaming with patients, their patients' families, and professional associates.

Create and sustain a therapeutic and ethically sound relationship with patients.

Everyone with whom I work needs to introduce himself or herself by name and position. We have a short period of time in which we must gain the trust and respect of the patient. If we just barge into the patient's room with no regard, the patient will not have a good first impression of us. Common courte-

sies, such as listening to all in the room and answering questions, puts the patient at ease.

Use effective listening skills and elicit and provide information using effective nonverbal, explanatory, questioning, and writing skills.

We have to ask directed questions. Many times, we have emergent situations in which we get only the most basic of information: last ate, allergies, and so on. If we ask these questions – and look the patient in the eye – then it could mean a world of difference to the patient. Of course, we are doing a hundred other things: putting monitors on, starting a line, and so on.

Work effectively with others as a member or leader of a health care team or other professional group.

On labor and delivery, we work very closely with the obstetricians, and we become aware of many idiosyncrasies, for better or worse. The case began with the slowest – truly slowest – obstetrician in the hospital. At the 1.5-hour mark, I suggested that we get another obstetrician to help, or else my anesthetic would run out (remember that I had done an intentional spinal, so I did not have an epidural to redo) – a big worry because the patient had a class 3–4 airway. The patient was operated on in a regular bed that did not go up and down and managed to have an anesthetic that did last. The anesthesiologist has to have a good rapport with the obstetrics team – here a second obstetrician was clearly needed, and my suggestion worked well enough to have the obstetrician say, "Yes, please call her in."

Systems-based practice

Residents must demonstrate an awareness of and responsiveness to the larger context and system of health care and the ability to effectively call on system resources to provide care that is of optimal value.

Understand how their patient care and other professional practices affect other health care professionals, the health care organization, and the larger society and how these elements of the system affect their own practice.

The patient was operated on in a regular bed that did not go up and down, and this complaint of mine to the RNs and director of obstetric anesthesia enabled the unit to change the type of operating room tables available so that no other team would have to endure what I had endured. It was an impossible situation in which to operate, but we made do at the time. Even placement of the spinal was challenging because I am tall and had to bend down; normally, I would bring the bed up, but this one only went so high.

Know how types of medical practice and delivery systems differ from one another, including methods of controlling health care costs and allocating resources.

Review of the literature showed us that there are more and more morbidly obese pregnant patients around the country, and it was good to see how each institution deals with this patient population, thus the idea to see patients in a clinic beforehand, for evaluation.

Practice cost-effective health care and resource allocation that does not compromise quality of care.

Standard cost-effectiveness should be used. This would mean not opening up additional epidural kits if this can be avoided. The best action would be to open an additional larger epidural needle as it is needed. Thus we use only what we need and will have the others for a rainy day or another day with a similar potential disaster case.

Advocate for quality patient care and assist patients in dealing with system complexities.

Sometimes we can be the only voice of reason for the patient. A calm voice that is reassuring and can state the facts in a nonjudgmental tone will help patients and their families make informed decisions regarding their care. This patient allowed me to reattempt an epidural once everything was explained to her. The day crew had tried to explain everything earlier, just before the change of shift, but was it done well? Maybe the team was looking just to go home. We owe it to our patients, though, to explain all, even at the end of the day. We have to repeat information as necessary – this is difficult material to process.

Know how to partner with health care managers and health care providers to assess, coordinate, and improve health care and know how these activities can affect system performance.

This baby was not in distress and did not have any apnea. I still like to know how these babies are doing and will follow up with the neonatal intensive care unit team afterward, just so I know how all is going for the baby and family. The baby girl had a 9, 9 Apgar, which is a scale signifying heart rate, respiratory effort, muscle tone, reflex, irritability, and color. It is measured at 1 and 5 minutes (less than 7, then continued every 5 minutes up to 20 minutes). There are limitations – Apgar is useful in predicting short-term mortality for groups of infants with low birth weight. It has a low value in predicting the survival of an individual. Primary apnea occurs after the initial attempts to breathe (stimulation or tapping feet can cause resumption of breathing). Secondary apnea occurs with continued oxygen deprivation – the baby gasps several times and then enters secondary apnea (stimulation does not restart breathing). I also followed up with postpartum on the patient. She did not even get a postdural puncture headache. As one of the senior anesthesiologists who trained me stated, "It's better to be lucky than good."

Additional reading

1. Hawkins J. Labor and delivery management of the morbidly obese patient. IARS 2008;57:6.

2. Mhyre J. Anesthetic management for the morbidly obese pregnant woman. Int Anesth Clin 2007;45:51–70.

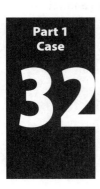

Kidney transplant

Syed Azim and Louis Chun

The case

A 61-year-old male with a history of end-stage renal disease secondary to long-standing diabetes and hypertension, on hemodialysis for 5 years, presents for deceased-donor renal transplantation.

Patient care

Residents must be able to provide patient care that is compassionate, appropriate, and effective for the treatment of health problems and the promotion of health.

Communicate effectively and demonstrate caring and respectful behaviors when interacting with patients and their families.

No doubt this is a big day for the patient, as he is about to not only go under anesthesia, but also receive an organ that could potentially alter the rest of his life, for better or worse. Building rapport and showing confidence in your ability to take care of the patient in the operating room (OR) cannot be overemphasized. Let him know that you will need to place multiple intravenous (IV) lines, a central venous catheter, an arterial catheter, and a Foley catheter. By the time he wakes up, he should feel like a Christmas tree.

Gather essential and accurate information about their patients.

When was his last dialysis? This gives an indication of whether he might be dry as a prune (immediately postdialysis) or plump as a tomato (just before dialysis). Where is his fistula (if any)? You would never want to place monitors or establish access on that extremity. What is his exercise tolerance or cardiac status? This will help guide our anesthetic induction and maintenance.

Make informed decisions about diagnostic and therapeutic interventions based on patient

---

information and preferences, up-to-date scientific evidence, and clinical judgment.

A patient with end-stage renal disease (ESRD) on hemodialysis presents many challenges, which include if and when to transfuse blood, how to correct metabolic acidosis if you decide to, and what to do with hyponatremia/hypernatremia. Remember, the deceased-donor kidney is on the watch. You may just have to work with whatever numbers you have in front of you as you prepare to wheel the patient to the OR.

Develop and carry out patient management plans.

Have drips ready to go, (e.g., antibiotics, gancyclovir, methylprednisolone, and alemtuzumab). At some point, you will need heparin. You may also use Benadryl to prevent allergic reactions; albumin, mannitol, and furosemide to flush the new kidney; and sodium bicarbonate and calcium chloride to counteract the effects of hyperkalemia after restoring blood flow to the new kidney. Usually, these patients are chronically anemic. It is imperative to have blood ready to be transfused.

Counsel and educate patients and their families.

Organ transplant surgeries seem always to occur at the most unexpected (and inconvenient) of times (e.g., when the schedule for the day is packed to the point where the laparoscopic appendectomy is to follow three emergency laparotomies and an intubation of a patient with epiglottis, or when you are cozying up on that favorite couch in the call room at 1:00 A.M. waiting for the organ – and patient – to arrive). It is therefore easy to lose sight of the importance of informing the patient and family just what to expect during and after surgery.

Use information technology to support patient care decisions and patient education.

Review all available laboratory values, including Chem8, complete blood count (CBC), chest X-ray, and electrocardiogram results. Check a finger-stick glucose prior to starting.

Perform competently all medical and invasive procedures considered essential for the area of practice.

Perform induction and intubation, followed by establishment of an arterial line (on the extremity without the arterial-venous fistula) to monitor beat-to-beat variations in blood pressure and a central line to monitor fluid status.

Provide health care services aimed at preventing health problems or maintaining health.

The survival of the graft kidney depends, in part, on the timely administration of antibacterial, antiviral, and immunosuppressive agents. We can do our part by getting those drugs in the patient intraoperatively.

Work with health care professionals, including those from other disciplines, to provide patient-focused care.

Your transplant surgeons need your help as much as they need the help of their scrub and circulating nurses. The surgeon may let you know when to give the heparin and when to get the blood pressure up to ensure perfusion to the new kidney. Also, you may need to ask the circulating nurse to send off multiple ABGs, and when you notice that the H&H confirms that the pallor of the patient's fingers is not the latest fashion statement on nail polish, you may ask the nurse to fetch blood in the refrigerator. Can you spell T-E-A-M-W-O-R-K?

Medical knowledge

Residents must demonstrate knowledge about established and evolving biomedical, clinical, and cognate (e.g., epidemiological and social-behavioral) sciences and the application of this knowledge to patient care.

Demonstrate an investigatory and analytic thinking approach to clinical situations.

Always expect the worst and hope for the best. As you begin this case, think about what could go wrong in the operating room. The patient will likely have abnormalities in platelet function and may present with bleeding diathesis. Compounding it to chronic anemia, and you could have a recipe for disaster. Every now and then, check how much blood was lost in the suction canisters and lap pads, and make sure you have blood ready to go.

Metabolic acidosis can be a chronic problem in these patients. With metabolic acidosis comes hyperkalemia, which, by the way, could be exacerbated by a number of things, including hemorrhage, massive blood transfusion, and the establishment of perfusion to the new kidney (acidosis). So how do you recognize hyperkalemia? You may want to occasionally check the electrocardiogram (EKG) monitor for the earliest signs, that is, peaked T-waves, flattened P-waves, prolonged PR, and a widened QRS complex.

Know and apply the basic and clinically supportive sciences that are appropriate to their discipline.

The kidney is a vital part of homeostasis, affecting multiple organ systems. Knowing the altered physiology of a patient with ESRD helps prepare for the critical stages of surgery. Common problems associated with ESRD include electrolyte imbalance and cardiovascular and hematologic dysfunction.

Practice-based learning and improvement

Residents must be able to investigate and evaluate their patient care practices, appraise and assimilate scientific evidence, and improve their patient care practices.

Analyze practice experience and perform practice-based improvement activities using a systematic methodology.

As you work through a case like this, you realize how overwhelming things can get, especially if there is an unanticipated glitch along the way. It is therefore important to develop a systematic approach to the steps taken from the moment the patient enters the OR to the point at which he settles down in the recovery room. Institution-specific protocols call for certain types and dosages of antibiotics, antivirals, and immunosuppressants to be administered, requiring the use of multiple lines. Developing a way to avoid tangling the spaghetti is helpful, to say the least. As the surgery progresses, having an idea of the timing of giving certain medications is crucial. With proper preparation and practice, experience, and practice-based improvement activities, there should be little variation in the way this surgery is handled, even among different clinicians.

> Locate, appraise, and assimilate evidence from scientific studies related to their patients' health problems.

Know what is recommended. For example, how would you carry out your maintenance anesthetic? A number of different combinations of inhaled and intravenous medications have been used with reasonable safety margins. General anesthesia is preferred. Desflurane, isoflurane, and sevoflurane can all be used, although there may be some concern with renal toxicity from the use of sevoflurane due to production of fluoride and compound A. Opioids other than morphine and meperidine, which have metabolites dependent on renal clearance, should be safe. Ideally, a muscle relaxant not dependent on renal clearance, such as atracurium or cisatricurium, should be used.

> Obtain and use information about their own population of patients and the larger population from which their patients are drawn.

Review the latest on anesthetic management of renal transplantation.

> Apply knowledge of study designs and statistical methods to the appraisal of clinical studies and other information on diagnostic and therapeutic effectiveness.

Is there any evidence to what is being done? For example, is an arterial line absolutely necessary for a kidney transplant procedure? The answer is no – there is no proof that arterial line placement improves graft outcome. However, it seems beneficial to have continuous blood pressure monitoring, particularly after revascularization of the transplanted kidney, because hypotension can lead to delayed graft function and/or renal vein thrombosis.

> Use information technology to manage information, access online medical information, and support their own education.

Again, review the latest literature.

Professionalism

Residents must demonstrate a commitment to carrying out professional responsibilities, adherence to ethical principles, and sensitivity to a diverse patient population.

> Demonstrate respect, compassion, and integrity; a responsiveness to the needs of patients and society that supersedes self-interest; accountability to patients, society, and the profession; and a commitment to excellence and ongoing professional development.

Again, although this may seem like another 4-hour haul for you in the middle of the night, when you wish you were snoozing away, try to think about it from the patient's perspective. As you would on a typical midmorning routine, you should be prepared to handle a bag of emotions at the bedside and demonstrate the appropriate respect, compassion, and responsibility that your patient demands.

> Demonstrate a commitment to ethical principles pertaining to provision or withholding of clinical care, confidentiality of patient information, informed consent, and business practice.

Review informed consent, double-check on surgery site, and be cognizant that there are others around you as you discuss details of your patient's medical record in the holding area. Also, make sure the surgeon has seen the patient prior to taking him to the OR.

> Demonstrate sensitivity and responsiveness to patients' culture, age, gender, and disabilities.

What may transcend all cultures, ages, gender, and disabilities is the notion of treating your patients as you would wish to be treated.

Interpersonal and communication skills

Residents must be able to demonstrate interpersonal and communication skills that result in effective information exchange and teaming with patients, their patients' families, and professional associates.

> Create and sustain a therapeutic and ethically sound relationship with patients.

Hand washing is an important habit to develop, especially when seeing patients who are potentially immunocompromised, as in this case in the postoperative period.

> Use effective listening skills and elicit and provide information using effective nonverbal, explanatory, questioning, and writing skills.

The patient will likely have many questions, some of which you may not be able to answer in detail. Although the patient may be emotionally prepared to undergo surgery (as he may have had a few years to ponder on this while being on dialysis), many patients may still have a zillion thoughts going through their heads. You may even be asked a question more appropriately answered by the surgeons, in which case, you should respectfully defer to your colleagues.

> Work effectively with others as a member or leader of a health care team or other professional group.

The significance of working effectively with other members of the OR staff should be reiterated. In addition, as you transition to the recovery room, your input may be requested not only by the recovery room staff, but also by urology, nephrology, and intensive care unit personnel.

Systems-based practice

Residents must demonstrate an awareness of and responsiveness to the larger context and system of health care and the ability to effectively call on system resources to provide care that is of optimal value.

> Understand how their patient care and other professional practices affect other health care professionals, the health care organization, and the larger society and how these elements of the system affect their own practice.

There are many levels of coordination involved in transplanting a deceased-donor kidney into a recipient. It is important to understand that viable organs are scarce resources that should be handled with the utmost diligence. From a societal perspective, many individuals are on a waiting list to receive a kidney, and the ultimate measure of success may mean an improved quality of life for a prolonged period of time. You have a chance to contribute to the likelihood of success by being vigilant in the OR and by following necessary infection precautions when seeing your patient.

> Practice cost-effective health care and resource allocation that does not compromise quality of care.

Intraoperatively, one may consider using isoflurane as this is relatively inexpensive and provides adequate anesthesia for a lengthy case such as this one. From a long-term perspective, length of graft survival is important to overall health care cost. Thus improving overall outcome means maintaining a blood pressure that will optimize perfusion to the graft without compromising the anastomoses.

> Advocate for quality patient care and assist patients in dealing with system complexities.

Understand the immediate postoperative concerns for this patient and be prepared to react appropriately in certain situations. For example, how do you deal with steroid-induced psychosis? What is the optimal blood pressure for this patient? What do you do when urine output is not responding to fluid challenges? Knowing what to do beforehand allows for a smoother postoperative course and a potentially better surgical outcome.

> Know how to partner with health care managers and health care providers to assess, coordinate, and improve health care and know how these activities can affect system performance.

The immediate postoperative period is important in terms of laying out goals, standards, and protocols for the care of the patient. Usually, medication orders will be clearly preprinted, and fluid management is focused on urine output assessment. Communication with the urology and nephrology teams is imperative.

Additional reading

1. Lemmens HJ. Kidney transplantation: recent developments and recommendations for anesthetic management. Anesthesiol Clin North Am 2004;22:651–662.

2. SarinKapoor H, Kaur R, Kaur H. Anaesthesia for renal transplant surgery. Acta Anaesthesiol Scand 2007;51:1354–1367.

3. Halloran PF. Immunosuppressive drugs for kidney transplantation. N Engl J Med 2004;351:2715–2729. Erratum, N Engl J Med 2005;352:1056.

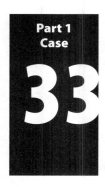

Contributions from Stony Brook University under Christopher J. Gallagher

Electrical glitch

Daryn Moller and Joseph Conrad

The case

A previously healthy 58-year-old female with a family history of breast cancer noted a lump in her left breast on self-examination. Following a positive biopsy and an in-depth discussion with her surgeon, the decision was made to proceed with bilateral total mastectomy with left sentinel lymph node biopsy.

After a smooth induction, easy intubation, and 90 minutes of general anesthesia with oxygen, desflurane, and fentanyl, the surgeon has nearly completed dissection of the first breast. In your vigilance, you glance at your anesthesia machine and notice the digital display has gone dark, the bellows are not moving, and there is no evidence of fresh gas flow.

Patient care

Residents must be able to provide patient care that is compassionate, appropriate, and effective for the treatment of health problems and the promotion of health.

> Communicate effectively and demonstrate caring and respectful behaviors when interacting with patients and their families.

The patient is asleep, and you have your hands full, so your caring behavior will be exactly that – caring for the patient. There will be plenty of time after the operation for respectful discussion of the day's events with the patient and her family.

> Gather essential and accurate information about their patients.

With your preoperative assessment complete and the patient under general anesthesia, information gathering is limited to physical exam and available monitors. In this case, the oxygen sensor, gas analyzer, and end-tidal capnography are lost with the machine. The pulse oximeter, blood pressure cuff, electrocardiogram, and temperature probe function will depend on the nature of the electrical failure. If the problem is limited to the machine, these monitors should continue to function; a problem with the electrical supply could affect these monitors. Your Foley catheter should function appropriately.

> Make informed decisions about diagnostic and therapeutic interventions based on patient information and preferences, up-to-date scientific evidence, and clinical judgment.

As it stands, the patient remains anesthetized and intubated, but without any fresh gas flow, ventilation, or volatile anesthetic. On top of that, patient monitoring has been compromised. Intervention will concentrate on these areas.

> Develop and carry out patient management plans.

With an airway already established, breathing is top priority. For ventilation without a ventilator, Ambu-bag is the answer. If possible, a portable ventilator will solve this problem as well, but will obviously take time.

As the patient is still in the middle of an operation, she will need anesthesia. The options are limited to intravenous (IV) anesthetics, so an infusion should be started as soon as possible. If the electrical supply to the room is intact, your infusion pumps will work without a problem. Even in a temporary blackout, their battery backup should still do the job. In case of apocalypse, total intravenous anesthesia (TIVA) can be done the low-tech way, with a bag of propofol on a microdrip IV set.

Monitoring will be a problem. Electrocardiogram and pulse ox are easily replaced by battery-powered units, and blood pressure can be done manually. However, an end-tidal CO_2 monitor may be hard to come by; you may have to make do with auscultation and observation of chest wall motion for the short term.

The oxygen sensor and gas analyzer may simply be unavailable.

With basic life support reestablished and all available monitors in place given the circumstances, the next step is to determine whether to abort the operation. In an elective case such as this, the safest situation might be to have the surgeon close at the next possible opportunity.

Counsel and educate patients and their families.

Clearly the anesthesiologist's opportunities to counsel and educate patients undergoing general anesthesia are limited to the preoperative and postoperative periods. Preoperative counseling should include discussions of reasonably foreseeable risks and their management. Unforeseeable events, such as total malfunction of the anesthesia machine, are better left to the postoperative period.

Use information technology to support patient care decisions and patient education.

While the loss of machine function represents an acute problem and intervening to stabilize the patient leaves little time for immediate information gathering, the anesthesiologist's thorough knowledge of the machine and operating room (OR) environment will allow effective decision making.

Perform competently all medical and invasive procedures considered essential for the area of practice.

Competent performance in this case requires quick, rational judgment. As in any case, you must realize that there is indeed a problem, identify and prioritize the relevant issues, and then address those issues. This means skillful use of hand ventilation and proper preparation of necessary infusions and monitors to expedite patient care.

Provide health care services aimed at preventing health problems or maintaining health.

Once a situation such as this arises, the anesthesiologist maintains the patient's health by reestablishing adequate resuscitation and monitoring. Again, in an elective case such as this, preventing health problems and maintaining health may best be carried out by aborting the procedure.

Work with health care professionals, including those from other disciplines, to provide patient-focused care.

Patient safety and care in the OR depends on teamwork and communication among the anesthesiologist, surgeon, and OR staff, even under optimal conditions. When adverse circumstances do arise, the anesthesiologist should communicate clearly with the rest of the team what needs to be done to alleviate the problem.

Medical knowledge

Residents must demonstrate knowledge about established and evolving biomedical, clinical, and cognate (e.g., epidemiological and social-behavioral) sciences and the application of this knowledge to patient care.

Demonstrate an investigatory and analytic thinking approach to clinical situations.

Once the patient is stable, an attempt should be made to determine the underlying nature of the problem and its implications for the rest of the case. Where was the malfunction that caused the anesthesia machine to stop working? If the digital display fails and the machine continues to work, that is likely a problem limited to the display itself. That the whole machine shut down indicates either a problem in the machine's power supply or a problem with the electrical supply to the OR. Multiple circuits in the OR help to localize the problem. If the anesthesia machine, electrocautery, the surgeon's stereo, and everything else in the room craps out simultaneously, the problem is likely outside the OR and nothing you can fix. If your machine is the only piece of equipment in the room to fail, you should check that it is plugged into an uninterruptible power supply, that is, a power supply with a backup. An interruptible power supply, one that can go off and stay off, may be identical to the uninterruptible socket, and machines have been plugged into the wrong supply. You should never assume that somebody probably checked it; you may be the first to diagnose this problem in your own OR.

Know and apply the basic and clinically supportive sciences that are appropriate to their discipline.

You don't need a biomedical engineering degree to be a competent anesthesiologist, but you should know enough about your anesthesia machine to perform basic troubleshooting. The high-yield solution is to perform a complete machine check every day, asking yourself at each step, "What might go wrong, and how will I fix it?"

Practice-based learning and improvement

Residents must be able to investigate and evaluate their patient care practices, appraise and assimilate scientific evidence, and improve their patient care practices.

> Analyze practice experience and perform practice-based improvement activities using a systematic methodology.

Again, the best systematic approach to machine-related problems in the OR is thorough knowledge of the machine and the OR environment, reviewed daily through the machine check. When you do have a problem with a machine, you must address it. While you may not have the means or expertise to remedy every problem, you should contact someone who can. Between your hospital's biomedical engineering department and the machine's manufacturer, you will eventually find someone who can fix the glitch.

> Locate, appraise, and assimilate evidence from scientific studies related to their patients' health problems.

The literature on power failure in the OR is in somewhat short supply relative to other clinical parameters. However, patient care in this setting should be based on the published data and recommendations in more broadly applicable areas.

Monitoring is founded on the American Society of Anesthesiology (ASA) standards for basic monitoring. This begins with qualified anesthesia personnel, followed by assessment of oxygenation, ventilation, circulation, and temperature. Beyond that, the anesthesiologist must be familiar with the planned procedure and the patient's comorbidities as they relate to the anesthetic plan.

> Obtain and use information about their own population of patients and the larger population from which their patients are drawn.

Again, the anesthesiologist's knowledge base derives from attentive assessment of each patient, combined with a knowledge of the current literature pertaining to the patient's primary disease process and comorbidities.

> Apply knowledge of study designs and statistical methods to the appraisal of clinical studies and other information on diagnostic and therapeutic effectiveness.

Once again, in the face of equipment failure, there is not much time for a perusal of the literature, and it would be difficult to anticipate this type of event the night before, while reading up on your cases. However, once you have run into this type of difficulty, you should be acutely interested in how others have approached similar circumstances, and it is likely that whatever reports you do find about similar cases will stick in your mind better, having faced the problem firsthand. You should examine how other clinicians have approached these problems in the past and compare their methods with your own.

> Use information technology to manage information, access online medical information; and support their own education.

While the literature on power failure and similar problems is limited to case reports and letters, it is likely that any problem you face will not be the first of its kind and that someone, somewhere has faced the same issues and lived to describe the experience. The best way to access the world's clinical experience is via the Internet, and this should be a regular part of every clinician's practice.

Professionalism

Residents must demonstrate a commitment to carrying out professional responsibilities, adherence to ethical principles, and sensitivity to a diverse patient population.

> Demonstrate respect, compassion, and integrity; a responsiveness to the needs of patients and society that supersedes self-interest; accountability to patients, society, and the profession; and a commitment to excellence and ongoing professional development.

Responsiveness to the needs of the patient is neatly summed up in the motto of vigilance. The anesthesiologist must function as the physician in the OR, attending to the anesthetized patient's needs while the surgeon addresses a specific pathology. In this way, the anesthesiologist is uniquely accountable to the patient because no other group of physicians has more direct and immediate control of their patients' physiology. In this case, the vigilant anesthesiologist immediately recognizes a compromise in the patient's respiration and quickly addresses it, while protecting her from the harm of pain and intraoperative awareness.

Demonstrate a commitment to ethical principles pertaining to provision or withholding of clinical care, confidentiality of patient information, informed consent, and business practice.

As in any case, the physician must honor the patient's privacy and autonomy by keeping information confidential and ensuring preoperatively that the patient knows what to expect from the perioperative experience.

Demonstrate sensitivity and responsiveness to patients' culture, age, gender, and disabilities.

These general principles should influence every physician-patient interaction, if slightly more subtly in the operative setting. The anesthesiologist should be familiar with the patient's disabilities, including medical, surgical, and substance history, and these should influence intraoperative decision making. For example, females should be expected to have a higher rate of postoperative nausea and vomiting, patients with hypertension will more likely have labile blood pressures requiring tighter pharmacologic control, and persons of increased age will have decreased requirements for inhalational anesthetics.

However, most of the immediate maneuvers in the case of a machine failure should be applicable to any patient. While the anesthesiologist should have an idea of the patient's respiratory reserve, any patient for whom the ventilator fails should be immediately switched to hand ventilation, if necessary, with an Ambu-bag, regardless of the state of health.

Interpersonal and communication skills

Residents must be able to demonstrate interpersonal and communication skills that result in effective information exchange and teaming with patients, their patients' families, and professional associates.

Create and sustain a therapeutic and ethically sound relationship with patients.

The anesthesiologist's interaction with the patient may be brief relative to that of other physicians, but the relationship should not suffer for that fact. From the preoperative assessment, the physician should encourage the patient to be open and honest to optimize the assessment and should, in turn, be honest with the patient about plans and expectations for the coming procedure, including reasonably foreseeable risks.

While the risk of failure of an anesthesia machine or other mechanism in the OR would not typically be addressed, the physician should make every effort to reassure the patient that when adverse events do occur, they are handled as effectively as possible, with the goal of patient care in mind.

Use effective listening skills and elicit and provide information using effective nonverbal, explanatory, questioning, and writing skills.

Following failure of your machine and subsequent stabilization of your patient, document! In the case of an adverse event or near-miss, the events should be recorded as accurately as possible for future review and improvement.

Work effectively with others as a member or leader of a health care team or other professional group.

The machine stopped working, and you are formulating your plans while hand-ventilating. If you are manually ventilating your patient, then no one in the OR is performing a more critical task. Now is the time to assert yourself as "doctor of the operating room." You will need the assistance of the surgeon and the OR staff, and likely outside help, to care for your patient effectively. Call on individuals and assign tasks just as you would in an advanced cardiac life support (ACLS) code. As professionally as possible, determine with the surgeon whether and how to proceed with the remainder of the operation. If conditions are temporarily unsafe to continue, ask him or her to pause. If conditions cannot be improved, alert the surgeon that the case must end as soon as possible.

Systems-based practice

Residents must demonstrate an awareness of and responsiveness to the larger context and system of health care and the ability to effectively call on system resources to provide care that is of optimal value.

Understand how their patient care and other professional practices affect other health care professionals, the health care organization, and the larger society and how these elements of the system affect their own practice.

The anesthesiologist must be aware of the effect of his or her own actions on other physicians, particularly the surgeon in the room. Honest and respectful communication sets the tone for a good working relationship and can facilitate proper patient care.

Practice cost-effective health care and resource allocation that does not compromise quality of care.

In this relatively long case, perhaps a more cost-effective inhalational anesthetic than desflurane might have been considered.

Advocate for quality patient care and assist patients in dealing with system complexities.

Make the most of the precious few minutes spent with the patient during the preoperative assessment. Inform patients of what to expect.

In the OR, be attuned to potential problems in the system. Try to look critically at aspects of patient care usually taken for granted. If a defect is identified in the machine you were using for this case, look at your next machine to see if the same defect is present. If the machine was simply plugged into the incorrect power supply, see to it that other machines are properly set up.

Know how to partner with health care managers and health care providers to assess, coordinate, and improve health care and know how these activities can affect system performance.

If you notice problems or ambiguities that might lead to compromised patient care, address these concerns to the proper authority, whether it be the OR coordinator, engineering, or a quality assurance body.

Additional reading

1. Chawla AV, Newton NI. Machine and monitor failure from electrical overloading. Anaesthesia 2002; 57:1134–1135.

2. Yasney J, Soffer R. A case of power failure in the operating room. Anesth Prog 2005;52:65–69.

3. Welch RH, Feldman JM. Anesthesia during total electrical failure, or what would you do if the lights went out? J Clin Anesth 1989;1:358–362.

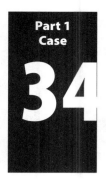

Contributions from Stony Brook University under
Christopher J. Gallagher

34 What do you mean you stop breathing in your sleep?

Deborah Richman and Vishal Sharma

The case

Your patient is a 45-year-old, hard-drinking, hard-smoking, and loud-snoring construction worker fresh from the work site. Appropriately attired in steel toe boots, muddy jeans, and a classic yet form-fitting flannel shirt, he and his wife stop by the preoperative assessment clinic before heading to the steakhouse for a 16-ounce T-bone with many, many sides. His abdomen cascades down his waistline, and his cough reminds you of a bulldozer moving gravel. The patient is scheduled for shoulder arthroscopy within 2 weeks secondary to a fall he suffered 1 month prior. You ask him about his accident, and he tells you that he fell asleep on his lunch break and hit his shoulder against the table. His past medical history is nondescript; he has no medical problems, takes no meds, has no allergies, had no previous surgeries, drinks about a six pack a day, and smokes about a half pack of cigarettes a day. He has chronic shoulder pain, for which he initially saw the orthopedist, who recommended that he have shoulder arthroscopy after magnetic resonance imaging revealed a slight rotator cuff injury. During your interview, a nurse asks for your assistance, and you briefly step out of the room. When you return to your office less than 5 minutes later, your patient is slouched over, snoring louder than Homer Simpson after a night at Al's Tavern. You ask him about his sleep, and he relates to you that he frequently wakes up at night short of breath, has morning sleepiness, falls asleep at work all the time, and has noticed that he has been having headaches more frequently. His wife states that he has snored forever, and sometimes in the middle of the night, he'll wake up "huffing and puffing."

You examine him and notice that he is a middle-aged, obese white male with nicotine-stained fingers on his right hand. He has a short, thick neck. His heart sounds are normal and his lungs are clear. His vitals reveal an elevated blood pressure of 155/84, a heart rate of 65, and a respiratory rate of 10. His weight is 143 kg, and his height is 180 cm (body-mass index = 44). An electrocardiogram shows sinus rhythm, with peaked P-waves.

You review his screening worksheet: no allergies are listed, but surprise, surprise – his STOP screen has four out of four positive answers!

Patient care

Residents must be able to provide patient care that is compassionate, appropriate, and effective for the treatment of health problems and the promotion of health.

Communicate effectively and demonstrate caring and respectful behaviors when interacting with patients and their families.

The concerns here are multifocal. In addition to obesity, the patient demonstrates signs and symptoms of obstructive sleep apnea (OSA) but has a recent injury that has him needing surgery to repair it and hasten his return to active work. So he has two issues that need to be addressed and may not be prepared for the first: a sleep consult and workup to get in the way of the second – his surgery.

OSA is characterized by repetitive obstruction of the airway during sleep with apnea lasting more than 10 seconds.

Why is this clinically significant for anesthesiologists and the patient? OSA is associated with significant perioperative morbidity and mortality. OSA is associated with increased risk of difficult intubation, postoperative hypoventilation and apnea, and arrhythmias as well as medical comorbidities such as hypertension, heart disease, obesity, and pulmonary hypertension. It is important in this situation to express concerns about undiagnosed and untreated OSA and to refer these patients to experts knowledgeable about sleep-related disorders to reduce their overall risk from developing complications during surgery and later down the road.

175

Although this gentleman seems less worried about his overall fitness than Lance Armstrong, it doesn't necessarily mean that he wouldn't be concerned about the possibility of having a disorder of sleep. You must educate the patient about your concerns of OSA, obesity, and cigarette smoking and inform the patient about medical care from which he may benefit, even if the patient seems apathetic about his own well-being.

Gather essential and accurate information about their patients.

History and physical have given us a clinical diagnosis. We need to assess our patient for end organ damage from his clinical sleep apnea and hypertension. Basic testing includes the following:

1. a hemoglobin as an assessment of chronic hypoxemia
2. renal function secondary to hypertension
3. electrocardiogram looking for evidence of ischemia, left ventricular hypertrophy, and right heart strain
4. resting room air oxygen saturation

Any abnormalities here would suggest further investigations – possibly echocardiogram and arterial blood gases, and of course, the aforementioned sleep consult.

Make informed decisions about diagnostic and therapeutic interventions based on patient information and preferences, up-to-date scientific evidence, and clinical judgment.

This patient is being evaluated in the clinic well in advance of his surgery, and steps should be undertaken to optimize him for his surgery. The definitive test for OSA remains the polysomnogram.

Develop and carry out patient management plans.

Formal diagnosis of OSA, initiation of treatment preoperatively, and a specifically tailored anesthetic plan will offer the patient the lowest risk perioperatively:

Appropriate continuous positive airway pressure (CPAP) treatment should be instituted to achieve the following:

- decreased airway edema and easier intubation
- decreased sympathetic tone and lower cardiovascular risk

- less postoperative (opiate- and sedative-aided) apneas with extubation to CPAP

The patient should also receive counseling regarding weight loss, exercise, and smoking cessation and control of systemic hypertension.

In terms of surgical venue, high-risk patients are not appropriate for free-standing ambulatory surgicenters (American Society of Anesthesiologists [ASA] guidelines). Additionally, the CPAP machine should be brought on the day of surgery for use in the recovery period.

Shoulder repairs are generally done under general anesthesia in combination with regional anesthesia (interscalene nerve block). This is especially important in the OSA patient – any possible avoidance of opiates and sedatives is good.

Obese patients with sleep apnea are at increased risk for difficult intubation. Advanced airway equipment may be needed and staff experienced in its use should be available. Postop CPAP availability as well as postop monitoring and ventilation facilities and opiate and benzodiazepine antagonists should be at hand.

ASA guidelines recommend that patients with OSA be monitored for 3 hours longer than their non-OSA cohorts in recovery, and any episode of desaturation warrants another 7 hours in a monitored bed. For ambulatory patients, it is best to book them early in the day to prevent overnight admission for this indicated monitoring.

Counsel and educate patients and their families.

The risks of untreated OSA should be explained to the patient so that he can make an informed decision on whether to continue with diagnostic testing and therapy. With OSA, he is at risk for heart disease, stroke, or death.

Use information technology to support patient care decisions and patient education.

There are numerous resources online for patients to utilize to gain information on the diagnosis and treatment of OSA. It is important that you direct the patient to Web sites with useful information and not Web sites steered toward home remedies and miracle drugs that simply have not been proven to work or that might be dangerous. One excellent resource for patients is WebMD (http://www.webmd.com), a patient-centered Web site with medical information on a vast array of medical topics designed to inform patients. Another is the Web site of the American Sleep Apnea Association (http://www.sleepapnea.org), which provides useful information and written literature on OSA and its treatment.

Medical knowledge

Residents must demonstrate knowledge about established and evolving biomedical, clinical, and cognate (e.g., epidemiological and social-behavioral) sciences and the application of this knowledge to patient care.

> Demonstrate an investigatory and analytic thinking approach to clinical situations.

Further findings to be looked for on physical exam are signs of pulmonary hypertension and hypoxemia, such as clubbing, cyanosis, ruddy facies, loud P2, RV heave, and right heart failure (enlarged liver, distended neck veins, and peripheral edema). These advanced findings would warrant further investigation with arterial blood gases and echocardiogram.

The STOP questionnaire, developed by Chung et al. and published in the *Journal of Anesthesiology* [5], confirms our suspicion. STOP corresponds to the following questions:

1. Do you *snore* loudly (louder than talking or loud enough to be heard through closed doors)?
2. Do you often feel *tired*, fatigued, or sleepy during daytime?
3. Has anyone *observed* you stop breathing during your sleep ("Honey, you stop breathing at night")?
4. Do you have or are you being treated for high blood *pressure*?

When incorporating other factors, such as body-mass index, age, neck circumference, and gender, the STOP-Bang screen has a very high sensitivity for detecting patients who have OSA and serves as an effective screening tool.

Polysomnography (PSG) incorporates electroencephalogram monitoring, chest and abdominal pressure for respiratory effort, an electrooculogram for NREM sleep versus REM sleep, capnography for airflow determination, pulse oximetry for the detection of oxygen saturation or desaturation, and an electrocardiogram for the determination of arrhythmias. After the sleep study, all these raw data are converted into a sleep report, which confirms the presence of OSA and quantifies its severity. Benumof and colleagues reported on the interpretation of a sleep study in "The New ASA OSA Guidelines," published in 2007: "the results of a sleep study are reported as events and indices. An apnea event is no airflow for more than 10 seconds; an hypopnea event is a tidal volume less than 50% of the control awake value for more than 10 seconds; a desaturation event is a decrease in the SpO_2 greater than 4% and an arousal event can be clinical (vocalization, turning, extremity movement) or a burst on the EEG. Indices are events per hour; the apnea hypopnea index (AHI) is the number of times the patient was either apneic or hypopneic per hour; the oxygen desaturation index is the number of times the patient had a decrease in SpO_2 greater than 4% per hour and the arousal index is the number of times the patient aroused per hour. The severity of OSA is most universally expressed in terms of the apnea hypopnea index, in which 6–20 is mild, 15–40 is moderate, and >40 is severe and is scored 1, 2 and 3 respectively."

Using these data, the sleep physician will then decide whether to place the patient on therapy for OSA, which includes CPAP. CPAP has been the mainstay of treatment for patients with OSA, but it is only in severe OSA that it has been shown to have significant benefit. CPAP is administered via an oral/nasal or oronasal face mask. Surgical intervention is sometimes necessary for patients with severe OSA and patients who have OSA symptoms that are refractory to high levels of CPAP and anatomy amenable to surgical intervention.

Use the PSG results to arrive at an OSA score, and use this for clinical decision making. The score consists of the sum of two components:

Component 1: severity of OSA – 1 = mild, 2 = moderate, and 3 = severe
Component 2: the higher of the following two scores

Postop opiate need	Surgical invasiveness/anesthesia
0 = None	0 = None/local anesthesia
1 = Low dose oral	1 = Superficial/regional anesthesia
2 = High dose oral	2 = Peripheral/GA
3 = Parenteral/neuraxial	3 = Airway/major/ abdominal/GA

Practice-based learning and improvement

Residents must be able to investigate and evaluate their patient care practices, appraise and assimilate scientific evidence, and improve their patient care practices.

Analyze practice experience and perform practice-based improvement activities using a systematic methodology.

Incorporate the STOP questionnaire in preoperative screening to readily detect patients with undiagnosed OSA.

Locate, appraise, and assimilate evidence from scientific studies related to their patients' health problems.

Several studies were used in this case.

Professionalism

Residents must demonstrate a commitment to carrying out professional responsibilities, adherence to ethical principles, and sensitivity to a diverse patient population.

Demonstrate respect, compassion, and integrity; a responsiveness to the needs of patients and society that supersedes self-interest; accountability to patients, society, and the profession; and a commitment to excellence and ongoing professional development.

Inform the patient of your suspicions of undiagnosed sleep apnea and the risks both perioperatively and long term. Offer advice on how to proceed as well as evidence-based information as to the importance of following this up preoperatively.

Demonstrate a commitment to ethical principles pertaining to provision or withholding of clinical care, confidentiality of patient information, informed consent, and business practice.

Ask the patient's permission to refer him to a sleep center or suggest that the patient ask his personal physician to refer him.

Should the patient elect to defer sleep evaluation, respectful discussion of an appropriate anesthesia plan and the increased risks, including that of admission and possible postoperative ventilation, is appropriate – patients have a right to informed refusal of testing or procedures (autonomy is one of the four principles of medical ethics).

Demonstrate sensitivity and responsiveness to patients' culture, age, gender, and disabilities.

Don't threaten him with, "If you don't get your sleep apnea treated, you may get a head injury next time!"

Interpersonal and communication skills

Residents must be able to demonstrate interpersonal and communication skills that result in effective information exchange and teaming with patients, their patients' families, and professional associates.

Use effective listening skills and elicit and provide information using effective nonverbal, explanatory, questioning, and writing skills.

Document clearly your thoughts in the chart, including reason for referral, expected change in management, and the calculation of the OSA score. Also include risks and benefits discussed with the patient.

Work effectively with others as a member or leader of a health care team or other professional group.

Book this patient first case in the day of his ambulatory surgery. Send appropriate information to the sleep center, including urgency, as it is a preoperative assessment. Keep the surgeon informed of the need for further testing, possible previously unknown risks involved, and the need for change of venue or anesthesia plan.

Systems-based practice

Residents must demonstrate an awareness of and responsiveness to the larger context and system of health care and the ability to effectively call on system resources to provide care that is of optimal value.

Understand how their patient care and other professional practices affect other health care professionals, the health care organization, and the larger society and how these elements of the system affect their own practice.

OSA still remains underdiagnosed and poorly treated because of the issues with testing and treatment. Sleep studies are not readily available in all parts of the country, and CPAP can be costly, uncomfortable, and embarrassing, causing patients to discontinue therapy.

> Practice cost-effective health care and resource allocation that does not compromise quality of care.

Having this patient canceled on the day of surgery because of lack of optimization or admitted postoperatively has high economic impact on the institution, the patient, and his insurance. It may also cost the family time off work.

Remember, too, that if he were having a carpal tunnel release (CTR), a preop sleep study would not change management, except for early booking, which can be done anyway with the clinical suspicion of OSA. The maximum OSA score for CTR surgery would be 4, so it is acceptable to proceed in a free-standing ambulatory center, and the procedure is done under local anesthesia with minimal sedation. Using a sleep consult/study spot for a CTR would use up the urgent slots in the sleep clinic, making them unavailable to other patients like our Mr. Jolly, whose management depends on the severity of his OSA.

> Know how to partner with health care managers and health care providers to assess, coordinate, and improve health care and know how these activities can affect system performance.

It is not enough to just screen for OSA (or other common diseases that impact perioperative outcomes). One has to have an organized and easily negotiable referral system for these patients to get the indicated workup without extensive delays in surgery or cost to the patient or institution.

The patient did indeed have severe OSA with an apnea-hypopnea index of 37 and oxygen desaturations down to 82%. His surgery was performed early in the morning in the main operating room with interscalene block and general anesthesia. He was extubated to his CPAP machine and discharged home after an uneventful 6-hour stay in recovery.

He and his wife now sleep peacefully at night.

Additional reading

1. Chung SA, Yuan H, Chung F. A systemic review of obstructive sleep apnea and its implications for anesthesiologists. Anesth Analg 2008;107:1543–1563.

2. Benumof JL, The new ASA OSA guideline. ASA Refresher Courses in Anesthesiol 2007;35:1;1–13.

3. Gross JB, Bachenberg KL, Benumof JL, Caplan RA, et al. Practice guidelines for the perioperative management of patients with obstructive sleep apnea: a report by the American Society of Anesthesiologists Task Force on Perioperative Management of Patients with Obstructive Sleep Apnea. Anesthesiology 2006;104:1081–1093.

4. Joshi GP. Ambulatory surgery for the patient with sleep apnea syndrome. ASA Refresher Courses Anesthesiol 2007;35:97–106.

5. Chung F, Yegneswaran B, Liao P, et al. STOP questionnaire: a tool to screen obstructive sleep apnea. Anesthesiology 2008;108:812–821.

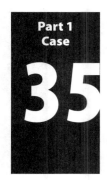

35

Contributions from Stony Brook University under Christopher J. Gallagher

Please prevent postop puking

Neera Tewari and Vedan Djesevic

The case

Mrs. B, a 52-year-old woman with a strong family history of breast cancer, underwent a workup that revealed a carcinoma of the right breast, and she is now scheduled for a right mastectomy. After seeing her chart the day before her proposed surgery, I noticed that she had no other significant medical problems. The challenge for me would be to prevent postoperative nausea and vomiting. The common thread in her surgical history was postoperative nausea and vomiting (PONV) – I was ready to face this challenge and provide this patient with a nausea-free anesthetic.

On the morning of surgery, I met Mrs. B. She was a pleasant lady with big blue eyes and curly blond hair. I immediately noticed that she was anxious and uneasy because she was constantly massaging her fingers throughout our conversation. Being a biochemist and having gone through two surgeries prior to this one, she was well aware of the risks of anesthesia and, more important, the postoperative nausea with which she was always afflicted.

Patient care

I knew I was going to have a challenge coming to work, but I didn't realize I would be facing an extensive family history of postoperative nausea and vomiting. I reassured her that I would do everything in my power to make this a vomit-free experience. It was important for me that I gain her trust right before the operation and let her know that I was well aware of her concerns and fears. Not only was she having an important surgery, but her postoperative comfort level was essential, as well.

I inquired extensively about her surgical and family history. She told me, "Doctor, I had PONV after my tonsillectomy with ether, my mother had it after her cholecystectomy with halothane, and my grandmother had it during her labor with chloroform. I want this to be the first operation without it. Please!"

I reassured Mrs. B that I would do everything in my power to decrease her chance of getting PONV again. I let her know that I would administer a volatile-free anesthetic, supplemented by a number of antiemetic medications, and minimize the use of perioperative opioids. Her anesthetic would be a total intravenous infusion of propofol, and she would get aprepitant, dexamethasone, and ondansetron perioperatively. I also let her know that I would speak with her surgeon about using local anesthetics at the surgical site to minimize narcotic use.

I explained to her my multifaceted approach to combat nausea and vomiting, but unfortunately, I couldn't guarantee it – I could only try my level best. She seemed relieved and was very happy to be included in the plan. "Usually 'they' don't explain all this," she stated.

Medical knowledge

Mrs. B was at high risk for PONV because she had multiple risk factors for postoperative nausea and vomiting. She had a history of PONV, and she was a nonsmoker and of female gender. In addition, the surgery was going to be longer than an hour, and it was breast surgery, both of which are surgical risk factors for PONV. Some of the anesthetic risk factors that contributed to her PONV in the past were use of nitrous oxide, use of volatile anesthetics, and the administration of intraoperative and postoperative opioids. I explained all these factors to her but also let her know that, on a positive note, many new antiemetic therapy regimens have been developed in recent years.

Practice-based learning and improvement

Right before we went into the operating room, I gave Mrs. B a pill called Emend (aprepitant), a new

181

neurokinin antagonist that significantly reduces postoperative nausea and vomiting at 24 hours and 48 hours after surgery. After the Emend, I gave her a good dose of benzodiazepines to calm her anxiety and worries. For her induction and maintenance of anesthesia, I decided to use propofol. I placed a laryngeal mask airway. I avoided nitrous oxide and inhalational anesthetic and minimized my intraoperative opioids. I asked Dr. S, her surgeon, to infiltrate a fair amount of local anesthetic to decrease the need for postoperative opioids. In addition, following the newest guidelines for management of postoperative nausea and vomiting, I gave Mrs. B a steroid (4 mg of dexamethasone) at the beginning of the surgery and a serotonin antagonist (4 mg of ondansetron) and an antidopaminergic drug (0.625 mg of droperidol) toward the end of the procedure. To minimize my use of opioids,

I gave Mrs. B a dose of a potent nonsteroidal anti-inflammatory drug (30 mg of ketorolac), as well.

Professionalism

It was very comforting to see Mrs. B emerge from her surgery comfortable and without any nausea or vomiting. She was pain-free and at ease. She was pleased and surprised that we were able to curb her genetic predisposition toward postop nausea. It was a rewarding day for me, knowing that I used my knowledge and professionalism to combat one of the oldest complications postsurgery.

Note in this case how we "cut to the chase" on four of the six core clinical competencies. By now (you've gone through 38 cases), you should be "thinking competencies" and be able to do this yourself.

Additional reading

1. Gan TJ, Meyer T, Apfel C, et al. Society for Ambulatory Anesthesia guidelines for the management of postoperative nausea and vomiting. Anesth Analg 2007;105:1615–1628.

2. Diemunsch P, Gan TJ, Philip BK, et al. Single-dose aprepitant vs ondansetron for the prevention of postoperative nausea and vomiting: a randomized, double-blind phase III trial in patients undergoing open abdominal surgery. Br J Anaesth 2007;99:202–211.

**Part 1
Case**

36

Contributions from Stony Brook University under Christopher J. Gallagher

Mr. Whipple and the case of the guy who likes to mix a few vikes with his vodka

Misako Sakamaki and Brian Durkin

The case

You are consulted the week before surgery by the surgical oncologist about "another one" coming for surgery for pancreatic cancer. You remember fondly the "last one," who drove everyone crazy, from the preoperative admission area nurses to the guy who held open the hospital door as he left for home and let it slam him in the rear. He had his big life-saving cancer surgery and was lucky to get out of the hospital alive – and that meant that someone had to keep the staff from killing him. This is the dreaded narcotic user and abuser who will tax your professionalism to the nth degree. You remember those days back in high school, when they showed those black-and-white movies about people who fell ill to the needle? Today, they don't dress as nice, may actually not use a needle, and may actually get their opioids from the same guy who gives you a flu shot. They live among us, and yes, they are often your patient.

The Whipple procedure (did Dr. Whipple succumb to pancreatic cancer? I think he did) is a long, tedious operation performed occasionally at your institution by a surgeon who likes to "keep the patient dry." "Don't follow those 'rules' you usually follow. Urine output is not that important. I don't want them to bleed too much." These are the words of this surgical oncologist, who also doesn't want you to use local anesthetic in the epidural for the first 24 hours postoperatively.

What are you to do for this patient? Can his postoperative pain be effectively managed?

Patient care

Residents must be able to provide patient care that is compassionate, appropriate, and effective for the treatment of health problems and the promotion of health.

Communicate effectively and demonstrate caring and respectful behaviors when interacting with patients and their families.

So it seems like this patient is one of those that leads you to say, "Is that him? Oh, no! Here he comes again … what do I do now?" When taking care of a so-called challenging patient like this one, it is particularly important to establish a good doctor-patient relationship. Gaining trust from a patient like this would be a first major step toward effective patient care (and will also make your perioperative life a little easier). After all, this patient has a cancer that is threatening his life, and now he has to undergo major surgery. He is most likely scared, anxious, and emotionally devastated. Be compassionate – he needs your help!

Gather essential and accurate information about their patients.

After establishing a good rapport with the patient, now it's time to get to know him. All we now know is that he has a major cancer and is a longtime narcotic user (is he really an "abuser"?). We need to know in detail about his other medical issues, cancer history (stage and prognosis), and pain management history. Is this patient a real narcotic abuser/seeker, or is he a pseudo-abuser – he may be not addicted, but actually undertreated (because his doctors are negatively biased against him and are denying adequate opioid coverage), and he is only seeking adequate pain relief. Talk to the patient and also contact his personal medical doctor, oncologist, and pain management specialist to get a full picture of this patient before you come up with an effective anesthetic plan.

We also need to know if he has any toxic habits: a patient with substance use disorders to alcohol, marijuana, or nicotine will show a higher incidence of dependence on other substances than the general population. In fact, nearly 70% of opioid addicts in the United States are dependent on either cocaine or other habituating substances. Opioid-dependent patients with superimposed cocaine dependence may present additional problems for us, including hemodynamic instability and extreme emotional lability.

Make informed decisions about diagnostic and therapeutic interventions based on patient information and preferences, up-to-date scientific evidence, and clinical judgment.

Assuming that this patient has no other medical issues, the main concern for him and his anesthesiologist is how to establish effective perioperative pain management. A patient like this usually has a very high tolerance to opioids, and he would not only require a very high dose of narcotics perioperatively, but may not even adequately respond to narcotics without significant unwanted side effects. I would talk to this patient about the use of neuraxial analgesia (thoracic epidural) for effective perioperative pain control. Discuss with the patient what the alternative option is (intravenous patient controlled analgesia) and explain the risks and benefits of each option. Make sure the patient has no contraindication to neuraxial anesthesia.

Develop and carry out patient management plans.

The plan is general anesthesia plus epidural anesthesia/analgesia and the use of a multimodal analgesia for the best perioperative course.

If there is no contraindication and the patient consents (and you *really* hope he does!), I would place a thoracic epidural catheter in this patient preoperatively. I would then dose his epidural catheter with local anesthetics prior to surgical incision. If the patient has not taken his usual dose of oral opioid on the morning of surgery, I would also administer the equivalent dose of opioid at the beginning of surgery.

Use multimodal/balanced analgesia: pain is mediated by various mechanisms; therefore, in addition to narcotics, we should be using different drugs targeting distinct mechanisms, for example, anti-inflammatories (nonsteroidal anti-inflammatory drugs, cyclooxygenase-2 inhibitor), N-methyl d-aspartate receptor antagonists (low-dose ketamine), and alpha-adrenergic mediated analgesias (clonidine).

Use information technology to support patient care decisions and patient education.

Even though there are no bibles or official guidelines for acute pain management in opioid-dependent patients, numerous clinical studies have been done, and there seems to be general consensus among the experts. Use evidence-based medicine.

Perform competently all medical and invasive procedures considered essential for the area of practice.

Place adequate intravenous access, a thoracic epidural catheter (without making a wet tap!), and an arterial line and secure the airway appropriately.

Work with health care professionals, including those from other disciplines, to provide patient-focused care.

Involve the surgeon, the pain management specialist, the oncologist, and possibly a psychiatrist prior to the patient's surgery to come up with the most effective plan. For example, talk to the surgeon preop and explain to him or her how important it would be to use epidural analgesia/anesthesia intraoperatively. We understand that surgeons are concerned with the possible hemodynamic changes associated with epidural sympathetectomy during the case. Discuss with the surgeons the risks and benefits of using an epidural catheter during the case. If hemodynamics are an issue, we can always administer narcotics without local anesthetic during the case.

Medical knowledge

Residents must demonstrate knowledge about established and evolving biomedical, clinical, and cognate (e.g., epidemiological and social-behavioral) sciences and the application of this knowledge to patient care.

Know and apply the basic and clinically supportive sciences that are appropriate to their discipline.

This is an opioid-dependent patient who is coming for a major abdominal surgery. First, adequate perioperative pain control is important, and not only for the patient's comfort – it would also affect the postop course: uncontrolled pain would place a patient at higher risk for postop cardiopulmonary complication and might prolong the patient's hospitalization.

While this patient would certainly require a much higher dose of narcotics perioperatively, this does not mean you just load him with buckets of intravenous narcotics. Narcotics have dose-dependent detrimental side effects such as nausea and vomiting, respiratory depression, and decreased gastrointestinal (GI) motility. This patient is undergoing major abdominal surgery – the use of mega-dose intravenous narcotics would slow down his GI recovery. Also, use of high-dose narcotics can induce opioid-induced hyperalgesia.

Neuraxial administration of opioids offers a more efficient method of providing postop analgesia than parental or oral opioids. Epidural doses of morphine are roughly 10 times more efficacious than the same dose of morphine given parentally. Therefore significantly greater levels of analgesia can be delivered to those patients recovering from more extensive procedures where postop parental opioid doses would be expected to be very high.

Use of neuraxial analgesia/anesthesia has also been shown to be beneficial for cancer-related surgery by decreasing the incidence of cancer recurrence. This is believed to be due to suppression of the stress response.

Nonopioid analgesic adjuvants may also be used to reduce opioid dose requirements and provide multimodal analgesia. Nonopioid analgesics include anti-inflammatory drugs, low-dose ketamine (0.5 mg/kg), and alpha-adrenergic-mediated analgesia (clonidine).

Practice-based learning and improvement

Residents must be able to investigate and evaluate their patient care practices, appraise and assimilate scientific evidence, and improve their patient care practices.

Locate, appraise, and assimilate evidence from scientific studies related to their patients' health problems.

There have been only a small number of published reviews that address the treatment of acute pain in patients with substance abuse disorders, and fewer have focused specifically on perioperative pain management in opioid-dependent patients.

Professionalism

Residents must demonstrate a commitment to carrying out professional responsibilities, adherence to ethical principles, and sensitivity to a diverse patient population.

Demonstrate respect, compassion, and integrity; a responsiveness to the needs of patients and society that supersedes self-interest; accountability to patients, society, and the profession; and a commitment to excellence and ongoing professional development.

Respect the patient and be compassionate. Your patient might be a drug addict, but he is your patient, and he needs professional help from you. He deserves the best care, just like any other patient.

Demonstrate a commitment to ethical principles pertaining to provision or withholding of clinical care, confidentiality of patient information, informed consent, and business practice.

Make sure the patient has informed consent. This means that the patient should have an understanding of the risks and benefits of each therapeutic option and alternative. Follow health insurance portability and accountability regulations for patient confidentiality. When filling out your billing forms, be ethical – bill only what you did.

Demonstrate sensitivity and responsiveness to patients' culture, age, gender, and disabilities.

Talk to the patient and try to understand why he is doing what he is doing – why is he taking so much pain medication? What is his understanding of his illness, and how is it affecting him physically, emotionally, and socially?

Interpersonal and communication skills

Residents must be able to demonstrate interpersonal and communication skills that result in effective information exchange and teaming with patients, their patients' families, and professional associates.

Create and sustain a therapeutic and ethically sound relationship with patients.

Always address patients by name (not just, "Hi, sir"), introduce yourself, shake hands, look professional (no coffee-stained coat!), and give the patient your undivided attention.

Use effective listening skills and elicit and provide information using effective nonverbal, explanatory, questioning, and writing skills.

To establish effective anesthetic and perioperative plans, we need to know the patient in full picture. We need to get the information we need so that we can provide the best care for the patient. Ask proper questions and listen to what the patient says. Some patients don't know the direct answers to your questions, but they may give you clues.

Practice cost-effective health care and resource allocation that does not compromise quality of care.

Good patient care ultimately leads to cost-effective health care. In this case, effective perioperative pain management would reduce the length of postanesthesia care unit time, fasten postsurgical recovery, and thereby minimize the length of intensive care unit stay.

Additional reading

1. Mitra S, Sinatra R . Perioperative management of acute pain in the opioid-dependent patient. Anesthesiology 2004;101:212–225.

Part 2

Contributions from the University of Medicine and Dentistry of New Jersey under Steven H. Ginsberg

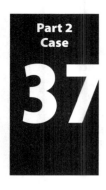

37

Burn, baby, burn
Anesthesia inferno

Jeremy Grayson and Stephen Lemke

The case

It was pediatric ear-nose-throat (ENT) day, and my first case was a 6-year-old girl with obstructive sleep apnea for tonsillectomy and adenoidectomy. While I was setting up the room, "Disco Inferno" was playing on the radio, and I struggled to contain my urge to dance. After greeting my patient and her family in the holding area and taking a thorough history and physical, we proceeded to the operating room. Following a boring mask induction with oxygen, nitrous oxide, and sevoflurane, Mom gave her munchkin a kiss and was escorted back to holding. We intubated using a 5.5-mm uncuffed endotracheal tube, confirmed proper placement, and auscultated a leak over the trachea at 20 cm of water. "Music, please!" exclaimed the surgeon. I dialed up isoflurane in a 50-50 mixture of oxygen and nitrous oxide and sang along – "We didn't start the fire; it was always burning since the world was turning" – and before I knew it, the first tonsil was out. Suddenly, there was a loud pop, and my patient's mouth looked like the Fourth of July.

Patient care

Residents must be able to provide patient care that is compassionate, appropriate, and effective for the treatment of health problems and the promotion of health.

Communicate effectively and demonstrate caring and respectful behaviors when interacting with patients and their families.

Establishing good rapport is critical, especially for pediatric anesthesia. Goal number one: get Mom and Dad to confidently put their child's life in my hands. I'm keenly aware of this fact as I approach the patient and her family. Right now, my attending is still yawning and wiping the crust from his eyes. It's my time to shine. I got a good night's sleep, shaved, and even brushed my teeth. I smile as I enter the room and confidently shake both parents' hands while introducing

myself. I take a thorough history, keeping in mind that not everyone is a doctor. I limit the amount of medical jargon but also don't dumb it down too much, as either extreme can be offensive. Based on the conversation, I adjust my vocabulary accordingly. Goal number two: try not to freak out the little girl. This can be a challenging task, to say the least. I blew up a latex glove, adorned it with a smiley face, and let her play with it as I washed my hands. I sat down on the bed next to her and put my stethoscope on her stuffed giraffe. Then I let her listen. "Decreased breath sounds on the right," she said (OK, maybe she didn't). Finally, making sure my stethoscope was nice and warm, I listened to her heart and lungs. By the time my attending showed up, the patient was happily playing with her glove, and the parents were pretty sure we weren't going to kill their daughter. Mom's happy, Dad's happy, and the patient is happy...mission accomplished.

Gather essential and accurate information about their patients.

So far, it may seem as though I have accomplished nothing. Not true, my friend. I blew up a balloon and played with a stuffed animal. I also carefully gathered all the information needed to plan my anesthetic. She – let's just call her Suzie, so I can stop saying "she" – is 6 years old, weighs 20 kg, was a full-term vaginal delivery; Suzie has no medical problems or recent illnesses, has never had surgery, and has no family history of problems with anesthesia. I also found out that Suzie snores like a 747 and has been sleepy and daydreaming at school, which, according to Mom, is why she needs a tonsillectomy. On physical exam, I noted no obvious anatomic abnormalities other than two big, meatball-sized, grade +4 kissing tonsils.

Make informed decisions about diagnostic and therapeutic interventions based on patient information and preferences, up-to-date scientific evidence, and clinical judgment.

It sounds like Suzie has obstructive sleep apnea, so I peruse the chart to look for a sleep study. Indeed, polysomnography confirms the diagnosis. Since I'm a stellar resident (just ask me), my attending assumes that I've read the most recent American Society of Anesthesiologists guidelines pertaining to perioperative management of obstructive sleep apnea and congratulates me for not heavily sedating the kid, predisposing her to airway obstruction and apnea in the holding area. I smile and nod, and whisper to the nurse, "Cancel the Versed" as he walks away. Just kidding, I didn't order Versed; the great rapport I established with Mom, Dad, and Suzie will be premedication enough. I did, however, read all about tonsillectomy and adenoidectomy and was well prepared for the case. I also read about airway fire, although it is rarely seen with this particular surgery. I know that it requires three components: ignition (such as an electrocautery device), fuel (tonsillar tissue, gauze, etc.), and an oxidizing agent (oxygen or nitrous oxide).

Develop and carry out patient management plans.

Although I hadn't planned on setting my patient ablaze or losing my composure, both happened in that order. The fire abated as quickly as it started, and the surgeon pulled out the electrocautery device with a hunk of flaming tonsillar tissue. I immediately stopped fresh gas flow by disconnecting the breathing circuit, extubated, then reintubated with a size 5 cuffed tube. Together with the ENT surgeon, we surveyed the damage. Although the pharyngeal mucosa was clearly *en fuego*, the patient was hemodynamically stable and the airway was secure, so the surgery was completed. Postop, even with the cuff deflated, there was no audible leak. I obviously couldn't extubate. Suzie was transferred to the prenatal intensive care unit (PICU) for further care.

Counsel and educate patients and their families.

Before the surgery, Mom and Dad wanted to know why Suzie couldn't eat breakfast and were also concerned about anesthesia awareness. I explained the naught per oris guidelines and how pancakes are bad for the lungs. I assured them that I would carefully monitor her vital signs and use a bispectral index monitor. After the surgery, we had a lot of explaining to do. Along with the surgeon, my attending and I discussed the day's events with the parents. We explained why Suzie was still sedated and intubated and promised them that we would take the tube out once the swelling subsided to the point that there was a leak around the endotracheal tube.

Use information technology to support patient care decisions and patient education.

When my attending was a resident, around the time Lincoln was shot, people didn't have tonsils, let alone the Internet. The night before the case, I did a literature search to look up the latest tonsil gossip and, of course, check out what was going on with Britney Spears. Just before fire erupted, I could've been surfing the Web on my phone.

Perform competently all medical and invasive procedures considered essential for the area of practice.

I had all necessary, and potentially necessary, equipment ready to go. This means a proper laryngoscope blade, endotracheal tube, breathing circuit, and bag. All medications were drawn up according to Suzie's weight, with a 21-gauge needle on those that could be injected intramuscularly. I also looked up which drugs could be given through the endotracheal tube. I calculated her fluid requirements, checked the monitors and equipment, put the IV in a vein and the endotracheal tube in the trachea – twice – and demonstrated how to deal with an airway fire. I believe I performed all procedures competently, although I'm slightly biased.

Provide health care services aimed at preventing health problems or maintaining health.

As a general rule, I try not to set my patients on fire. Besides that, I give antibiotics when appropriate, wash my hands, use clean equipment, and keep my patient warm (I'll admit, usually not this warm). Lighting the kid on fire segues perfectly with trying to get Dad to quit smoking. I'm pretty sure I shouldn't bring this up now, but the health impacts of secondhand (and even thirdhand, as I just learned on my iPhone) smoke on kids are well documented, and this subject should be broached prior to her leaving the hospital.

Work with health care professionals, including those from other disciplines, to provide patient-focused care.

Any case in which we share the airway with surgery demands complete collaboration. Once a fire occurs, we must decide together whether it's safe to continue the case and also how to manage Suzie postoperatively. After agreeing to keep her intubated and sending her to the PICU, I remained involved with her care. With surgery, nursing, and respiratory therapy present, I spoke about the implications of the airway fire to make sure we were all on the same page.

Medical knowledge

Residents must demonstrate knowledge about established and evolving biomedical, clinical, and cognate (e.g., epidemiological and social-behavioral) sciences and the application of this knowledge to patient care.

> Demonstrate an investigatory and analytic thinking approach to clinical situations.

What could've happened here? As I mentioned previously, three components must be present for fire to occur: fuel, an ignition source, and an oxidizing agent. Although I had no control over the first two, I could've limited my FiO_2 and turned off the nitrous oxide after induction. Apparently, the oxygen index of flammability, or the percentage required to support combustion, is between 25% and 30%. I auscultated a cuff leak over the trachea at 20 cm of water. Last night, I read in an article by Mattucci and Militana [4] that with a cuff leak of less than 12, the pharyngeal concentrations of nitrous oxide and oxygen are equal to that of the inspired mixture. If the leak is greater than 12, the pharyngeal gas concentration equals that of room air. In other words, with a cuff leak of 20, it's unlikely that this could be the culprit. What I neglected to do is recheck for a leak after the ENT surgeon put in the mouth gag and repositioned the head. This, too, can increase the leak.

I also knew not to extubate her at the end of the case without a leak around the endotracheal tube. Now pay attention: in a child, the narrowest portion of the funnel-shaped airway is at the cricoid cartilage, and the lack of a leak meant that on extubation, her airway could close up or get really, really narrow where the tube was once stenting it open. Airway swelling is worse in children as every millimeter of swelling, in an already narrow airway, increases resistance, and this resistance is inversely proportional to the radius of the lumen to the fourth power for laminar flow and to the radius of the lumen to the fifth power for turbulent flow. How's that for droppin' some knowledge!

> Know and apply the basic and clinically supportive sciences that are appropriate to their discipline.

Being familiar with the anatomy of the pediatric airway is very important for this case. In kids, again, the narrowest part of the airway is at the cricoid cartilage. For this reason, endotracheal tube sizing is critically important. Too large a leak may make ventilation difficult and put everyone in the operating room to sleep. Too small a leak can place the child at risk for postextubation stridor. Classic teaching is to refrain from using cuffed endotracheal tubes in kids less than 8 or 9 years old. However, I read a study that found no difference in the incidence of long-term sequelae or postextubation stridor in PICU patients with cuffed versus uncuffed tubes. Instead, the author believes the occurrence of mucosal edema to be more closely related to using too large a tube or having a long surgery. In light of this, I reintubated with a cuffed endotracheal tube, trying to create a less combustible surgical environment equivalent to room air.

Practice-based learning and improvement

Residents must be able to investigate and evaluate their patient care practices, appraise and assimilate scientific evidence, and improve their patient care practices.

> Analyze practice experience and perform practice-based improvement activities using a systematic methodology.

At this point in my residency, I've done roughly 30 tonsillectomies and was beginning to feel pretty cozy. Although I've never said "in my vast experience" or "in my practice" to my attending, I have indeed begun to cultivate my own style. I have seen all too often the emergence delirium that can be caused by maintenance with sevoflurane. Last time I gave too much narcotic, this time I roasted my patient. Without a doubt, the traumatic events of today are forever burned into memory and will affect my practice tomorrow. Just when I thought I couldn't be any more of an obsessive-compulsive control freak, so that others may learn vicariously through me, we hosted an interdepartmental meeting involving anesthesia, ENT, operating room staff, and PICU staff to discuss the case. It was hoped that this would facilitate safer care in the future.

> Locate, appraise, and assimilate evidence from scientific studies related to their patients' health problems.

In my reading, I found that there are two main reasons for doing a tonsillectomy in a child: chronic pharyngitis and obstructive sleep apnea. Knowing how both conditions can affect anesthetic management is crucial. If Suzie's obstructive sleep apnea was associated with other comorbid conditions or syndromes, I would've used information technology to ensure that I was prepared to deal with those issues. After the case, I changed my pants and did a literature search to see how others have dealt with this issue. I was delighted that I remembered to stop fresh gas flow, disconnect the circuit, extubate, and then reintubate.

> Obtain and use information about their own population of patients and the larger population from which their patients are drawn.

"In my vast experience" with tonsillectomies, I have cared primarily for ASA-I and -II patients and, occasionally, a child with Down's syndrome. We are very fortunate in that we treat a very ethnically diverse group of patients. As you might expect, many kids with obstructive sleep apnea are obese. This is the perfect opportunity to educate parents about the benefits of healthy eating, exercise, and weight loss.

> Apply knowledge of study designs and statistical methods to the appraisal of clinical studies and other information on diagnostic and therapeutic effectiveness.

I have to be honest, whenever I hear terms like *Kruskal-Wallis test* or *chi squared*, I vomit a little into my mouth. Well, get your ondansetron, because in the age of the six Core Clinical Competencies and evidence-based medicine, understanding basic statistical analysis is a must for truly being able to interpret journal articles and studies. Speaking of vomiting, in my literature search, I found that prevention of postoperative nausea and vomiting is key for tonsillectomies.

> Use information technology to manage information, access online medical information, and support their own education.

My dad is a highly intelligent man but can barely use a cell phone. He despises technology. Being a "millennial resident," I've acknowledged technological advances as my friend. Playing Tiger Woods's golf in the operating room is just bad form, but being able to access the seemingly infinite resources on the Web has revolutionized medicine.

(*First author's note*: Tiger Woods golf may be losing some popularity for other reasons, as well).

Professionalism

Residents must demonstrate a commitment to carrying out professional responsibilities, adherence to ethical principles, and sensitivity to a diverse patient population.

> Demonstrate respect, compassion, and integrity; a responsiveness to the needs of patients and society that supersedes self-interest; accountability to patients, society, and the profession; and a commitment to excellence and ongoing professional development.

We should always be cognizant of this. Before seeing the patient, I remembered that asking the nurse if my patient was a FLK (funny-looking kid, for those of you not hip to the lingo) is unprofessional. I also tried not to ignore Suzie during the initial encounter or tell her to suck it up when she started crying on the operating room table. When the Bovie exploded, I didn't tell the surgeon that his mistake was going to cost me my 12:00 tee time at Beth Page Black or that it would take me a couple months to get back there. I did my best to deal with the situation in a respectful manner, realizing that I'm a patient advocate as well as part of the perioperative team. Later, I reported the event to the anesthesia quality assurance committee so that we could review the case at our next meeting and also make it the topic of an upcoming multidisciplinary conference.

> Demonstrate a commitment to ethical principles pertaining to provision or withholding of clinical care, confidentiality of patient information, informed consent, and business practice.

While flipping through the chart, I noticed that this patient was self pay. However, I did not walk out of the holding area and tell the medical student to "take care of this one; apparently it's on the house!" or announce it to everyone, infuriating the Joint

Commission for Accreditation of Hospitals. I didn't replace my sevoflurane vaporizer with enflurane or use cheaper drugs because of the patient's socioeconomic status. I've already taken my cultural competency classes for the year and know this would not be ethical. After the case, I explained to the parents what happened and helped them understand why Suzie would remain intubated until the airway edema resolved.

Demonstrate sensitivity and responsiveness to patients' culture, age, gender, and disabilities.

Again, I took my cultural competence classes for the year, so I know that if the family only spoke Spanish, for example, it would be inappropriate to communicate without an interpreter. I also know that using the patient's 14-year-old brother as the interpreter is inappropriate. Our hospital has official translators on staff to provide that service, and if, for some reason, the only Icelander is not available to translate for young Björk and her mom because she's back in Reykjavik on holiday, I know that the telephone interpreter is available 24/7/365!

Interpersonal and communication skills

Residents must be able to demonstrate interpersonal and communication skills that result in effective information exchange and teaming with patients, their patients' families, and professional associates.

Create and sustain a therapeutic and ethically sound relationship with patients.

Before meeting Suzie and her parents the morning of surgery, I stopped by the bathroom and made sure I looked as professional as possible. I didn't want to walk in looking like I spent the night sleeping on 42nd Street, hair tussled and smelling like a distillery. Nothing instills fear in a parent like a hungover, dirty resident.

Use effective listening skills and elicit and provide information using effective nonverbal, explanatory, questioning, and writing skills.

When speaking with my patient and her family, I purposely made eye contact with Suzie and both parents. To show them that my head was in the game,

I nodded compassionately when they spoke. When Mom asked me how the anesthesia works and how I know how much to give, I didn't reply, "Why, are you some sort of amateur pharmacologist who spent last night huffing butane out of a brown paper bag?" I gave a basic explanation and was prepared to tailor the discussion based on verbal and nonverbal cues, being mindful not to scare little Suzie. Aside from taking a detailed history and physical, I also wrote a legible, full account of the airway explosion, including how it was dealt with and the rationale for keeping Suzie intubated until the swelling resolved.

Work effectively with others as a member or leader of a health care team or other professional group.

When fire broke out, I had to act decisively, with confidence and without hesitation. I knew it was my job to stop gas flow, disconnect the breathing circuit, extubate, and resecure the airway. Along with the surgeon, my attending and I surveyed the damage and made a joint decision to continue with the case. Later, I called the pediatric intensivist to give a detailed report of the transpired events and to ensure that a bed would be ready for Suzie. Continuity of care was further established as my attending and I transported her to the PICU and gave report to all residents, fellows, nurses, and respiratory personnel who would be involved. Finally, I visited her on a daily basis until discharge so that I could see the effects of my care beyond the operating room.

Systems-based practice

Residents must demonstrate an awareness of and responsiveness to the larger context and system of health care and the ability to effectively call on system resources to provide care that is of optimal value.

Understand how their patient care and other professional practices affect other health care professionals, the health care organization, and the larger society and how these elements of the system affect their own practice.

This is one reason I visited Suzie postoperatively. Not only did I have a vested interest in her health, but I was also interested to see how the PICU team would manage her care. I learned that although airway fire is a rare complication, it has serious effects, not just for the health of our patient, but also for the entire system. This unplanned admission was expensive and consumed many valuable resources. Complications directly, and indirectly, contribute to the ever escalating cost of health care and insurance.

Practice cost-effective health care and resource allocation that does not compromise quality of care.

Giving a cost-conscious anesthetic should always be a consideration, as long as care is not compromised as a result. I try never to draw up unnecessary drugs, and if possible, I try to use a generic version, as long as its efficacy and safety are proven. Using low flows of oxygen and nitrous oxide is a great way to conserve inhaled anesthetic. Especially for this case, giving prophylactic antiemetics can decrease the likelihood of postoperative nausea and vomiting and potential issues with hemostasis (which could lead to the dreaded postoperative tonsillectomy bleed, the management of which I have read about in many other texts), which may accompany vomiting. As we all know, intractable nausea and vomiting is a major cause for unplanned hospital admission.

Advocate for quality patient care and assist patients in dealing with system complexities.

For the anesthesia team, our role with respect to this competency is to talk to parents about the unforeseen electrocautery explosion as well as the unplanned, yet necessary, overnight intubation and to educate them about what to expect during Suzie's hospital stay.

Know how to partner with health care managers and health care providers to assess, coordinate, and improve health care and know how these activities can affect system performance.

As mentioned earlier, notifying the PICU team about a surprise admission to their service is the first step in transferring care. In addition, social workers should be available to assist Mom and Dad with their needs, including logistical and psychological support, during this unforeseen stressful time.

Additional reading

1. American Society of Anesthesiologists. Welcome! 2009. Available from: http://www.asahq.org/publicationsAndServices/sleepapnea103105.pdf.

2. Barash PG, Cullen BF, Stoelting RK. Clinical anesthesia. 5th ed. Philadelphia: Lippincott Williams & Wilkins; 2006.

3. Cote CJ, Todres ID, Lerman J. A practice of anesthesia for infants and children: expert consult. New York: Elsevier Health Sciences; 2008.

4. Mattucci KF, Militana CJ. The prevention of fire during oropharyngeal electrosurgery. Ear Nose Throat J 2003;82:107–109.

5. Roland KN, Chidiac EJ, Zestos MM, Ahmed Z. Electrocautery-induced fire during adenotonsillectomy: report of two cases. J Clin Anesth 2006;18:129–131.

Contributions from the University of Medicine and Dentistry of New Jersey under Steven H. Ginsberg

CABG

John Denny and Salvatore Zisa Jr.

The case

A 62-year-old male is admitted for coronary artery bypass grafting (CABG). His history is significant for stable angina, hypertension (HTN), hyperlipidemia, and type II diabetes. He reports, "My sugar got out of control. I used to take the pills but now I take the shots."

After an uncomplicated three-vessel CABG, you breathe a sigh of relief as the blood pressure (BP) stabilizes at 105/60. The surgeon asks you to give the protamine, and you humbly comply. As you begin to tidy up your lines, you glance up at the monitor and notice that the BP is now 60/30 and shows no signs of going up. Another 30 seconds pass, and the BP is still heading down. You also notice that the peak inspiratory pressure on your ventilator has jumped from 25 to 50! *Help!*

Patient care

Residents must be able to provide patient care that is compassionate, appropriate, and effective for the treatment of health problems and the promotion of health.

Communicate effectively and demonstrate caring and respectful behaviors when interacting with patients and their families.

Although at this point, the best way to demonstrate caring and respect is to quickly diagnose and treat the problem at hand; you did meet the patient the night before surgery and discussed the anesthetic plan with him. He is a simple man, with whom you sat for 20 minutes and answered all his questions about anesthesia and "incubation." You respectfully and politely explained that he will remain intubated for some time after the operation immediately postop. After explaining everything in simple terms, the patient and family felt comforted by your visit.

Gather essential and accurate information about their patients.

This is no time for a chart review and a rectal exam. We must figure out what is going on *now* and act immediately if we are to beat back the grim reaper on this case. You take a quick glance at the field to make sure the surgeon has not poked a hole in the aorta or the PA, or any blood-containing chamber, for that matter. No blood pouring from the chest! Your transducers are zeroed, and all your equipment is working. You quickly recall from your diligent preoperative evaluation that this patient has been on NPH insulin, and you just gave protamine!

Make informed decisions about diagnostic and therapeutic interventions based on patient information and preferences, up-to-date scientific evidence, and clinical judgment.

You quickly surmise that this must be a protamine reaction. After all, you have been reading the literature and recall that there is approximately an 8- to 10-fold increased risk of a major protamine reaction in patients receiving NPH insulin. Your clinical judgment says act now, or the patient will forever rest in peace. You make an informed decision based on the MAP of 40 that it is time to undertake a therapeutic intervention.

Develop and carry out patient management plans.

Systemic hypotension within 10 minutes of giving protamine suggests protamine as the cause. Specific therapy depends on associated hemodynamic events. If simply due to rapid administration, BP will usually respond to giving volume.

Complete vascular collapse due to anaphylaxis can only occur with previous exposure to protamine. Bronchospasm usually coexists. Stop protamine, if not already given. Discontinue anesthetic agents and ventilate with 100% FiO_2. EPI, EPI, where art thou – my epinephrine, that is. Contractility and systemic vascular resistance (SVR) have suffered, so reach for the big guns. Reassess and reassess after each intervention, but don't lose your cool – the next few seconds can be life or death. If rapid volume administration and epinephrine are not corrective, prompt, full reheparinization and going back on bypass are necessary. Subsequently, add H1 and H2 blockers, bronchodilators, and steroids.

Normal pulmonary artery pressures with low BP suggest either that protamine was given too quickly or that an anaphylactoid reaction occurred. Anaphylactoid reactions are nonimmunologic and thus do *not* require previous exposure to the antigen. IgG antibodies to protamine and the heparin-protamine complexes can activate the *complement* system and generate fragments called *anaphylatoxins*. The complement activation generates thromboxane, causing acute pulmonary vasoconstriction. These complement-mediated reactions can range from a little fall in BP to severe pulmonary vasoconstriction, acute RV failure, and cardiovascular collapse. The RV obstruction produces a systemic fall in BP, requiring inotropic support. Inotropes, such as milrinone, will support the failing RV, while facilitating flow across the pulmonary vasculature. Systemic hypotension can be a problematic side effect requiring pressors. Nitric oxide can be useful. With severe hemodynamic deterioration, unresponsive to more conservative measures, full reheparinization and return to cardiopulmonary bypass (CPB) may be necessary.

Counsel and educate patients and their families.

This patient needs to be told of his life-threatening reaction and requires outpatient follow-up with an allergist and possibly skin testing. This can be done during the postoperative visit, as part of our perioperative physician model of delivering care.

Use information technology to support patient care decisions and patient education.

You review the preoperative catheterization, electrocardiogram, labs, and echo, if available. This is valuable information that can paint a picture for you as to how frail or robust the patient is and should not be overlooked. The hospital intranet and the Web can offer valuable access to medical information. Of particular relevance to cardiac surgery are echocardiography Web sites.

Perform competently all medical and invasive procedures considered essential for the area of practice.

Cardiac surgery and big lines go hand in hand. Establish large-bore intravenous access, an arterial line, and an introducer in a central vein to start. Secure the airway. Do the transesophageal echo exam, maintain the patient, and transition to CPB. Technical skill and attention to detail are essential to ensure a good outcome. When the resident does many invasive procedures during residency, the Residency Review Committee will become happier and happier with the resident's core competency in procedures.

Provide health care services aimed at preventing health problems or maintaining health.

At this point, the only thing we need to prevent is the patient's death. However, you did remember to give the antibiotics prior to skin incision, right? Those sternal wound infections can be nasty. Furthermore, future hospital (and physician) reimbursement will be penalized when so-called preventable surgical wound infections occur.

Work with health care professionals, including those from other disciplines, to provide patient-focused care.

Right now, this patient's survival will require 100% focus and effort on the part of the entire operating room team. Anesthesia, perfusion, and the surgeon will interact and react to each other's coordinated efforts to try to bring this crisis under control. Part of residency training is learning to resolve the inevitable differences of opinion that will occur in such a crisis, without unfavorably impacting patient care. If only the Core Clinical Competency writers could see us now – they would be so proud.

Medical knowledge

Residents must demonstrate knowledge about established and evolving biomedical, clinical, and cognate (e.g., epidemiological and social-behavioral) sciences and the application of this knowledge to patient care.

Demonstrate an investigatory and analytic thinking approach to clinical situations.

Hmmm, let's think this through. The blood pressure tanked soon after giving an exogenous polypeptide. A quick survey to rule out other causes like bleeding or an equipment malfunction turned up empty (don't forget to make sure your transducers are zeroed). Could it be air shot down a coronary? This certainly can cause ventricular dysfunction but is usually limited to the distribution of the affected vessel, not like the global insult we are seeing here. The temporal relation to the administration of a medication, the dramatic change in the patient's condition, and the knowledge of prior exposure to the substance seals the deal. We must be dealing with an anaphylactic reaction.

Perhaps the most important analysis one can make here is to recognize this as anaphylaxis. If a return to CPB was necessary, it would have required more heparin. As indicated earlier, you now must decide whether the risk of further protamine administration, and the risk of repeating this scenario, outweighs spontaneous resolution of the effects of heparin and its associated increased risk of bleeding. If this is truly anaphylaxis, the latter may be justified. Round two of protamine versus heart may be the fatal knockout blow.

Know and apply the basic and clinically supportive sciences that are appropriate to their discipline.

It's a good thing you didn't fall asleep during that endocrine lecture in medical school as you recalled that the *P* in NPH stands for protamine (neutral protamine hagedorn). The protamine is complexed with regular insulin so that when it is injected subcutaneously, it slows absorption, giving you intermediate-acting insulin. You remember this well because you were kind of grossed out to learn that protamine is actually made from salmon testes! Your extensive basic science training taught you all about how prior exposure to these proteins forms antiprotamine IgE, just waiting for you to come along and give some protamine and set off an immunological firestorm.

Practice-based learning and improvement

Residents must be able to investigate and evaluate their patient care practices, appraise and assimilate scientific evidence, and improve their patient care practices.

Analyze practice experience and perform practice-based improvement activities using a systematic methodology.

Analyzing our practice experience begs the question, could things be done differently to avoid such occurrences in the future? Is this a common occurrence, or was this an idiosyncratic reaction limited to this patient? At the end of the day, do you leave the hospital saying, "Well, that was interesting," and return the next day as if it never happened? Not if we are following our clinical competencies. Look at these issues as they occur in your practice systematically, and review the published data to avoid the morbidity and potential mortality from reoccurring.

Should patients at increased risk be pretested by an allergist or premedicated to reduce the likelihood of a catastrophic reaction? Only patients with a prior history of an adverse response to protamine merit special treatment.

Locate, appraise, and assimilate evidence from scientific studies related to their patients' health problems.

A look at the literature suggests that the incidence of such adverse reactions can vary from 0.06% to 10.6%. They have been reported in patients with fish allergy, in those previously exposed to protamine (the diabetic taking NPH), and in vasectomized and infertile men. Why, you may wonder? The all-knowing literature says that these men develop antibodies to protamine due to sperm released into the bloodstream. Thankfully, catastrophic reactions to protamine during cardiovascular surgery are estimated at only 0.13%.

Use information technology to manage information, access online medical information, and support their own education.

If any of the preceding is to be done, we must be proficient at utilizing the Internet and electronic resources.

Professionalism

Residents must demonstrate a commitment to carrying out professional responsibilities, adherence to ethical principles, and sensitivity to a diverse patient population.

Demonstrate sensitivity and responsiveness to patients' culture, age, gender, and disabilities.

Be professional and include all of the preceding considerations. Enough said!

Interpersonal and communication skills

Residents must be able to demonstrate interpersonal and communication skills that result in effective information exchange and teaming with patients, their patients' families, and professional associates.

Create and sustain a therapeutic and ethically sound relationship with patients.

As anesthesiologists, we have to gain the patient's trust in a short period of time. Knowing the patient's issues by prior chart review, being informed of the procedure to be done, and possessing the ability to answer all the patient's questions thoroughly go a long way here.

Work effectively with others as a member or leader of a health care team or other professional group.

Working together with the operating room team is essential as procedures become more and more complex. Poor communication can lead to errors and, ultimately, harm to the patient.

Systems-based practice

Residents must demonstrate an awareness of and responsiveness to the larger context and system of health care and the ability to effectively call on system resources to provide care that is of optimal value.

Practice cost-effective health care and resource allocation that does not compromise quality of care.

Here is something we can control as anesthesia providers. Do I choose the expensive desflurane or the cheap isoflurane? Use the cheap pancuronium or expensive rocuronium? In cases in which the patient will be kept intubated, cheap, longer-acting agents suffice. Those "routine" CABG patients on the fast track may need more expensive agents to allow quicker wake-up, but remember that the quicker they get out of the expensive intensive care unit, the more money the hospital saves.

We should be aware of the cost of the agents we use and keep this in mind as we tailor the anesthetic to each individual patient's surgery.

Advocate for quality patient care and assist patients in dealing with system complexities.

While he or she is under anesthesia, we are the patient's advocate. Do what's right for the patient to ensure a safe anesthetic.

Additional Reading

1. Panos A, Orrit X, Chevalley C, Kalangos A. Dramatic post-cardiotomy outcome, due to severe anaphylactic reaction to protamine. Eur J Cardiothorac Surg 2003;24:325–327.

2. Weiler JM, Gelhaus M, Carter J, et al. A prospective study of the risk of an immediate adverse reaction to protamine sulfate during cardiopulmonary bypass surgery. J Allergy Clin Immunol 1990;85:713–719.

3. Levy J, Zaidan J, Faraj B. Prospective evaluation of risk of protamine reactions in patients with NPH insulin-dependent diabetes. Anesth Analg 1986;65:739–742.

4. Levy J, Franklin N. Anaphylaxis during cardiac surgery: implications for clinicians. Anesth Analg 2008;106:392–403.

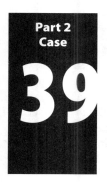

Contributions from the University of Medicine and Dentistry of New Jersey under Steven H. Ginsberg

The Da Vinci Code for anesthesiologists

Steven H. Ginsberg, Jonathan Kraidin, and Peter Chung

The case

This case involves a 52-year-old gentleman of Indian descent with no significant past medical history. He seems to be extremely anxious and is surrounded by family. He has a good airway and plans to have robotic prostatectomy. He is 5 foot 10 inches and 82 kg in weight.

Patient care

Residents must be able to provide patient care that is compassionate, appropriate, and effective for the treatment of health problems and the promotion of health.

Communicate effectively and demonstrate caring and respectful behaviors when interacting with patients and their families.

After you speak to the patient and his family in the holding area and go over his past medical history, you tell them about the anesthetic plan for the day. You describe the two intravenous lines that you will place, how you will keep him warm, and how you will remove the "breathing tube" at the end of the case. You let him know that he may be swollen in the face or arms after the surgery due to the positioning. He may actually look a bit bug-eyed with those edematous sclera (don't forget that when there is swelling on the outside, there may be swelling around the airway). The brother (the cardiologist) wants to know why he would be swollen. You let him know that the facial and airway swelling may occur because of a decrease in venous return because of the patient positioning.

They want to know why the steep Trendelenburg position is needed. You let them know that for the surgeon to get the view he needs, he will need the head of the table down at a steep angle, leaving the legs up and spread eagle. If there are any other questions about it, the surgeon can better explain things related to the surgery.

The brother asks why you didn't mention a Swan Ganz, as he wanted. You let him know that in someone with a healthy heart, it is not indicated, and that the latest reports show that robotic prostatectomy has significantly less blood loss than a conventional, open prostatectomy.

The brother really wants a "cardiac anesthesiologist," and you tell him that your attending and you work with his doctor all the time and are very comfortable and proficient at taking care of patients having this procedure.

Don't say what you're thinking: leave the anesthesia to me. You obviously should stick to the exercise treadmill.

When the patient asks you to come closer so that he can whisper his concern for his ability to "pee" and, more important, get a "hard on" after the surgery, you call the surgeon, who is the best person with whom to have this conversation. Usually, this conversation has already occurred, and the surgeon has mentioned what you have read: that there is great nerve sparing and less of an occurrence of impotence with robotic surgery compared to open prostatectomies.

Gather essential and accurate information about their patients.

You tell your attending about your concerns for this patient and family. You have made them much more comfortable about the surgery with your interview, and now you would like to give the patient an anxiolytic prior to going into the operating room. You wouldn't mind giving a little something to the cardiologist brother, but you don't mention this because of your sensitivity to him and the family. Now you're thinking if you were even permitted to have that conversation with our government and hippopotamus (HIPAA). Speaking of silly regulations! Of course! The patient was present, and if he had any objection to it, he would have mentioned it.

Develop and carry out patient management plans.

I can't really measure urine, and the patient's arms are tucked – should we need access, how about a CVP and an arterial line to manage volume status and draw some labs if the patient gets into trouble? Your attending states that back in the day (2002, at our institution), when the urologists were still on the learning curve of robotic surgery, invasive monitoring was indicated in a patient like this, who is otherwise healthy, but now they actually seem to know what those controls and joy sticks do so that they're not running into trouble. Know your surgeon, know your case, know your ability – my attending speaks wisely.

After performing an uneventful induction, you tell your attending your plans for the care of this patient. You mention that you will assist in placing the patient's arms at his side, while padding the elbows and leaving the palms in rolled towels to maintain a neutral position. You will make sure that nothing is tangled and that the strap that is placed over the patient's chest is not too tight.

You explain that the purpose of this strap is to maintain the patient's position on the operating room table in this totally unnatural upside down position. You tell your attending that the history of using the shoulder braces for this purpose has caused more harm than good, with shoulder nerve and brachial plexus injury.

You are using an underbody warming blanket and one wrapped around the patient's torso. Somehow you are hoping to keep this patient warm, when he has been naked for the last 45 minutes of positioning for this operation. He better be warm after surgery, or the insurance company won't pay a dime. Oh, yeah, he's not Medicare, and this isn't a patient who is part of the SCIP (Surgical Care Improvement Project) initiative, so we are OK with the insurance. You say that you won't use a lot of fluids at the beginning of the case, unless they are needed to maintain blood pressure, because the fluid may affect visualization of the surgical field while using the robot as well as to minimize facial and laryngeal swelling.

After that prostate is out, I am going to catch up with 1–2 L of those fluid warmers, or he'll be shivering like there's no tomorrow in the recovery room.

Counsel and educate patients and their families.

Patients are often worried about recall of surgical events, so you let the patient know that this is very rare and that you take particular precautions to see that it doesn't happen by using a special monitor to measure the depth of sleep. This stuff isn't perfect, so there is always a chance of recall, particularly if the surgeon hits something bad and the blood pressure falls so much that the only way to save the patient from Mr. Death is to turn the anesthesia off.

You kindly and patiently answer any questions and let the family know about the recovery room course and how you will be there throughout the surgery, and that your attending will be with you intermittently and will be continually supervising your care. You let the patient know that you will visit with him the day after surgery.

Use information technology to support patient care decisions and patient education.

You have searched the anesthesia, urological, and laparoscopic surgical literature and discussed with your attending the common problems that are seen with these types of cases. Of course, there is not much out there, and the other hospitals don't even have protocols for this stuff. Some of the things that you discuss include facial and airway swelling due to the decreased venous return from the insufflation of pressurized gas in the abdomen, corneal abrasion, and lower extremity weakness after surgery because of the low flow state that can occur with prolonged lithotomy and Trendelenburg position. You discuss the need to keep Trendelenburg to a minimum and still be able to do the procedure effectively. The procedure is in its infancy, and there aren't any blinded, controlled-outcome studies; it is clearly better retrospectively at decreasing blood loss and hospital length of stay. There was a recent review which stated that there may be a greater incidence of impotency and urinary dysfunction in the robotic group although ethically this study cannot be done in humans. Patients should check with their surgeons for their particular rates of morbidity as they vary greatly with experience. Although you couldn't find any precise information, you learned that obese patients will be harder to ventilate and oxygenate during this surgery. You explain that you will see a great V/Q mismatch in steep Trendelenburg and will have a decreased functional residual capacity with increased airway pressures. So basically, if you're short and fat, we're going to have problems – but you knew that when you ate the two pizzas for dinner.

Perform competently all medical and invasive procedures considered essential for the area of practice.

In addition to the standard basic American Society of Anesthesiologists monitors, bispectral index, and nerve stimulator, you would consider invasive monitors based on the experience and skill level of the surgeon and on the medical status of the patient. You have performed a smooth induction without any complications and plan to be vigilant with respect to patient positioning throughout the case.

Provide health care services aimed at preventing health problems or maintaining health.

As soon as we are ready in the operating room, I call my attending, and the surgical and anesthesia attendings do a time-out, in which they confirm the patient's name and type of surgery with the circulating nurse. This is to make sure that the wrong person didn't sneak in and get a prostatectomy. Nowadays, this is so nonchalant that no one really listens, and while it is designed to prevent an error, one may occur anyway. I'll have to discuss my concerns with the head nurse and my attending. This is another way to partner with health care management (in a later competency).

I have read the institutional policy on robotic surgery, which mentions that it should not be performed after 4 hours and in patients who have major health issues or in patients who have a body-mass index (BMI) greater than 20% of their expected BMI. All criteria have been met; however, you are concerned about the length of the surgery. What if the surgeon decides not to pay attention to that policy this week? Who am I going to call? My attending is a wimp and the fourth attending on this case. I don't know what to do.

I tell the surgeon that the abdomen has been insufflated for almost 5 hours and that he will have to stop surgery. He wants to know why, and you explain that we set up this policy to limit patient morbidity and mortality and that he must deflate the abdomen and let the patient come out of Trendelenburg for at least 30 minutes. What you really tell him is that the patient will get a compartment syndrome of his legs and they'll have to be amputated. He won't be able to walk, and

we won't extubate him until tomorrow. He's got a lot of "splaining to do, Lucy." You will do a blood gas at that time and a lactate level, and maybe a creatinine kinase and urine myoglobin, if you are really worried. If the patient is still stable and the surgeon can finish the surgery in under an hour, then he can continue.

Work with health care professionals, including those from other disciplines, to provide patient-focused care.

I have worked closely with the urological team on this case, and we have communicated throughout the procedure and addressed each other's needs as they pertained to our patient. I even held up a calendar and flipped some of the pages to let the surgeon know that he should hurry it up a bit. This patient gave me a benign medical history, so I did not have the need to discuss things further with his primary care physician, although I did have an in-depth conversation with his brother the cardiologist. At that time, I explained the lack of medical necessity for invasive monitoring for this procedure and his brother's care.

Medical knowledge

Residents must demonstrate knowledge about established and evolving biomedical, clinical, and cognate (e.g., epidemiological and social-behavioral) sciences and the application of this knowledge to patient care.

Demonstrate an investigatory and analytic thinking approach to clinical situations.

They started the robotic surgery, and the patient's blood pressure is on the high side. What did you learn in your reading? That's right. These patients get hypertension, and it's not just from a reflex reaction from the decreased venous return. Their catechols rise, and they have an increase in vasopressin, too. So how about some more anesthetic, or maybe start some nitro.

You know what? I'll sneak some nitrous; let's see if it seeps into the field and catches a spark. That would be some neat little explosion in this guy's gut. That'll take his mind off the cancer.

There's decreased venous return because of the five harpoons in his abdomen, which are insufflating gas into it at a pressure of 15–20 mmHg!

Know and apply the basic and clinically supportive sciences that are appropriate to their discipline.

The patient didn't have hypertension at the beginning of the case or at any other time in his life. So what are we doing here? We have an increase in SVR from the decrease in venous return, I can't give any volume, and they're putting all that gas in the belly. Don't they know what it will do to him?

Practice-based learning and improvement

Residents must be able to investigate and evaluate their patient care practices, appraise and assimilate scientific evidence, and improve their patient care practices.

Analyze practice experience and perform practice-based improvement activities using a systematic methodology.

There are no sinks in the operating rooms, but I better make sure that I keep my hands clean at all times. Oh, no! Did I forget the antibiotics? Do I come clean or just give them now and write them on the record at the beginning of the case? I think we give too many antibiotics. In another couple of years, they won't work for anyone.

They keep bugging me about wearing my scrubs to work, but I haven't seen any study that shows that it matters.

In the last one of these cases, I got in trouble for letting the CO_2 get too high. This time, I think I'll hyperventilate a bit once they start insufflating the abdomen. Maybe I'll use pressure support ventilation for those high airway pressures.

I remember how my attending is a stickler for that twitch monitor. Check the twitches whenever you relieve someone or take a break. You don't want to look like an idiot with a moving patient. Two twitches are fine with this procedure.

Literature search and current institutional practice and experience, and guess what? I won't have to set up a triple transducer and look for those cables and constantly level the thing, like they did at the start of the century, when they used an arterial line, introducer, and Swan!

Locate, appraise, and assimilate evidence from scientific studies related to their patients' health problems.

Tell the surgeon up front about your concerns about steep Trendelenburg and the case reports you have read. It is good to keep communicating. Is this a Core Clinical Competency, too?

Tell him why you want his help with the two warming blankets so that maybe next time, it will become routine. That is, if he cares at all.

Obtain and use information about their own population of patients and the larger population from which their patients are drawn.

The last time I did one of these, I didn't use fluid warmers and was OK until I gave that final liter – the patient woke up shivering. I almost thought he was having a seizure. It made the prior 4 hours of excellent care go out the window.

K.I.S.S. Keep it simple, stupid! Just two intravenous lines, some propofol, sux, and put the tube in. Keep him warm and limit the fluids. Stop trying to read and play with yourself with the lights off. Try to stay awake.

Apply knowledge of study designs and statistical methods to the appraisal of clinical studies and other information on diagnostic and therapeutic effectiveness.

We are presently studying the last 400 of these cases to see if there were any problems and their trends. We already see a shorter hospital stay, no one is getting addicted because they don't need much pain relief, and the patients have great erections. What more can you want?

They're also not peeing on the floor as much and can go back to work sooner, which is good because … wait until they get the bill.

In about a year, we can start to look at 10-year data on the robot and see how we are doing. It's still gonna cost some serious bucks to buy it, maintain it, use it, and train people for it.

Use information technology to manage information, access online medical information, and support their own education.

I checked all the labs last night on the hospital computer and did that full literature search before we started. The surgeon even threatened to call administration because I was delaying his case. That's the only way I'm going to learn anything in this program, while my attending is checking his e-mail in his office.

Professionalism

Residents must demonstrate a commitment to carrying out professional responsibilities, adherence to ethical principles, and sensitivity to a diverse patient population.

> Demonstrate respect, compassion, and integrity; a responsiveness to the needs of patients and society that supersedes self-interest; accountability to patients, society, and the profession; and a commitment to excellence and ongoing professional development.

Maybe if the attendings stop talking about charity care and Medicare reimbursement, I can concentrate on the real reasons for being here because I really do care about what I am dong, as long as I don't have to work more than 80 hours this week. What about my attending? How many hours is he working?

I am looking forward to a smooth wake-up and seeing this guy in a few days to see how happy he is. I have learned from my prior patient populations that they feel really good after this procedure. I just hope the brother the cardiologist isn't there.

> Demonstrate a commitment to ethical principles pertaining to provision or withholding of clinical care, confidentiality of patient information, informed consent, and business practice.

That's a lot of requirements from me! Let's start with not mentioning the brother to the other residents over lunch. Of course, if anything goes wrong or off the beaten path, they'll hear from me at our morbidity and mortality conference, where I will have to cross out his name and refer to him as the patient, and not as the "prostate."

What about the ethics when they ask me if the surgeon is any good and I know that he shouldn't operate on my pet? I still haven't figured that one out. My attending does refuse to work with certain surgeons because of their lack of ability.

I told the patient about many of the issues in my preop speech. I'm not going to tell him that he could die from this anesthesia stuff unless he asks. I told him that I could hurt a tooth or cut a gum.

> Demonstrate sensitivity and responsiveness to patients' culture, age, gender, and disabilities.

I know not to say things like "you're old enough to be my grandfather," "is that your wife...oops, daughter?" or "where did you get that accent and can someone translate for me?"

Our patient is really concerned about losing his erectile function; it is hoped that this is a conversation the surgeon had with the patient preop because it is not meant for the day of surgery. You must show compassion and sensitivity at this point. Don't say that there are other things in life, and be happy if they get the cancer.

Interpersonal and communication skills

Residents must be able to demonstrate interpersonal and communication skills that result in effective information exchange and teaming with patients, their patients' families, and professional associates.

> Create and sustain a therapeutic and ethically sound relationship with patients.

This is where the preop comes in handy. I spent time with the patient and his family. I patiently answered all their questions – even the ones from the brother the cardiologist. I deferred to the surgical team on the questions that should have been left for them to answer and helped relieve some of the patient's anxiety related to the procedure and his hospital course.

> Use effective listening skills and elicit and provide information using effective nonverbal, explanatory, questioning, and writing skills.

In the holding area, despite our different backgrounds and ages, I was able to touch base with this patient and occasionally pass a joke that made him laugh during this serious time.

> Work effectively with others as a member or leader of a health care team or other professional group.

207

I effectively communicated with the surgical team about my concerns related to this procedure at the beginning of the case. They clearly understood and listened and seemed to have the same concerns. I probably don't need to show them the calendar to let them know how long they are taking!

Systems-based practice

Residents must demonstrate an awareness of and responsiveness to the larger context and system of health care and the ability to effectively call on system resources to provide care that is of optimal value.

Understand how their patient care and other professional practices affect other health care professionals, the health care organization, and the larger society and how these elements of the system affect their own practice.

Doing robotic surgery can be very expensive, and I always wonder if the cost outweighs the benefit. Our society really can't afford all the latest gadgets and techniques, and it is frustrating to me that the costs are never contained. It costs over a million dollars just to purchase the robot. The procedure also takes longer than an open prostatectomy. I wonder if they can really get all the margins cancer-free with the robotic procedure?

I am also glad that this surgeon is not new because more patients would get hurt with his "learning curve." Do the patients actually know this information? Probably not.

Practice cost-effective health care and resource allocation that does not compromise quality of care.

The patients certainly have to eat that terrible hospital food for 1–2 fewer days, but the surgery costs more.

Although in some countries, the breathing circuit will be cleaned and reused, we won't even think about that in the United States. I can make sure that I use inexpensive inhalants for the long cases and reserve the expensive, short-acting ones for the short ambulatory cases. I always try to use inexpensive narcotics such as morphine.

We got that sheet with prices of drugs at the beginning of the year; I always try to refer to it. Whenever I have a clean, drug-filled syringe at the end of the case, I try to bring it to my next assignment. I think that pharmacy can do a better job of limiting and controlling the extra medications than I can.

Unfortunately, these multidose vials always get thrown out and don't get made in smaller-dose vials. I only draw up the amount of paralytic that I plan to use. For example, I drew up into two 5-cc syringes that 10-cc (mg) of rocuronium at the beginning of the case. I wish there was an inexpensive way to reuse the clean items that are thrown out at the end of the case.

Advocate for quality patient care and assist patients in dealing with system complexities.

The other day, I saw a bewildered patient wandering around the hospital. I approached him and said, "You look lost. Can I help?" I brought him to his destination. Our system can be very overwhelming for us as well as our patients.

I tried to explain why I needed an additional electrocardiogram (EKG) this morning – because the faxed copy from the patient's primary doctor could not be read. I didn't really have a good answer when the patient asked me about the bill for the extra EKG, although I do think that the hospital charges might be bundled – they don't really tell the residents anything about this.

I took the extra time this morning to make sure that an additional torso warming blanket was placed prior to the drapes being applied and that all the pressure points were protected. This is part of my routine; sometimes the surgeon yells when it takes too long, and I hope that I have an attending who backs me up.

I use eye patches, but it is important to check frequently for and avoid surgical equipment, robotic arms, and cables lying across the patient's face. I check the patient's arms and face throughout the procedure, keeping his safety in mind. *Safety first!*

Know how to partner with health care managers and health care providers to assess, coordinate, and improve health care and know how these activities can affect system performance.

I told the head nurse that we can use the room a little better for robotic surgery by moving some of the equipment slightly, and we can try this the night before the case. I actually felt good that my input mattered here. We even talked about getting the patient charts the day before so that the patient didn't have to come in so early prior to his surgery. If I had his phone number, I could call the patient the night prior to surgery to help make him more comfortable.

Additional reading

1. Miller RD. Miller's anesthesia. 7th ed. New York: Elsevier Health Science; 2009;2128, 2389–2403.

2. Phong SVN, Koh LKD. Anaesthesia for robotic-assisted radical prostatectomy: considerations for laparoscopy in the Trendelenburg position. Anaesth Intensive Care 2007;35:281–285.

3. Berryhill R, Jhaveri J, Yadav R, et al. Robotic prostatectomy: a review of outcomes compared with laparoscopic and open approaches. Urology 2008;72:15–23.

4. Box GN, Ahlering TE. Robotic radical prostatectomy: long-term outcomes. Curr Opin Urol 2008;18:173–179.

5. Danic J, Chow M, Alexander G, Bhandari A, Menon M, Brow M. Anesthesia considerations for robotic-assisted laparoscopic prostatectomy: a review of 1,500 cases. J Robotic Surg 2007;1:119–123.

6. Joseph JV, Leonhardt A, Patel HRH. The cost of radical prostatectomy: retrospective comparison of open, laparoscopic, and robot-assisted approaches. J Robotic Surg 2008;2:21–24.

7. Hu J, Gu X, Lipsitz S, et al. Comparative Effectiveness of Minimally Invasive vs, Open Radical Prostatectomy. JAMA 2009;302(14).

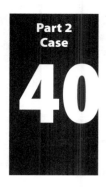

Contributions from the University of Medicine and Dentistry of New Jersey under Steven H. Ginsberg

Transhiatal esophagectomy
Do you have the stomach for it?

Jonathan Kraidin, Steven H. Ginsberg, and Tejal Patel

The case

A 64-year-old man required an esophagectomy to remove a cancerous section. The procedure involves removing the distal esophagus, ripping a pathway through the mediastinum from the abdomen to the neck, and finally, mobilizing the stomach through that path for attachment to the proximal esophagus.

During the part of the case when the surgeon had his hand blindly dissecting through the mediastinum, the pressure fell. The pressure continued to fall, and the heart rate rose as blood began to pool in the chest. We quickly realized that a blood vessel had been ripped and that the patient would soon be dead.

(*First author's note*: This is similar to an earlier case. Let's see how these authors write up the core clinical competencies from their point of view.)

Patient care

Residents must be able to provide patient care that is compassionate, appropriate, and effective for the treatment of health problems and the promotion of health.

> Communicate effectively and demonstrate caring and respectful behaviors when interacting with patients and their families.

This pertains to getting a good history and performing a good physical. Remember, this is an interaction between you and the patient; this is a time for you to get information and to answer questions and relieve patient-family anxiety. Prepare the patient for the intravenous (IV) access lines, arterial line, and possibility for postoperative ventilatory support.

The patient also needs to know, in the kindest of ways, that this is not a small operation and that there is a risk of blood loss. This way, the patient understands why large-bore IV access is required, and if peripheral access is unacceptable, the patient knows why central access is a necessity. One can also be considerate

by offering patient controlled analgesia (PCA) or an epidural for postoperative pain management, which the patient should more than appreciate.

> Gather essential and accurate information about their patients.

Information gathering is of the utmost importance, starting with the baseline hemoglobin. If the patient is starting out with anemia, one should not hesitate to start transfusing the patient to a reasonable level once the case begins. If an epidural is planned, one should query the patient about the use of blood thinners such as Plavix and Coumadin. He might think you are strange to ask about garlic supplements, but these, too, can cause significant bleeding. A good PT/INR (prothrombin time/international normalized ratio), PTT (partial prothrombin time), and platelet count are a good idea, too.

Even though you might be concerned about intraoperative bleeding, do not forget about the rest of the vital systems. Inquire about cardiac, pulmonary, and kidney function. Check the airway while you are at it. You don't want to be so worried about potential problems, only to be blindsided by a difficult intubation. Your colleagues would have a good laugh at that one!

> Make informed decisions about diagnostic and therapeutic interventions based on patient information and preferences, up-to-date scientific evidence, and clinical judgment.

The most salient feature about this case is the chance for a catastrophic bleed if the surgeon violates the aorta, pulmonary vessels, or vena cava. Knowing this, it does not take a genius to understand the need for large-bore IV access. A double lumen tube is also needed to drop a lung so the surgeon can explore either chest cavity, looking for the source of bleeding, should this become necessary.

In addition, one needs to insert an arterial line in either arm. When the surgeon is ripping (and I mean ripping) a pathway through the mediastinum, he will be compressing the heart and vena cava. One needs to know exactly how the blood pressure is responding for quick intervention.

Develop and carry out patient management plans.

Don't stand there looking at the patient. Get those lines placed! Make sure that there is an arterial line transducer set up; get those warming blankets, and while you're at it, call for the bronchoscope and check that it works before you start the case. If you have never had a broken bronchoscope or one with poor fiber optics, then you have not done enough of them.

Counsel and educate patients and their families.

One needs to discuss with the patient and family the potential for receiving copious amounts of fluids and blood products, and if large amounts of fluids are given, the patient may wake up on a ventilator.

The patient has a choice for postoperative pain relief. The resident should ascertain the patient's preference toward intravenous narcotics or a thoracic epidural.

Use information technology to support patient care decisions and patient education.

Look at the lab work to determine if you need to alter your management plans. If the patient has not been eating, he may have a volume contraction; if he has been losing blood, he could be anemic. Is his potassium elevated such that it would preclude the use of succinylcholine or make an arrhythmia more likely? How is the patient's cardiac function? If the history or electrocardiogram are suggestive of ischemia, the patient might need an angioplasty or stent before undergoing this stressful operation.

Let's not forget about the coagulation studies. A thoracic epidural would be an excellent choice for pain management, and many patients will express an interest. However, one can only place one if the potential for harm is minimal. The patient must not have a history of any bleeding disorders, and coagulation studies must be normal. The patient should not have received low molecular weight heparin within the last 24 hours, and Plavix must have been stopped for 10 days. Also, check if the surgeon is going to use subcutaneous heparin. This will have to be given at least

an hour *after* the epidural is placed, and not before placement.

Perform competently all medical and invasive procedures considered essential for the area of practice.

When you are thinking about an epidural, make sure the team and patient know that if there is significant bleeding during the case, and the patient develops a coagulopathy, clotting studies must be close to normal before the epidural can come out. Epidural hematomas can form from removing a catheter in this situation. Consider treating any underlying condition, and think about giving platelets, fresh frozen plasma (FFP), and cryoprecipitate if they are indicated. When the epidural is removed, perform neurological checks frequently for the first 12 hours.

Provide health care services aimed at preventing health problems or maintaining health.

There is a saying I like with regard to taking care of patients: no one is your friend. What does this mean? Does it mean to be antisocial? No.

Think of how one perceives taking care of a friend. One cuts corners and bends some rules. Maybe we will do one less blood draw to save our friend from a needle stick. Maybe 9 days off Plavix is enough because we want our friend to have the best pain relief. This is wrong, and this is how mistakes are made. Treat everyone the same, prince and pauper alike. Think of how your friend will feel if he gets that epidural, and then gets an epidural hematoma because you made an exception for him.

Work with health care professionals, including those from other disciplines, to provide patient-focused care.

We need to look at the patient as a whole. Is there any other pertinent history? How is the patient's heart? This is a very physiologically stressful procedure, and one should make sure the heart is up to the challenge. If there are symptoms suggestive of ischemia, a stress test might be in order so we can determine if we need to optimize coronary perfusion. This would be a good time to call your friend the cardiologist.

If there are no contraindications for the procedure, don't neglect your surgical colleague. Keep up with the status of the case and anticipate potential events. Crack a few jokes with the team if you wish, but ask now and then how things are going and if more blood loss or mediastinal manipulations are anticipated.

Medical knowledge

Residents must demonstrate knowledge about established and evolving biomedical, clinical, and cognate (e.g., epidemiological and social-behavioral) sciences and the application of this knowledge to patient care.

> Demonstrate an investigatory and analytic thinking approach to clinical situations.

While the surgeon was creating a path through the chest for the neoesophagus, the blood pressure fell. This is normal for this case and could be due to compression of the heart and vena cava, or it could be a vagal response. However, the blood pressure should rise when the surgeon stops the dissection. In this case, the blood pressure continued to fall and blood continued to fill up the suction canisters. In a very short time, there were liters of blood in them.

One needs to think fast about the causes for acute hypotension. One also needs to plan ahead and have blood in the room. Think of the horse and not the zebra. The surgeon had his hand digging through the chest, ripping the tissues to make some space. The blood pressure is low and the heart rate is high. Oh, and there are three liters of blood in the suction canisters, and the volume of blood is growing. Chances are really good that a blood vessel got ripped and the patient does not have long before complete exsanguination.

> Know and apply the basic and clinically supportive sciences that are appropriate to their discipline.

Vital organs need oxygen. The blood carries oxygen, which crosses the cell membranes when there is a sufficient pressure. No blood means no oxygen and cell death. In other words, the patient needs blood, and a lot of it.

One needs to communicate over the drapes there yonder and update the surgeon about the hemodynamic situation. What is he doing about it? Does he have control of the bleeding? Does he need more help? Does he have to do a thoracotomy or sternotomy? If the surgeon needs to do a thoracotomy, then we need to isolate one of the lungs with that double lumen tube. Now the double lumen tube placement makes sense because the last thing the surgeon needs while combing through a chest full of blood is a lung popping up in his face.

Practice-based learning and improvement

Residents must be able to investigate and evaluate their patient care practices, appraise and assimilate scientific evidence, and improve their patient care practices.

> Analyze practice experience and perform practice-based improvement activities using a systematic methodology.

I have usually found in my experience that a patient who loses more than 40% of his blood volume will be dead if nothing is done about it. Furthermore, I have found in my experience that the best remedy for blood loss is giving packed red blood cells. If the cancer is not a contraindication, cell-salvaging techniques diminish the number of autologous units the patient requires.

Whether or not this patient lives, one needs to ask if there was adequate IV access from the beginning. Should a central line have been placed? Could the surgeon have used a different surgical approach to avoid the situation?

In an ideal world, you would have a surgeon who never makes mistakes and patients who have no comorbid conditions. Alas, this blissful fantasy is not for this world. Surgeons do make mistakes, and patients do have other problems, but we deal with them. However, if the surgeon happens to make a lot of unnecessary mistakes, maybe one needs to set up a meeting with the surgical and anesthesia departments to see how one can improve the situation.

> Locate, appraise, and assimilate evidence from scientific studies related to their patients' health problems.

After doing the case and taking a few days of a much needed vacation, consider doing a literature search. You might want to call one of your colleagues at another institution to see how the cases are done there.

> Use information technology to manage information, access online medical information, and support their own education.

Sometimes it is a good idea after a long, bloody case to step back and research how other institutions do the same thing. Maybe they use a thoracic approach, instead of an abdominal one.

Professionalism

Residents must demonstrate a commitment to carrying out professional responsibilities, adherence to ethical principles, and sensitivity to a diverse patient population.

Demonstrate respect, compassion, and integrity; a responsiveness to the needs of patients and society that supersedes self-interest; accountability to patients, society, and the profession; and a commitment to excellence and ongoing professional development.

If you have read *The Hitchhiker's Guide to the Galaxy*, a running theme is *don't panic*. You may be wading though puddles of blood, but yelling, screaming, and barking orders to staff members won't make the problem go away. Stay calm. Think calmly. Be calm. This, of course, doesn't mean to lay down, kick up your feet, and order that piña colada. You still need the 20 units of blood, FFP, and platelets, but you can get them without freaking out at everyone.

Interpersonal and communication skills

Residents must be able to demonstrate interpersonal and communication skills that result in effective information exchange and teaming with patients, their patients' families, and professional associates.

Use effective listening skills and elicit and provide information using effective nonverbal, explanatory, questioning, and writing skills.

One needs to always pay attention to one's surroundings. You need to know where the surgeon is in the operation so you can anticipate potential problems. When the surgeon says that there is significant bleed-

ing, you should not think he is cracking a joke just to see your facial expression.

These listening skills are useful preoperatively, too. When eliciting the patient's history, pay attention to any signs suggesting that this may be a more difficult case. Maybe the patient received radiation therapy to the chest, resulting in fibrous strictures.

Work effectively with others as a member or leader of a health care team or other professional group.

As mentioned before, communication is of paramount importance. Maybe more help can be procured by asking for it. Have someone watch the vitals while products are given. Direct someone to give pressors, as needed. Inquire with the surgeon about his progress; maybe he can temporarily pack the area to allow you to catch up with the blood therapy.

Systems-based practice

Residents must demonstrate an awareness of and responsiveness to the larger context and system of health care and the ability to effectively call on system resources to provide care that is of optimal value.

Understand how their patient care and other professional practices affect other health care professionals, the health care organization, and the larger society and how these elements of the system affect their own practice.

After you give 28 units of blood products and your patient survives pulseless electrical activity, you better tell the ICU about all the troubles you encountered in the OR. Give them a phone call and give a detailed report. Tell them about the operative course and the patient's current status. Inform them what products and fluids the patient received and the current hemodynamic status. Postoperative ventilation will be given, so have those ventilator settings ready.

How is your patient going to affect these professionals' practice? It's going to give them a lot of work! But hey, they're here to work, too.

Contribution from the University of Texas M.D. Anderson Cancer Center under Marc Rozner

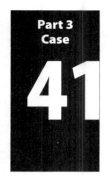

Part 3 Case

41

Contribution from the University of Texas M.D. Anderson Cancer Center under Marc Rozner

Never yell fire in a crowded OR

Charles Cowles and Marc Rozner

The case

You are counting the days left in your residency, and the staff running the board grants a bit of leniency from the typical CA-3 day of doing a single-lung transplant on the guy with malignant hyperthermia. The case given to you is a wide local excision of a suspicious lesion on the face. Meeting the patient for the first time right before the procedure, you find that he is a jovial chap who weighs in at about 250 pounds, and if he were to slap on a white beard, he could play Santa without any extra stuffing needed. He has the surgeon's initials drawn right by the little dot residing about one-third of the way between the ear and the nose. Sally, his wife, pipes in during your preop assessment to remind you that he snores really badly at night.

Dr. Pyro, the plastic surgeon, meets you in the room and tells you that this will be a really quick case and a "little sedation" is all he needs. "Five minutes tops," he says.

You get started with a bit of propofol and midazolam, but within a minute, the patient drops his sats to 92%. He is snoring away; some people saw logs when they sleep, and your patient does it with a chainsaw. Dr. Pyro tells you he can't work with all that snoring, so you slip in a nasal airway and crank up the oxygen on the face mask. All is now good.

The excision is over and Dr. Pyro leaves it to his trusty resident to "dry up and close," while he goes to talk with the family. The resident, Dr. Crispers, has one little bleeder he needs to zap with the Bovie, which he does.

Now there is a loud pop, a sizzle, and a swoosh. You look up and the oxygen mask, drapes, and patient are on fire. It looks like someone dropped a lit match on a BBQ pit after a drenching with lighter fluid. The scrub tech throws water on the inferno, the nurse pulls off the drapes, and you think to disconnect the oxygen tubing and shut off the gas. The fire is out, the patient has an oxygen mask melted to his face, and he is screaming. It

comes to your mind, "I hope Dr. Pyro hasn't told the family that everything is OK."

Patient care

Residents must be able to provide patient care that is compassionate, appropriate, and effective for the treatment of health problems and the promotion of health.

Communicate effectively and demonstrate caring and respectful behaviors when interacting with patients and their families.

You might have chosen anesthesiology because you are not the social butterfly and prefer to hang around the comatose, but when dealing with patients who are awake, you will have to dust off those people skills that you sold to the department chair during interview season. Explaining "what to expect" to the patient prior to the administration of any drugs, and the likely events that will take place during the case, is important to a successful sedation case. Telling patients that it is normal to hear noises, smell smoke (to a degree), and feel pressure will help to soothe them and reassure them that everything is going as planned.

If an unanticipated event occurs, you may want to incorporate the TEAM approach in breaking bad news to the family. Specifically,

Tell the truth

Empathize (eye contact, emotion, evidence of compassion)

Apologize (with appropriate context, i.e., for the inconvenience, discomfort, unanticipated outcome, and for a mistake if one occurred)

Manage (this is really key: explain to the patient and family what will happen next to deal with the unanticipated outcome)

The experts who analyze anesthesia-related closed claims, which are derived from direct feedback from

217

the patient or family members involved, suggest this TEAM approach (R. A. Caplan, personal communication, April 30, 2009).

Gather essential and accurate information about their patients.

Follow up on that preop lead that Sally was mentioning: does the patient snore and stop breathing at night? Was he ever formally evaluated for obstructive sleep apnea (OSA)? Is a copy of the sleep lab assessment available? These data might give you some clues to the degree of difficulty in managing this patient. See if plans should be altered for narcotic use and suggest the need for additional postoperative observation time.

Make informed decisions about diagnostic and therapeutic interventions based on patient information and preferences, up-to-date scientific evidence, and clinical judgment.

Even in "simple MAC" cases, the anesthesiologist needs to know the application of complex patient management issues spanning across several specialties. This includes practice advisories and guidelines from our own specialty, such as the American Society of Anesthesiologists, as well as other professional organizations, such as the American College of Cardiologists/American Heart Association, who provide guidelines for perioperative evaluation. If your attending asks about the differences between a guideline, standard, statement, and advisory, you might explain that standards provide rules or minimum requirements for clinical practice; a guideline assists the anesthesiologist in making decisions; statements are the opinions, beliefs, and best medical judgments of a group like the ASA House of Delegates; and finally, advisories are systematically developed reports to assist clinical decision making. However, all the guidelines in the world cannot substitute for clinical judgment.

Develop and carry out patient management plans.

There may not be a better instance of the need for planning than in cases deemed a high-risk procedure for fire. The ASA classifies these cases as the use of oxidizers in the proximity of an ignition source. The oxidizers can be either oxygen or nitrous oxide. Ignition sources commonly used in the operating room (OR) are the electrosurgical unit (ESU), a cautery or the Bovie, lasers, high-intensity laparoscope lights, and

the lit cigarette of a surgeon (just kidding – I was testing to see if you were still awake). The plan for a high-risk procedure involves educating yourself in the exit routes to be used in case of fire, the medical gas cutoff location, the location of the nearest fire extinguisher, and the location of one of those little red fire pull boxes for the alarm.

Because an ESU might be used to control bleeding, and you will probably need to use oxygen supplementation, this case becomes a high-risk procedure for an intraoperative fire. You should have a fire timeout prior to the start of the procedure, at which time, everyone in the OR should be given a specific task in case a fire occurs. The surgeon should be aware that if the patient requires more than 30% FiO_2 to maintain adequate oxygen saturation, then the airway will need to be secured with a laryngeal mask airway or endotracheal tube prior to the use of an ESU.

Also, in this case, your plans for the use of narcotics may need to be altered given the history of possible OSA. The postoperative recovery of this patient may require monitoring in postanesthesia care unit for a longer period of time than usual and may require the use of a continuous positive airway pressure machine during the recovery phase. It should be clear by now that this is not the case to be booked at 5:00 P.M. on Friday, unless you really have nothing to do this weekend.

Counsel and educate patients and their families.

You don't need to show your patient pictures of disfigured faces with oxygen masks melted into them, but you want to make the patient aware of how the anesthetic plan may change, depending on how the patient responds to sedation and if cautery is used. A brief mention of the fact that if sedation is not tolerated, then the airway may need to be secured with an ETT of LMA for safety and medical management would be satisfactory to most patients and families.

Use information technology to support patient care decisions and patient education.

To maintain that superstellar "gunner" reputation, you could look at a resource like guideline.gov the night before a case. This is the site of the National Guideline Clearinghouse, with links to most any guideline relevant to health care, and there are probably a few included that aren't relevant, just for fun. If you are able see the patient in a preop clinic (I know you are thinking that *anesthesiology* and *clinic* are two words, like *government* and *help*, that should never be in the same sentence), you might want to hand the patient and family a few well-established Web sites to research the anesthesia plan they have been provided before they search and find something like iwasawake-formyentiresurgery.com.

> Perform competently all medical and invasive procedures considered essential for the area of practice.

Like all the rest of your patients, you should aim well in IV and LMA/ET placement. Should a fire occur in or around a patient's airway, the patient should undergo a formal airway assessment, preferably by rigid bronchoscopy. In some facilities, the anesthesiologist may be the only one experienced in bronchoscopy.

> Provide health care services aimed at preventing health problems or maintaining health.

Well, the big picture here is to be ever so respectful of the fire triangle, which consists of heat, fuel, and oxidizer. That will avoid a health problem of grand magnitude. Also, give the preop antibiotics in a timely fashion and position the patient to prevent aspiration. Let's move on.

> Work with health care professionals, including those from other disciplines, to provide patient-focused care.

There are not many better opportunities to play in the sandbox with the surgeons, nurses, scrub techs, and even firefighters than in a procedure that could set the patient blazing. Good teamwork leads to good outcomes, even under fire (pun intended). Many institutions utilize crew resource management adapted from the aviation industry. Under this model, all "crew" members have the ability to bring a potentially unsafe practice to the attention of the crew leader. The procedure cannot continue further until the problem is directly addressed or a protocol is followed. In this case, if the anesthesiology resident thinks the situation is headed toward ignition of the patient, he or she can alert the surgeon that a high-risk situation exists. If the surgeon blows the resident off, then the anesthesiology resident can evoke a further assessment of the situation based on an algorithm like "patient needs oxygen, 'check,' the patient does not have secured airway,

'check,' cautery is going to be used near the oxygen source, 'check,' so now we have assessed the potential for a high-risk procedure." Of course, it would probably be wise to be "working with" your supervising attending at this point.

Also in this situation, a fire time-out should be initiated. This time-out will provide information and assignments so that everyone in the OR understands the serious nature of the problem and gets assigned a specific task to complete, like throwing saline on the fire, pulling the tube, shutting off gas flow, grabbing fire extinguishers, and removing the drapes. Note that there is no correct order in which these events should be carried out. Time should not be wasted deciding what should be done first, especially with a lit ET tube. Remember, the goal is quick extubation and to quickly turn off the gas supply. No set order needed, just "get-r-done."

Finally, make every effort to quickly notify your surgeon if an intraoperative or postoperative complication should arise. No one likes surprises in the surgical environment. If the patient management is more complex than usual, you may want to ask the surgeon to hang around in case of complication. It will give you an extra set of hands and will keep the surgeon from rushing out to the family with the "everything went fine" speech.

Medical knowledge

Residents must demonstrate knowledge about established and evolving biomedical, clinical, and cognate (e.g., epidemiological and social-behavioral) sciences and the application of this knowledge to patient care.

> Demonstrate an investigatory and analytic thinking approach to clinical situations.

For this case, the risk of fire can be reduced if one recognizes that this is a high-risk procedure (where an ignition source may come in proximity to an oxidizer-enriched atmosphere, thereby increasing the risk of fire). The obese patient with a history of snoring may require supplementation of oxygen if sedated, especially if narcotics are used. This should prompt the analytical thinker to secure the airway with a LMA or ET tube to contain the oxygen, preventing oxidizer enrichment of the surgical field where cautery is used. Since this is a high-risk procedure with respect to fires, you should hold a fire time-out (discussed earlier). This will define your role and the roles of others should fire break out.

Recall that the key difference between monitored anesthesia care and conscious sedation is that anesthesiology professionals can convert the "monitored anesthetic care" to a general anesthetic, if needed, for the given clinical situation. Conscious sedation is provided by non-anesthesia-trained personnel and incorporates a "ceiling," where any procedure has to be aborted if sedation fails to provide the desired clinical effect (i.e., the patient is jumping off the table).

Know and apply the basic and clinically supportive sciences that are appropriate to their discipline.

There is a bit of overlap here with the management plans stated earlier and elsewhere, but let's have a course in fire basics. When the elements of fuel, oxidizers, and heat come together, they experience a chemical reaction, and voilà! Fire! In the OR (or anywhere you sell your services), these elements are quite abundant.

We begin with the racing car fuel used to clean your patient – the isopropyl alcohol–based prepping solutions. These solutions are highly flammable compounds that should be avoided to prevent converting your patient into a Sterno heater. If they are used, they must be allowed to dry fully. Draping and barriers should be configured to prevent pooling, either in natural recesses, like the umbilicus, or underneath the patient or in the table sheets. Consider that the flames of alcohol-based fires are very difficult to see because of the heat of the flame and the purity of the fuel, and the flame gets harder to see in the field with bright surgical lights. Of course, flesh, the plastic oxygen mask, the ET tube, or the LMA can be a fuel. Remember, in the presence of a high concentration of oxidizers, nearly *anything* can burn.

Speaking of oxidizers, we commonly use two in the OR: oxygen and nitrous oxide. They function equally in the role of filling one of the sides of the fire triangle. It is impossible to determine the concentration of oxidizers at the surgical site. For example, we can measure oxygen concentration as it leaves the delivery device as FiO_2, but once that is mixed with air, the concentration becomes unknown. So even though we can reduce oxygen flows and concentration, like when performing a tracheotomy, the actual oxygen percentage

in the field is unknown. Observational and bench studies have indicated that if the FiO_2 is kept below 30%, the dilution will result in an oxygen percentage presumably safe for procedures near an ignition source. But the safest course of action is either to isolate the oxygen within the airway using an ETT or LMA or to use 21% oxygen (like room air).

Finally, ignition sources such as the ESU (the Bovie), lasers, and even the tip of laparoscopes are used in nearly every case. The ESU tool should be returned to the holster between uses because the surface can be hot enough to ignite surgical drapes. The tip of the ESU should be cleaned of debris by using a scratch pad. Surgeons should notice if the spark at the ESU tip seems more intense than usual, indicating the likely presence of an oxidizer-enriched environment. Surgical scopes can generate enough heat at the tip or at the light source to ignite paper drapes or alcohol preps. Laser use requires an entire set of operating rules to be followed, not the least of which is the use of the proper laser tube if the laser is used in the proximity of the endotracheal tube.

Practice-based learning and improvement

Residents must be able to investigate and evaluate their patient care practices, appraise and assimilate scientific evidence, and improve their patient care practices.

Analyze practice experience and perform practice-based improvement activities using a systematic methodology.

If the preceding case were to happen, all the operating room faculty and staff who were present should participate in an immediate debriefing, if possible. As time passes, the recollection of exact events begins to fade, so it is best if this is done as soon as possible. Support should be offered, if needed, to team members, especially if there is a catastrophic outcome. Participation in specialty-specific morbidity and mortality and interdisciplinary rounds is an important educational activity. Compare the facts and progression of your case to current standard of care, and review institutional policies to see if they can be improved or redesigned to facilitate safe and consistent care. Personally, you can review your actions to see what could have been done differently and how you can change your own practices based on this experience.

> Locate, appraise, and assimilate evidence from scientific studies related to their patients' health problems.

Not a lot can be found in the area of OR fires with respect to formal randomized control trials (RCTs). The institutional review boards seem unwilling to approve a protocol with "In arm number 1, we will set the patient on fire." But multiple case studies have been published and are interesting from the perspective of "Gee, I never thought of that happening." Learning from the mistakes or misadventures of others can certainly help your own practice. Also, review the literature and recommendations to see if they are scientifically valid and not based solely on the author's opinion.

> Obtain and use information about their own population of patients and the larger population from which their patients are drawn.

This can well be applied if you work in "America's Fattest City" or the "Sunshine Capital." Many specialty centers are known for obesity-related procedures, and MAC cases may create quite a challenge. Sun-related damage is one of the leading causes of investigation and removal of skin lesions. These cases are the ones in which the unknowing are led down the path of destruction by lighting up the electrocautery in proximity to an open oxidizer source such as an oxygen mask.

> Apply knowledge of study designs and statistical methods to the appraisal of clinical studies and other information on diagnostic and therapeutic effectiveness.

Even though no RCTs exist relating to proper management of OR fires, the ASA has published a practice advisory containing a robust literature search and analysis of the topic. It includes solid scientific principles, like the fire triangle, which have considerable applicable information.

> Use information technology to manage information, access online medical information, and support their own education.

For cases that are known high-risk procedures, online information is available from the Anesthesia Patient Safety Foundation (APSF), ECRI (a large nonprofit institute dedicated to testing and research to improve patient safety), and the previously mentioned guideline.gov. The ASA has an OR fire algorithm to review and post at anesthetizing locations. This, of course, should be done way ahead of time, not when you smell smoke.

Professionalism

Residents must demonstrate a commitment to carrying out professional responsibilities, adherence to ethical principles, and sensitivity to a diverse patient population.

> Demonstrate respect, compassion, and integrity; a responsiveness to the needs of patients and society that supersedes self-interest; accountability to patients, society, and the profession; and a commitment to excellence and ongoing professional development.

An extra minute or act of kindness with the patient and his family may leave an impression of professionalism that may serve you well if a complication arises. Accountability is a major component of being a physician. You assume responsibility for your patient's health and well-being in the operating room under your care. Accountability means total responsibility for your actions and dedication to safety because unlike others, you are assumed to have the intellect and power to change or stop what is not right. Integrity means that you are up front with all involved parties and that you are honest and not seeking to cover things up or shift the blame. A commitment to excellence even begins with your relationship with the surgeon; you should always introduce yourself and talk to the surgeon before the case, not just when problems arise.

> Demonstrate a commitment to ethical principles pertaining to provision or withholding of clinical care, confidentiality of patient information, informed consent, and business practice.

Even in surgery centers where high case turnover is expected, there may be cases that should not be performed due to patient safety concerns. Also, bad outcomes can result in media inquiry. However, even if your local investigative reporter prints the story "Death under the Knife: It Could Happen to You," confidentiality still must be maintained, even if you have to be the "no comment" guy. Like any case you perform, proper consent should be verified, and billing information should be kept factual.

> Demonstrate sensitivity and responsiveness to patients' culture, age, gender, and disabilities.

For this case, it might be wise to hang the old "patient is awake" sign on the door to keep your friends from stopping by and telling of their weekend exploits or the usual dark humor of the OR. We have all heard jokes and stories told in the OR at the expense of one or more of the mentioned categories. This is not good when the patient is wide awake and listening or, according to the "hearing is the last sense to go" theorists, even when he or she is asleep.

Interpersonal and communication skills

Residents must be able to demonstrate interpersonal and communication skills that result in effective information exchange and teaming with patients, their patients' families, and professional associates.

> Create and sustain a therapeutic and ethically sound relationship with patients.

Try to establish rapport with your patient early for a planned MAC case to get a feel for how social he or she will be. Some patients need a bit of reassurance, and others want constant attention. Some are easy and others are difficult, but all deserve your professional attention. Oftentimes, cues will need to be given during MAC cases to remind your patient to be quiet and still. It is also helpful to explain what is going on relative to the surgery. If there is an unexpected complication with a bad outcome, don't run from the situation. Instead, follow up with the patient and the family. Give them adequate time for questions and discussion, and let them air their concerns.

> Use effective listening skills and elicit and provide information using effective nonverbal, explanatory, questioning, and writing skills.

Follow up on those leads given by family as to medical history. Assessing the patient early on for nonverbal clues to nervousness, claustrophobia, cooperation, and fear may help you decide that MAC may not be the best option for the patient. Also, be and look professional because these actions will inspire patient con-

fidence in you. Be honest and up front with answers to any questions your patient may have.

Like any good physician, you should have evidence of a history and physical, anesthetic plan, and postop care plan. These items should be legibly documented into the patient chart, with minimal errors.

> Work effectively with others as a member or leader of a health care team or other professional group.

For this case, beginning with a fire time-out to alert the crew that this is a high-risk procedure and designating roles in case of fire set a professional example. Demonstrate your role as an expert consultant by asking the surgeon if cautery will be needed around the head and neck area so that he or she will understand the need to convert to a general anesthetic with a secure airway should the patient be unable to maintain an adequate oxygen saturation. If complications arise, lead the team through the situation, and also discuss complications with family members, Quality improvement initiatives, and risk management.

Systems-based practice

Residents must demonstrate an awareness of and responsiveness to the larger context and system of health care and the ability to effectively call on system resources to provide care that is of optimal value.

> Understand how their patient care and other professional practices affect other health care professionals, the health care organization, and the larger society and how these elements of the system affect their own practice.

One of the few things worse than a bad outcome is the associated bad press. Cases that make their way into the court of public opinion are not good for anyone, including you, your colleagues, your hospital, and your fellow anesthesiologists. Societies may have to address the area of concern and may initiate a task force to examine means to handle the problem. Be consistent in your commitment to always do the safe thing, which can lead to a paradigm shift from practices like oxygen supplementation in the uncontrolled airway and the use of alcohol-based surgical preps.

Practice cost-effective health care and resource allocation that does not compromise quality of care.

Safety can be accomplished by common practices and common sense, with a little bit of planning. You do not need expensive, well-dressed consultants with elaborate, multicolored reports to have a safe operating environment. Combining select representatives from a variety of specialties with staff who work in the OR to form a safety review committee will allow the assessment of various procedures, with the purpose of identifying whether improvements can be made. Even the Joint Commission wants one question to be answered in a sentinel event: why?

One should never compromise patient care or safety to achieve quick turnovers or financial gain. In the long run, it will cost you more and may even cost a life or your reputation.

Also, if you work at a location that performs many high-risk procedures, then you might want to assemble a cart for high-risk cases. The cart can include several bottles of saline, carbon dioxide (CO_2), a fire extinguisher, ETT rated for use with lasers, replacement tubes, masks, circuits, drapes, sponges, and even a rigid bronchoscope for airway assessment. Finally, a copy of the ASA Algorithm for the Management of OR Fires can be attached to the anesthesia machine for review during those 20-hour-long cases with nothing to do but stare at railroad track vital signs.

Know how to partner with health care managers and health care providers to assess, coordinate, and improve health care and know how these activities can affect system performance.

If you take the initiative in any topic, by learning a bit more than the average bear and presenting a lecture at a grand rounds, you will have taken the first step toward improving health care. From there, you can speak at other venues at your hospital and even at a medical or nursing school. Eventually, your local, state, and national societies will take notice, and you can progress to leadership within those societies. Share your thoughts with colleagues and help on committees, if you are so inclined. You can make a difference.

Additional reading

1. Caplan RA, Barker SJ, Connis RT, et al. Practice advisory for the prevention and management of operating room fires. American Society of Anesthesiologists Task Force on Operating Room Fires. Anesthesiology 2008;108:786–801.

2. Milliken RA, Bizzarri A. Flammable surgical drapes. Anesth Analg 1985;64:54–57.

3. Halstead MA. Fire drill in the operating room: role playing as a learning tool. AORN J 1993;58:697–706.

4. Greco RJ, Gonzalez R, Johnson P, Scolieri M, Rekhopf PG, Heckler F. Potential dangers of oxygen supplementation during facial surgery. Plast Reconstr Surg 1995;95:978–984.

5. Barker SJ, Polson JS. Fire in the operating room: a case report and laboratory study. Anesth Analg 2001;93:960–965.

6. Eade GG. Hazard of nasal oxygen during aesthetic facial operations. Plast Reconstr Surg 1986;78:539.

7. Howard BK, Leach JL. Prevention of flash fires during facial surgery performed under local anesthesia. Ann Otol Rhinol Laryngol 1997;106:248–251.

8. Reyes RJ, Smith AA, Mascaro JR, Windle BH. Supplemental oxygen: ensuring its safe delivery during facial surgery. Plast Reconstr Surg 1995;95:924–928.

9. Gross JB, Bachenberg KL, Benumof JL, et al. Practice guidelines for the perioperative management of patients with obstructive sleep apnea: a report by the American Society of Anesthesiologists Task Force on Perioperative Management of patients with obstructive sleep apnea. Anesthesiology 2006;104:1081–1093.

Part 4

Contributions from the University of Miami Miller School of Medicine under Michael C. Lewis

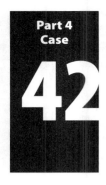

42 Nephrectomy

Contributions from the University of Miami Miller School of Medicine under Michael C. Lewis

Michael C. Lewis and V. Samepathi David

The case

A 50-year-old male with poorly controlled-insulin-dependent diabetes has an incidental computed tomography finding of a left renal mass. The patient is scheduled to undergo a laparoscopic-assisted left nephrectomy.

Patient care

Residents must be able to provide patient care that is compassionate, appropriate, and effective for the treatment of health problems and the promotion of health.

Communicate effectively and demonstrate caring and respectful behaviors when interacting with patients and their families.

Preoperative evaluation includes the following:

- Meet with the patient and family in a quiet room.
- Acknowledge everyone in the room.
- Empathize with the family's anxiety and lack of knowledge about medical care.
- In explaining the anesthesia use understandable language.
- Ask the patient and his family if they have any other questions.

Gather essential and accurate information about their patients.

This includes the following:

1. Familiarize yourself with the patient's chart (consultations, laboratory tests, etc.) prior to the preoperative interview. If necessary review previous medical records of the patient's care.
2. Speak directly with primary care and referring physicians regarding unresolved questions about a patient's medical history.

3. Request that a copy of the original test result be available in the patient's current chart.
4. Review previous medical records of the patient's care
   - Electronic medical record chart from Health Information Management Department

---

Make informed decisions about diagnostic and therapeutic interventions based on patient information and preferences, up-to-date scientific evidence, and clinical judgment.

Develop and carry out patient management plans.

Discuss with the patient and family the role you will execute in perioperative management:

1. Preoperative preparation and optimization of the patient begins with the preoperative interview on the day of surgery:
   - laboratory tests
   - fasting blood sugar
   - interval change in patient's medical status
   - regional analgesic blocks, invasive monitors, and venous access

2. Perform intraoperative monitoring, treatments, and interventions during induction, maintenance, and mergence.
3. Postoperative management includes the following:
   - acute pain management
   - patient controlled epidural analgesia
   - monitoring, treatments, and interventions in the postanesthesia care unit
   - repeat fasting blood glucose
   - complete blood count

Counsel and educate patients and their families.

---

1. Preoperative
   - Obtain informed consent by guiding the family through the risks and benefits of the options for anesthesia.
   - Discuss relevant information regarding practice guidelines.

2. Postoperative
   - Be honest and open when discussing patient harm that resulted from the administration of anesthesia.
   - Share expectations regarding further recovery from the effects of anesthesia.
   - Use family/patient-based questions that arise in the postoperative period as an opportunity to educate.

Use information technology to support patient care decisions and patient education.

During the preoperative interview, educate your patient and show him/her the guidelines and standards of care that are used during their care. These guidelines and standards of care are available on the computer.

Perform competently all medical and invasive procedures considered essential for the area of practice.

Prior to induction, the following should be considered:
- Intravenous catheters should be placed after disinfecting the skin.
- Protective gloves should be worn.
- All monitors should be applied in standard fashion.
- A good mask seal should be established during preoxygenation.

During induction and intubation,
- the patient's eyes should be protected from injury
- the "sniffing position" should be sought to improve intubating conditions and reduce injury to the teeth and tongue
- universal precautions should be practiced during placement of the arterial line and a second intravenous line
- all pressure points should be padded
- hospital policy of two-person cross-checking of blood prior to administration should be used

During emergence, use the train-of-four monitor to determine reversal of muscle relaxation prior to extubation.

Provide health care services aimed at preventing health problems or maintaining health.

- Administer prophylactic antibiotics 30 minutes prior to incision.
- Check serum blood glucose serially.

Work with health care professionals, including those from other disciplines, to provide patient-focused care.

- operating room nurses
- postanesthesia care unit nurses
- physician assistants
- consultant physicians
- pharmacists

Medical knowledge

Residents must demonstrate knowledge about established and evolving biomedical, clinical, and cognate (e.g., epidemiological and social-behavioral) sciences and the application of this knowledge to patient care.

Demonstrate an investigatory and analytic thinking approach to clinical situations.

Use a systematic and organized approach to differential diagnosis and treatment plans.

Know and apply the basic and clinically supportive sciences that are appropriate to their discipline.

- pharmacology
- anatomy
- physiology
- biology

Practice-based learning and improvement

Residents must be able to investigate and evaluate their patient care practices, appraise and assimilate scientific evidence, and improve their patient care practices.

Analyze practice experience and perform practice-based improvement activities using a systematic methodology.

1. continuing medical education

    a. ASA SEE Program
    b. difficult airway workshop
    c. regional anesthesia workshops
    d. ultrasound-guided techniques

2. individual quality improvement indicators

    a. reintubation rate
    b. postdural puncture headaches
    c. unrecognized difficult airways
    d. escalation in care
    e. unanticipated hospitalization
    f. postoperative hypothermia

3. corrective action

    a. CME
    b. video seminars
    c. apprenticeship

4. hospital committee involvement

    a. quality improvement committee
    b. performance improvement committee

Locate, appraise, and assimilate evidence from scientific studies related to their patients' health problems.

1. online sources

    a. PubMed
    b. Google
    c. American Society of Anesthesiology

2. reference textbooks

    a. coexisting disease

3. annual meeting syllabus

    a. abstracts
    b. poster presentations

4. correlate with existing practice guidelines and accepted practice standards

Apply knowledge of study designs and statistical methods to the appraisal of clinical studies and other information on diagnostic and therapeutic effectiveness.

Particularly important regarding patient management are the following:

- Does the benefit of an arterial line or central line placement outweigh the risk of its placement?
- Does an epidural for postoperative pain management lead to reduced hospital stay and reduced morbidity?

    1. degree of statistical significance
    2. sufficient power
    3. double blinded
    4. degree of randomization

Use information technology to manage information, access online medical information, and support their own education.

Access medical records and old charts.

Professionalism

Residents must demonstrate a commitment to carrying out professional responsibilities, adherence to ethical principles, and sensitivity to a diverse patient population.

Demonstrate respect, compassion, and integrity; a responsiveness to the needs of patients and society that supersedes self-interest; accountability to patients, society, and the profession; and a commitment to excellence and ongoing professional development.

- work ethic
- dependability
- motivation
- taking initiative

Demonstrate a commitment to ethical principles pertaining to provision or withholding of clinical care, confidentiality of patient information, informed consent, and business practice.

- HIPAA regulations
- informed consent prior to all procedures

Demonstrate sensitivity and responsiveness to patients' culture, age, gender, and disabilities.

- Respect religious preferences.
- Refer to patients by their surnames.

Interpersonal and communication skills

Residents must be able to demonstrate interpersonal and communication skills that result in effective information exchange and teaming with patients, their patients' families, and professional associates.

Create and sustain a therapeutic and ethically sound relationship with patients.

Preoperative evaluation involves the following:

- Meet with the patient and family (spouse, children, parents) in a quiet room.
- Acknowledge everyone in the room.
- Sympathize with the family's anxiety and lack of knowledge about medical care.
- Use simple terms and illustrations.
- Ask if they have any other questions.
- Maintain eye contact.
- Speak clearly.

Systems-based practice

Residents must demonstrate an awareness of and responsiveness to the larger context and system of health care and the ability to effectively call on system resources to provide care that is of optimal value.

Understand how their patient care and other professional practices affect other health care professionals, the health care organization, and the larger society and how these elements of the system affect their own practice.

In the following, I describe how these elements affect my practice:

- other health care professionals
  - increased requirement for subspecialty consultative services
    - establish patient-subspecialty physician relationship prior to surgery
    - encourage input from subspecialists as early as possible
    - ensure that all diagnostic test results are on the patient's chart, to avert potential delays in obtaining the results in the postoperative period
- health care organization
  - resource utilization

- prolonged hospitalization/delayed discharge limiting available bed space
- emergency room patient flow and intensive care unit (ICU)/PACU transfers
- optimization of comorbidities in association with their referring physician and other subspecialists
- appropriate invasive/noninvasive monitors to guide fluid administration
- frequent monitoring of blood sugar levels and hemoglobin
- regional anesthetic techniques for postoperative pain management, where applicable
- unplanned ICU admission, leading to an escalation in care
- postoperative recovery needs based on the preoperative assessment
- surgical ICU, MICU, critical care unit, step-down unit, telemetry
- increased laboratory and diagnostic testing
  - surgery postponed until the patient has been optimized
- increased exposure to morbidity
- nosocomial infections
  - perioperative glucose control
  - perioperative antibiotics administered according to hospital protocol
- iatrogenic injury
  - limit invasive procedures
  - ultrasound guidance, where appropriate
  - avoidance of escalation in care/prolonged hospital stay
- society
  - limited access to inpatient hospitalization and services
  - escalation in health care delivery costs

Practice cost-effective health care and resource allocation that does not compromise quality of care.

This includes the following:

- Follow evidence-based practice guidelines, preoperative assessment, and intraoperative management and monitoring.
- Use finger-stick glucose monitoring rather than repeated serum testing.
- Use PONV prophylaxis and prompt treatment.

- Reduce utilization of supplies.
- Maintain perioperative normothermia.
  - Reduce utilization of supplies.
  - Reduce hypothermia-related complications.
- Prepare/utilize only essential equipment and supplies in the operating room.
  - Reduce waste.

Advocate for quality patient care and assist patients in dealing with system complexities.

This involves the following:

- Maintain clear communication with patient and family.
  - Ensure that instructions are concise and devoid of complex medical terms.
  - Make them of aware of where the operating room is in relation to the recovery room, medical-surgical floor, and intensive care units.
  - In conjunction with the surgeon and other health care practitioners, keep the family informed of progress in the operating room and recovery room.
  - Remain visible to the family in the immediate postoperative period.

Know how to partner with health care managers and health care providers to assess, coordinate, and improve health care and know how these activities can affect system performance.

- surgical services
- infection control
- pharmacy and therapeutics
- performance improvement/quality assurance
- medical executive

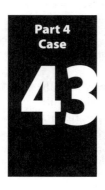

Contributions from the University of Miami Miller School of Medicine under Michael C. Lewis

43 Another day at the office…based anesthesia

Steven Gil and Nancy Setzer-Saade

The case

A 15-year-old girl is scheduled at an outpatient facility for colonoscopy with monitored anesthesia care. She has been complaining of diffuse abdominal pain for 6 weeks, intermittent diarrhea, and occasional blood per rectum. Her primary care provider feels she would benefit from lower endoscopy. The patient and her mother arrive at your practice's office on Tuesday. She missed school yesterday because of her symptoms.

Patient care

This young lady is suffering from a constellation of medical problems. While irritable bowel syndrome and Crohn's disease are possible diagnoses, other potential diseases must be considered and ruled out. It appears that her primary care provider, either her pediatrician or gynecologist, has excluded more common etiologies such as infectious or menstrual issues and has sought the help of a specialist in diagnosing her disease. Abdominal pain can be one symptom of a multitude of disease processes with anesthetic implications that affect her preop, intraop, and postop care. During your evaluation, consider that her problem might be more severe than previously considered; does she have a small bowel obstruction? Would this make her a candidate for an office-based procedure?

When you first address the daughter and mother, you introduce yourself and your role within the center. The mother is aggravated and demanding to know why her daughter is waiting for the procedure, why she had to do the colon preparation, and why her daughter could not eat anything this morning. The daughter is strangely quiet, preferring not to look you in the eye. You politely explain the reasons for all her concerns and ask that you be able to speak with her daughter alone for a few minutes so that you are able to talk and examine the daughter about her condition and the ensuing procedure scheduled for the morning. The mother seems apprehensive but acquiesces.

When she slowly walks away, the daughter does not say much. When the mother is outside the holding area, you introduce yourself again and state that everything discussed is confidential and will not be told to her mother. At this point, the girl starts whimpering. You ask what she is feeling. Suddenly, you are immersed within a story of how she and her boyfriend had been sexually active 6 weeks ago and that they had broken up this past weekend, when she told him she missed her period last week. She thinks she is pregnant and that this is causing her pain. You comfort the girl and slowly begin to consider your subsequent actions.

Interpersonal skill and communication

In anesthesia, we are accustomed to our patients being asleep (or pleasingly sedated), but in unexpected times, we may be faced with medicosocial problems more attuned to a primary care provider. It would be irresponsible of the doctor-patient relationship to abandon this girl in her time of need. This may have been the first time away from her mother that she has been able to speak to a medical professional honestly about her situation. The competencies deem that we be able to give compassionate care to our patients. Not every emotional medical problem can be solved with a benzodiazepine, and we need to ensure that the competencies address the compassion needed for patients in need of support.

Professionalism

Patient confidentiality is a basic tenet of the doctor-patient relationship and a precept of being a professional. Only when patients have complete trust in their medical provider can one assume that the provider is beginning to provide optimum health care. Requesting that the patient be allowed to speak with the physician without the mother present allowed a breakthrough in the treatment of her medical condition.

Systems-based practice

At some point, the acute care physician is ultimately unable to follow up on the long-term care of patients. Therefore other professionals will need to be consulted and introduced into the picture. The girl's primary care provider, a social worker, and the endoscopist are going to have long-term follow-up with this girl. It would be beneficial to recognize the utility of using a team of professionals to assist in this patient's care. We function within a system of providers; not one is perfectly situated to give all care, but all are able to ask for help to give a better outcome.

After discussing the girl's situation with her gastrointestinal physician, you decide to perform a pregnancy test, with the patient's permission. The patient has a urine test, which is negative, and you tell her the results. She is relieved, but realizing that her stomach pain is still prevalent, she is curious as to why she still feels ill. You therefore continue with her preoperative assessment. Other than a slight anemia, her evaluation is normal. You decide that she is optimized for MAC and that it is OK to proceed with the procedure. Her mother returns and is still upset over the delay. You tell her of the medical need to be thorough before colonoscopy. She is irate and wants to leave the center.

Interpersonal skills

You are in a very delicate situation of maintaining the doctor-patient relationship while supporting and explaining to the mother how the medical process works. Any irreverence, trust-destroying comments, or misunderstandings could be detrimental to the patient, her family, your employer, and your professional standing. Through practice and patience, one should be able to explain the necessity of the process, while maintaining respect for all those involved. Although the mother demands to know what her daughter told you, your first obligation is to your patient, the daughter.

Medical knowledge

Is the patient prepared for the procedure? What is your plan for anesthesia? Is her anemia a contraindication for this invasive procedure? Is your facility prepared for all types of complications? The patient is suffering from a storm of social and medical issues, but there was no absolute contraindication for proceeding with the endoscopy. Can you proceed?

After you apologize for the delay, the mother agrees to proceed. You start your anesthetic, and the procedure goes without complication. Some biopsies are sent, and a report will be given to the family at a follow-up clinic appointment later that week. The patient is now in the postanesthesia care unit and is suffering from intractable nausea and vomiting. You delay discharge and administer additional intravenous fluids, but she is not feeling better. Although the outpatient clinic staff is scheduled to go home, you are concerned about the patient's status and consider transferring her to the hospital for overnight hospitalization and rehydration. After you persuade the clinic staff to stay late, and after another dose of an antiemetic, the patient is feeling better and soon able to tolerate liquids. The patient and her mother express having a long and emotional day and thank both you and the clinic staff. The patient also thanks you for listening to her social situation earlier in the day. You promise to keep her story confidential. They leave the surgery center and will return later on that week for results of the study.

Practice based learning

You have had a patient who needed the complex care of many arms of the health care community. She began the day with psychosocial issues and a straightforward medical problem. Before the day was through, she ended with a resolution of part of her problem but the unveiling of a more complex issue, mainly, the possibility that she might need to be transferred to an upper-level facility for fluid replacement secondary to nausea and vomiting.

A couple days later, a colleague who witnessed the previous day's story pulls you aside and compliments you on your performance. You thank her and realize that although you are satisfied with the outcome, there is always room for improvement in any field of medicine.

Superficially, it seems that "all's well that ends well" with this case, but you wonder how you might have done better and might improve the experience for both the practitioners and patients in this setting in future similar circumstances. You contact your colleague who specializes in quality improvement for your group and suggest that you present this case at your next meeting for discussion. You realize that you would have had an uncomfortable predicament if the pregnancy test had been positive and that community resources to help in similar circumstances should be identified before the need arises.

The outpatient setting presents a unique set of problems, rewards, and complexities to the anesthesiologist. Although patients may present with more straightforward medical problems and be healthier overall than those in an inpatient unit, the anesthesiologist is more isolated and needs the adaptability to perform a multitude of multilevel perioperative functions compared to the large-practice, hospital-based group. The Core Clinical Competencies apply just as easily to this setting as any other situation resident physicians face every day. As the role of the anesthesiologist expands in different settings, we constantly explore how to apply these principles to our everyday practice and strive to implement them in future unknown circumstances.

Additional reading

1. Ross AK, Eck JB. Office based anesthesia for children. Anesthesiol Clin North Am 2002;20:195–210.

2. Matthes K. Gastrointestinal endoscopy in the office-based setting. In Shapiro FE, editor. Manual of office-based anesthesia procedures. Philadelphia: Lippincott; 2007:120–132.

3. American Society of Anesthesiologists. http://www.asahq.org/publicationsAndServices/ standards/12.pdf Accessed 10-12-2009.

4. Fletcher G, Glavin R. The non-technical skills of anesthetists. In: Greaves D, editor. Clinical teaching – a guide to teaching practical anaesthesia. Lisse, the Netherlands: Swets and Zeitlinger; 2003:53–62.

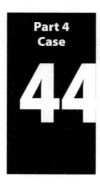

Part 4 Case

44 OB to the core

Contributions from the University of Miami Miller School of Medicine under Michael C. Lewis

Deborah Brauer and Murlikrishna Kannan

The case

A lazy Sunday evening, 7:00 P.M. Time for a shift change – funny how everything seems to happen around this time. The outgoing call team has had a very quiet day; debriefing of the day's events includes new cheat maneuvers on the play station. Thirty minutes into the call, the pager sounds – a request to preop a new patient.

The anesthesia resident ambles along and reaches the labor room. The obstetric resident quickly reaches out and hands you a few papers on the patient, which reveal the patient's history.

A 28-year-old primigravida at 36 weeks' gestation is admitted to the labor floor for an evaluation of hypertension to "rule out preeclampsia." Her medical history is significant for an aortic stenosis. She is currently under the care of the cardiologist, who has advised that she is medically optimized and that her exercise tolerance is relatively unimpaired, with her most recent echo estimating her valve area to be 1.0 cm² and her valve gradient to be 50 mmHg.

You stare at a nebulous mass of facts: aortic stenosis, preeclampsia, hemodynamics, pregnancy, CSEs, general anesthetics, obstetric drugs with cardiac side effects – an endless list, so let's start to simplify.

Patient care

Residents must be able to provide patient care that is compassionate, appropriate, and effective for the treatment of health problems and the promotion of health.

Communicate effectively and demonstrate caring and respectful behaviors when interacting with patients and their families.

Ascertain with whom you are speaking – the guy standing next to the moaning patient may be her son or husband – so do not put your foot in your mouth. You will probably never break enough ground to recover from mistakes like this.

Gather essential and accurate information about their patients.

Some of us are poor history takers, so our patients tend to be poor historians. Gather all essential and accurate information. Please be patient for this, though you want to scream out for help. Also, read the chart and collaborate with the obstetrician to supplement and enhance your understanding of your patient.

Make informed decisions about diagnostic and therapeutic interventions based on patient information and preferences, up-to-date scientific evidence, and clinical judgment.

If you do not know the answer to a patient question or you are unsure, say so! Don't guess or, still worse, tell her the completely wrong thing. You will have to eat your words. Determine what the patient wants and what she knows (some patients may know more than you, thanks to Google!).

Develop and carry out patient management plans.

The patient may have a lot of questions, too, so work it out – answer all her questions, while being sure to hear all her answers. Do not be rude and cut her sentences short during a conversation. Then, make a collaborative, informed decision for optimal management.

Counsel and educate patients and their families.

Be polite, make eye contact, smile, and show empathy – even though you quietly wish that this shift would magically end.

Perform competently all medical and invasive procedures considered essential for the area of practice.

Do an arterial line, but do it using a clean technique, possibly with local anesthesia. Explain why you are doing it, and avoid medical jargon while explaining. Performing an arterial line can be a lot of pressure because the patient sees your skilled hands at work, whereas during an epidural, you can hide behind the patient.

Provide health care services aimed at preventing health problems or maintaining health.

Does she need antibiotics prophylaxis for infective endocarditis? If unsure, check with her cardiologist; do not guess! More important, always follow the first principle: "first, do no harm." Do not start inserting PA catheters, even though you just did it the previous month in cardiac rotation. Your surroundings are completely different.

Work with health care professionals, including those from other disciplines, to provide patient-focused care.

This is the ultimate goal of the entire team. The aim is to have a healthy and happy mother and baby. Know important pager numbers and the extensions of those who may come in handy when you need help. Be kind and cordial at all times to all members of the health care team.

Medical knowledge

Residents must demonstrate knowledge about established and evolving biomedical, clinical, and cognate (e.g., epidemiological and social-behavioral) sciences and the application of this knowledge to patient care.

Know and apply the basic and clinically supportive sciences that are appropriate to their discipline.

The competency of medical knowledge in this scenario does not expect you to spew out all signs and symptoms of aortic stenosis and the minutiae of the effects of pregnancy and anesthesia on aortic stenosis. Residents need to *synthesize all information* presented by the patient with the facts spelled out by her lab tests.

This approach should be involved in analyzing all the patient's parameters. Residents need to understand what each parameter actually means. What does the valve size mean? What does that transvalvular gradient of 50 or 60 indicate? How would a diagnosis of

preeclampsia change your approach to this underlying condition?

Now, given all these parameters, the key is to anticipate the possible situations that could get our patient into trouble. Some of the important examples are given in the following list, but surely this list is not exhaustive. Build your own list, system-wise, if need be:

1. What are the patient's hemodynamic parameters, Hb/Hct, and echo findings?
2. What is the obstetric plan? Vaginal delivery or cesarean section? What is the anesthetic plan if a stat cesarean section becomes indicated?
3. Do they expect to use oxytocin or methergine or hemabate? What would be the effects of these drugs on SVR? If you're not sure, look it up.
4. Does the patient wish to have labor analgesia in the form of CSE or epidurals? It is preferable to get an arterial line? This will necessitate intensive care unit monitoring, so is there a bed available?
5. Does the obstetrician anticipate postpartum hemorrhage, any polyhydramnios, premature rupture of the membrane, placenta previa, or a multiple pregnancy, to list just a few possibilities?

So we reiterate: understand the significance of diagnostic values, anticipate circumstances and co-morbidities specific to the parturient, and devise an adaptable plan that will best accommodate the current as well as potential changing status of your patient(s).

Practice-based learning and improvement

Residents must be able to investigate and evaluate their patient care practices, appraise and assimilate scientific evidence, and improve their patient care practices.

Analyze practice experience and perform practice-based improvement activities using a systematic methodology.

So the case went on smoothly, but don't be too quick to pat each other on the back. The enemy of good is better, so reassess if anything can be done better in the future.

Whatever methodology suits you, adopt it. Discuss the case with peers and colleagues. You will get interesting views and some irritating Monday-morning quarterback reviews. Take both in stride; your best critic is your best friend (painful, but true).

Locate, appraise, and assimilate evidence from scientific studies related to their patients' health problems.

"Life is short, so learn from other people's mistakes." Nothing stresses the importance of reading journals and case reports than this saying. Cursing under your breath "damn, I should have read the case report well instead of watching the movie" will not bode well in private practice.

You will not have the time to use Google Scholar. Obstetric emergencies involve a great many *knee-jerk reactions*, reactions that have been passed down through generations because they work well, but without a scientific principle. Time is of the essence; do your homework when you have elective complicated cases. You can assimilate these experiences when dealing with emergencies. Do not count on your iPhone or Amazon's Kindle to spew out facts and myths to help you make an informed decision.

Apply knowledge of study designs and statistical methods to the appraisal of clinical studies and other information on diagnostic and therapeutic effectiveness.

Do you want to practice evidence-based medicine? Actually, you do not have a choice. So you will be better off if you are able to analyze whether you are reading a good study or not. You always thought, "If it is in a good journal, the study has to be good" – but did you realize that all these journals give retractions in small columns of pages of future issues?

Use information technology to manage information, access online medical information, and support their education.

If you are savvy in using iPhone and Twitter, you will be cool with this. For the rest of the population, you have to catch up or else be left far behind. More advancements are online than in print. Get to your university library and ask them to help you with this.

Professionalism

Residents must demonstrate a commitment to carrying out professional responsibilities, adherence to ethical principles, and sensitivity to a diverse patient population.

Demonstrate respect, compassion, and integrity; a responsiveness to the needs of patients and society that supersedes self-interest; accountability to patients, society, and the profession; and a commitment to excellence and ongoing professional development.

In short, be altruistic. Is this really possible? You will encounter patients across a spectrum, from the curious, to the unrealistic, to the hypochondriac. This is where the rubber meets the road.

You are leery of spinals and epidurals in this patient with tight aortic stenosis, but the patient requests a CSE. You should not try to talk her out of it, but rather, attempt to lay out facts and case reports, and allow her to make an informed choice. Try all this in 9 minutes; it is impossible, especially if you have not read the literature properly.

Demonstrate sensitivity and responsiveness to patients' culture, age, gender, and disabilities.

Remember that an Asian or Latin patient with aortic stenosis will be approached differently compared to a Caucasian. Understanding this might help you navigate your preanesthetic visit and titrate your talk based on patient needs. We are not asking you to be racially biased, but rather, to have understanding on a case by case basis and to tailor your interactions. This will help you to be an effective communicator.

Interpersonal and communication skills

Residents must be able to demonstrate interpersonal and communication skills that result in effective information exchange and teaming with patients, their patients' families, and professional associates.

Create and sustain a therapeutic and ethically sound relationship with patients.

Your obstetrician had 9 months to do this. You have probably 9 minutes or less. Because time is against you, act like you know what you are doing. Here we would like to reinforce what we said in the section about patient care: make eye contact; smile; and don't just hear, but listen. Use effective listening skills and elicit and provide information using effective nonverbal, explanatory, questioning, and writing skills.

Though the preceding sentence seems obvious, not doing this is the most common cause for medical lawsuits. It will be well worth your while to actually do this like a quick speech, pausing for moments of contractions.

> Work effectively with others as a member or leader of a health care team or other professional group.

You might think this is a no-brainer, but this might end up being as painful as stubbing your toe. Talk with other team members and establish a good rapport. Be sure to get a specific response from a specific provider to close the communication loop.

As an anesthesiology resident, you may have to take on the role of team leader. It may not be a frequent occurrence, but the willingness to take on a leadership role may be the difference between a living or dead patient. Situations like massive hemorrhage will need change of anesthetic plan, liaison with the blood bank, and planning for safe intensive care unit transfer.

Systems-based practice

Residents must demonstrate an awareness of and responsiveness to the larger context and system of health care and the ability to effectively call on system resources to provide care that is of optimal value.

> Understand how their patient care and other professional practices affect other health care professionals, the health care organization, and the larger society and how these elements of the system affect their own practice.

In obstetric anesthesia, it is important to understand what is going on in the obstetric world. It is important to understand how subtle changes in the local hospital can have wide ramifications to the practice of anesthesia. For example, hospitals might bring in a policy that the patient be given a dose of heparin soon after surgery to commence DVT prophylaxis. If you are using CSE, the accusing finger for delay in heparin dosing is toward anesthesia! Or if you are leaving the epidural catheter in the patient, removal is now an issue that has to be worked out. The resident will need to take active part in obstetric morbidity and mortality meetings to understand how things are viewed outside the anesthesia world.

> Practice cost-effective health care and resource allocation that does not compromise quality of care.

The patient's echo was done last year. Her clinical picture has not changed since that time. Repeating an echo may not be a worthwhile exercise, especially if the hospital has to pay more to get a tech to come and do it on a Sunday night. On the other hand, with the hemodynamic changes of pregnancy, an updated assessment may still be prudent. Residents will need to ask the important question, "Will performing this test tell me anything that I don't already know? If it will, how will that information affect my anesthetic plan?"

> Advocate for quality patient care and assist patients in dealing with system complexities.

Is this really my job? The answer is *yes*. If your hospital policy does not ambulate epidural patients, try to find out why. It may be because of lack of adequate staff to walk laboring mothers. Can the patient's family take care of this issue? Can the family understand their role? This involves breaking the mold and walking the fine rope between policy safety straps and improving patient experiences.

> Know how to partner with health care managers and health care providers to assess, coordinate, and improve health care and know how these activities can affect system performance.

The patient's experience can be enhanced by health care managers coordinating follow-up of this patient by all the involved specialties – cardiology, anesthesiology, and obstetrics – early on in her pregnancy. This will allow the patient to meet and get to know the team involved in her care and have a definitive plan for labor and delivery. Her file, which has logged all hospital visits, labs, imaging, and detailed discussion with the patient, can be pulled out. This avoids repetitive questioning, and outcomes are significantly better when the same teams work over a period of time.

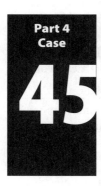

Contributions from the University of Miami Miller School of Medicine under Michael C. Lewis

Cut off at the knees

Ashish Udeshi

The case

Mr. J is a 67-year-old business executive and avid skier. He has a history of hypertension and diabetes and is scheduled to undergo his second total knee replacement. His prior surgery 5 years ago on the other leg resulted in intolerable postoperative pain and an extended hospital course due to the development of a deep vein thrombosis (DVT). To avoid a recurrence of these problems, Dr. Hammer (the orthopedic surgeon) wants his patient anticoagulated and mobilized as soon as possible after the procedure and requests an anesthesiologist with a working knowledge of regional anesthesia.

Patient care

Residents must be able to provide patient care that is compassionate, appropriate, and effective for the treatment of health problems and the promotion of health.

Communicate effectively and demonstrate caring and respectful behaviors when interacting with patients and their families.

Since the total knee replacement is an elective procedure, Mr. J and his family were scheduled to come to speak with the anesthesia team at the preoperative evaluation clinic. This visit occurred 1 week before the scheduled surgery. It was important to make sure that both Mr. J and his family could have the experience of speaking with the anesthesia team face-to-face concerning about his options and participate in the development of his anesthesia care plan.

Gather essential and accurate information about their patients.

His preoperative visit in our clinic kind of acts like a first date. It represents a time during which we have a chance to ask him a series of important questions that relate to our future (our anesthesia relationship).

Since this is his second time undergoing total knee replacement, it is helpful to know what type of anesthesia he received in his previous surgery. Mr. J had no idea what kind of anesthesia was used last time. He didn't even meet his anesthesiologist until minutes before his procedure. All he remembers is that he received some medications, a tube to help him breathe was inserted, and he was knocked out for the whole case. Finally, when he woke up, he was in the postanesthesia care unit with a lot of pain in his leg and was told to push a button for pain medication around the clock. This didn't work and only made him drowsy, nauseous, and itchy. He couldn't get out of bed until 3 days after surgery and somehow developed a clot that required him to be in the hospital for 2 weeks.

Make informed decisions about diagnostic and therapeutic interventions based on patient information and preferences, up-to-date scientific evidence, and clinical judgment.

With Mr. J's description of his past surgery, it seems he underwent general anesthesia and pain management was probably facilitated using a patient controlled analgesia (PCA) pump containing opioids. This wasn't totally effective. He was in significant pain, which, together with the side effects of the opioids, limited his ability to move and rehab quickly, leading to the potential of DVT formation.

Alternative options for postoperative analgesia available to us for this surgery include neuroaxial blockade, peripheral nerve blocks, or intraarticular local anesthetics.

Develop and carry out patient management plans.

While talking with Mr. J and his wife, we discuss the available options, including regional anesthesia, and the option of using peripheral blocks such as a femoral nerve block catheter in combination with a single-shot sciatic nerve block. We explain to him that these techniques can be used either in combination with general anesthesia or as the sole anesthetic technique and that the major benefit of a catheter placement either epidurally or on the femoral nerve lies in the extended pain control.

Counsel and educate patients and their families.

Mr. J responds and says, "I'm a pretty smart and educated man, but I don't speak doctor. Do you mind saying that in English?" It is clearly explained what an epidural catheter is, and how it will block the pain fibers in the areas of his surgery. He responds, "That makes sense, but what was the other thing you mentioned, some femoral thingy?" We explain to him that there are nerves in the thigh and knee that can be blocked specifically where he would feel the most pain. Since he is still at our preoperative evaluation clinic, we show him on a diagram on the wall where the femoral nerve is and exactly how we plan on blocking the areas it supplies. Additionally, we indicate that we can put a catheter in the area surrounding the nerve, which will deliver pain medication from a pain pump for 48 hours after the procedure. It is explained that one of the major benefits of this type of this technique is that it lacks central effects and won't make him drowsy, nauseous, or itchy. He says, "Thanks, doctor, that makes a lot more sense to me and my wife, but how about the blood clot? Dr. Hammer wants me to start taking blood-thinning pills right the next day after surgery and continue this for a few weeks." We explain to him that the medication is probably oral Coumadin, and we confirm this with a phone call to Dr. Hammer's office. After this explanation we jointly agree that a femoral catheter and a single-shot sciatic block represent the best choice because the femoral catheter can be left in place and removed 2 days after surgery, even with the blood-thinning medicine, whereas an epidural catheter would have to come out. Mr. J says, "That's great, doctors, but there has got to be some risk with these nerve blocks." It is explained that the risks of peripheral nerve blocks include nerve injury, local anesthetic toxicity, and hematoma. He is assured that these risks are rare. Mr. J responds, "I understand and I think I would like this technique, but during surgery, I don't want to hear or see a thing." We inform him that this can be accomplished either by making him sleepy or by completely putting him to sleep with a general anesthetic after the nerve blocks have been performed. Mr. J states, "That sounds fantastic, let's

go with the blocks and being completely out during surgery. I appreciate the explanation and look forward to seeing you next week."

Use information technology to support patient care decisions and patient education.

Looking at his prior medical records, we notice that he sees his primary care physician, Dr. Feel-Good, yearly. He suffers from hypertension and diabetes mellitus. His blood pressure has been controlled with low-dose metoprolol twice daily, and he takes metformin for glucose control. He also had an electrocardiogram (EKG), which showed mild left ventricular hypertrophy (LVH) and normal sinus rhythm, and his prior two-dimensional echo showed an ejection fraction of greater than 55%, with mild LVH. His laboratory results included a coagulation panel that was within normal limits. His chest X-ray was normal. Dr. Feel-Good has also provided him with medical clearance for the surgery.

Perform competently all medical and invasive procedures considered essential for the area of practice.

The following week, Mr. J and his wife arrive for the surgery and are in the holding area. His anesthesia plan is reviewed again. He signs his consent, with his wife as a witness. We take him to our regional block room and start an intravenous (IV) line and connect him to a noninvasive blood pressure cuff, O_2 saturation monitor, and EKG leads.

Provide health care services aimed at preventing health problems or maintaining health.

After placing the monitors, prophylactic antibiotics are administered. Dr. Hammer had ordered 1 g of vancomycin IV, and this is started about an hour before the patient is supposed to leave for the operating room, and an infusion is started at the appropriate rate.

An oxygen mask is placed on Mr. J's face. Mild sedation is produced with the administration of some IV midazolam. After performing a time-out to identify the patient and to verify the correct site and procedure, the operator disinfects the femoral crease area with chlorhexidine and then puts on a sterile gown and gloves. An assistant opens the femoral nerve block kit, which contains sterile drapes.

Work with health care professionals, including those from other disciplines, to provide patient-focused care.

Before we started giving the patient any anesthesia, we went to check with Dr. Hammer's team in the operating room to make sure that the surgical site had been marked and that there weren't any delays, and that we were still on the same page regarding Mr. J's surgery. We also verify with the nursing staff that all paperwork is complete, such as the surgical informed consent, and that the history and physical are updated.

Medical knowledge

Residents must demonstrate knowledge about established and evolving biomedical, clinical, and cognate (e.g., epidemiological and social-behavioral) sciences and the application of this knowledge to patient care.

Demonstrate an investigatory and analytic thinking approach to clinical situations.

Now that Mr. J and the entire operating room team are ready, it's time for us to carry out our detailed anesthetic plan. We have chosen to go with a regional technique, with the insertion of a femoral catheter that can aid in postoperative pain via a PCA pump, combined with a single-shot sciatic block as well as a general anesthetic for the duration of the procedure. With the combined technique, we can accomplish two important things for the patient.

The first is prolonged postoperative analgesia with the femoral catheter and a continuous infusion of local anesthetics that lasts for up to 48 hours or even longer. This will reduce the need for systemic pain medications such as opioids and consequently reduce their side effects such as drowsiness, itching, and nausea. The improved pain control will allow Mr. J to participate earlier and more effectively in his physical therapy and will get him out of bed faster, which should reduce his risk of DVT development. In addition, this technique does not interfere with Dr. Hammer's plan for immediate postoperative anticoagulation.

The second is that we can comply with the patient's wish of being "completely out" doing surgery. We can administer a general anesthetic technique in addition to the nerve blocks.

Know and apply the basic and clinically supportive sciences that are appropriate to their discipline.

Mr. J is mildly sedated, his vital signs are stable, and he is positioned supine on the stretcher, with his right femoral crease area disinfected and sterilely draped. Four major nerves innervate the lower extremities: the femoral (L2–L4), obturator (L2–L4), lateral femoral cutaneous (L1–L3), and sciatic nerves (L4–S3). The first three nerves are in the lumbar plexus, and the common peroneal and tibial nerves are continuations of the sciatic nerve from the sacral plexus. With the placement of the femoral catheter and the single-shot sciatic block, we are able to provide analgesia to the knee during the patient's surgery and can prolong these effects with the femoral catheter postoperatively for the femoral and lateral femoral cutaneous nerves.

The first step in placing this block requires us to remember the phrase we learned in first-year medical school, "NAVEL," which helps us identify that the femoral nerve is always lateral to the artery (lateral → medical, nerve, artery, vein, empty space, and lymphatics). The nerve is encased in a sheath that extends from the psoas muscle to just below the inguinal ligament. To find the femoral nerve, we palpate the femoral artery in the femoral crease. The femoral nerve is located about 1 cm lateral to the artery. After some local anesthetic infiltration of the skin, the nerve block needle (a 2-inch, 22-gauge stimulating needle) is advanced, and we look to see if there is any response. We notice an appropriate twitching in the quadriceps, or a "patellar snap." Now we reduce the stimulation to less than 0.5 mA, inject 1 mL of local anesthetic, and when we witness the disappearance of motor activity, we aspirate for blood (which is negative) and then inject 20–30 mL of local anesthetic. An indwelling catheter is then placed at this location. The patient is then turned into a lateral position, and a posterior sciatic nerve block using Labat's classic approach is performed.

Once the nerve blocks have been established, the patient is transferred to the operating room for the induction of the general anesthetic.

Interpersonal and communication skills

Residents must be able to demonstrate interpersonal and communication skills that result in effective information exchange and teaming with patients, their patients' families, and professional associates.

Create and sustain a therapeutic and ethically sound relationship with patients.

Right before general anesthesia is induced we reassure Mr. J. We also explain every step of the anesthesia induction and warn him about the burning sensation that is sometimes associated with propofol injection. After surgery, we will make sure that his pain is well controlled in recovery, and we will follow up on him daily on the floor to manage his postoperative pain and to ensure his progress.

Use effective listening skills and elicit and provide information using effective nonverbal, explanatory, questioning, and writing skills.

At the end of surgery, Mr. J regains consciousness, he is extubated, and transported to the recovery room. The patient is somewhat concerned now, because he can't move his toes. This concern exists despite the fact that he was informed in the preoperative visit that motor block can be associated with our nerve blocks and may last until the next day. We patiently explain this again to Mr. J and his family. The patient and his family are provided with an educational brochure on what to expect from a peripheral nerve catheter and an infusion of local anesthetics. In addition, we question Mr. J about whether he has any other complaints such as a sore throat or nausea, and we inspect the site of our nerve block catheter to make sure that Dr. Hammer and his team didn't pull the catheter out when they removed their drapes and the tourniquet. To make sure the nursing staff knows what's going on with the patient, we give a detailed report before we leave the recovery room and mention the nerve blocks. We also point out to the nursing staff that the nerve block procedure note is in the chart, and we fill out the infusion order form for our nerve block catheter.

Work effectively with others as a member or leader of a health care team or other professional group.

The next morning, when we visit Mr. J for the first time on the floor, the physical therapist had just arrived. He is new in our hospital and not familiar with nerve blocks and nerve block catheters, and is also a little bit concerned that Mr. J can't move his quadriceps too much, while his foot and lower leg have normal strength. We explain to him that this is quite normal but can be improved by reducing the infusion rate of the femoral catheter.

We also locate Mr. J's nurse before leaving the floor and make sure that she knows that we reduced the infusion rate and that Mr. J can have pain medications for breakthrough pain, as ordered. She is reminded that she can contact us at any time if there are any questions regarding Mr. J's care. Finally, we run into the intern working on Dr. Hammer's team. He confuses the femoral catheter with an epidural and wants to make sure that he can start the patient on oral Coumadin. We point the difference out to him and reinforce the importance of the DVT prophylaxis in Mr. J's case.

Systems-based practice

Residents must demonstrate an awareness of and responsiveness to the larger context and system of health care and the ability to effectively call on system resources to provide care that is of optimal value.

Understand how their patient care and other professional practices affect other health care professionals, the health care organization, and the larger society and how these elements of the system affect their own practice.

Mr. J continues to make great progress. He has been able to achieve a lot of flexion in his knee joint on the continuous passive motion machine and is actually able to walk on the second day after surgery. Owing to his rapid rehabilitation, he is able to leave the hospital on the third postoperative day, without experiencing any complications. He states that this second surgery was like "day and night" when compared with his prior experience.

Mr. J's case is a great example of how choosing an appropriate anesthetic plan can affect the outcome of a surgery and influence patient satisfaction and society. In this instance, reducing the patient's pain allowed him to have a shortened hospital stay and minimize excessive hospital costs. Other advantages include:

- The patient does not want postoperative pain or complications such as DVT and wants quick surgery with quicker rehab.

- The surgeon wants to work with someone who is efficient and who can also provide the patient with efficient pain control in the postoperative period.
- The hospital wants patients and surgeons to be satisfied and wants to avoid complications that would result in prolonged hospital stays.

Know how types of medical practice and delivery systems differ from one another, including methods of controlling health care costs and allocating resources.

Mr. J is so happy with "these blocks" that he has another idea. "My son is having ambulatory surgery in an outpatient surgical center next month on his shoulder. Anything that you guys would suggest so he can also have a pain-free experience?" We advise Mr. J that his son should discuss the option of an interscalene catheter placement with the anesthesiologist taking care of him. While an ambulatory center probably does not have an acute pain service following up on patients with nerve block catheters, patients can be sent home with this technique after appropriate instruction, and the follow-up can be done over the phone by the nurses in the ambulatory center. That saves resources, and the patients can still benefit from the advantages associated with the continuous nerve block technique.

Practice cost-effective health care and resource allocation that does not compromise quality of care.

By utilizing nerve block techniques for Mr. J's perioperative care, we were able to be very cost effective. He didn't require any expensive medications to treat nausea and/or vomiting in the recovery room, and also he didn't require pain medications. We did have expenses by using special nerve block needles, placing a nerve block catheter, and infusing local anesthetics. However, Mr. J was able to walk and leave the hospital in record time, without having another DVT, which represents a tremendous cost savings overall.

Advocate for quality patient care and assist patients in dealing with system complexities.

On the second postoperative morning, Mr. J tells us during our visit that the physical therapist hasn't shown up yet, as he had promised the day before. He is a little bit concerned because nobody seems to be able to tell him what's going on, and he is really looking forward to getting out of bed and trying to walk a short distance. We call down to the physical therapy department for the therapist and come to find that they are short staffed due to some unexpected illnesses. We remind the physical therapists of Mr. J, and they assure us that somebody will come in the afternoon to work with Mr. J. The patient is relieved to hear that he has not been forgotten after we explain the circumstances to him.

Know how to partner with health care managers and health care providers to assess, coordinate, and improve health care and know how these activities can affect system performance.

Every month, we attend the meeting of the Operating Room Committee, at which we discuss with hospital administration and our surgical colleagues how things can be made better in our hospital and for our patients. Once we presented scientific evidence on how beneficial regional anesthesia techniques and, consequently, improved pain management can be for our patients and the facility, they were all ears and supported our endeavor.

The main goal of any health care provider or institution is to provide top-quality care to patients. The only way to improve performance is to know what works and what you can do better next time. The best way to judge performance is to follow up with your patient. In this case, we followed up with Mr. J 3 months later. He was pleased to hear from us. He told us that he was progressing with his recovery and that he was looking forward to his next skiing trip over the coming winter.

Additional Reading

1. Raya J, Mikhail M. Anesthesia for orthopedic surgery. In: Morgan GE, Mikhail MS, Murray MJ, editors. Clinical anesthesiology. 4th ed. New York: McGraw-Hill; 2006: 848–860.

2. Peripheral nerve blocks. In: Morgan GE, Mikhail MS, Murray MJ, editors. Clinical anesthesiology. 4th ed. New York: McGraw-Hill; 2006: 324–348.

3. Hollman MW, Wieczorek KS, Smart M, Durieux ME. Epidural anesthesia prevents hypercoagulation in patients undergoing major orthopedic surgery. Regional Anesth Pain Med 2001;26:215–222.

Contributions from the University of Miami Miller School of Medicine under Michael C. Lewis

Neuro

Eric A. Harris and Miguel Santos

The case

The patient is a 29-year-old female with a 3-month history of worsening headaches. She had a witnessed seizure 2 weeks ago which prompted her to seek care in the emergency room. A magnetic resonance image (MRI) done at that time was suspicious for an intracerebral arteriovenous malformation (AVM). This diagnosis was confirmed by a cerebral angiogram performed 4 days after the MRI. The patient is now scheduled for endovascular embolization of the AVM in the neuroangiography suite, and she presents to the preoperative clinic as an outpatient 2 days before her scheduled surgery. She reports that she is otherwise healthy and denies tobacco, alcohol, or drug use. She has been taking phenobarbital 100 mg bid since her seizure.

Patient care

Residents must be able to provide patient care that is compassionate, appropriate, and effective for the treatment of health problems and the promotion of health.

Gather essential and accurate information about their patients.

Is there any other relevant medical history? This should include a full review of systems, a review of prior surgeries and anesthetic events, a review of the patient's medication regimen and allergy history, and a family history.

A thorough physical exam must be completed and documented. Special attention should be paid to the airway exam as well as a neurological exam to discover and document any deficits that might be attributable to the AVM .

Make informed decisions about diagnostic and therapeutic interventions based on patient information and preferences, up-to-date scientific evidence, and clinical judgment.

What laboratory studies are needed for this patient? Because the patient is young and otherwise healthy, coagulation studies are probably not necessary. A chemical profile and liver enzyme levels may be ordered at the discretion of the anesthesiologist; although phenobarbital can cause liver and kidney abnormalities, the short course that the patient has been on (2 weeks) makes these complications unlikely. A complete blood count is also debatable; while many practitioners insist on this study in female patients of childbearing age, this specific procedure does not place the patient at risk for blood loss. If intracranial bleeding does occur, it manifests more as an increase in intracranial pressure, rather than a decrease in circulating volume. A urine pregnancy test is recommended.

Counsel and educate patients and their families.

The patient states that she has not been sexually active for several months and refuses to submit to a pregnancy test. How do you proceed? The patient has the autonomous privilege of refusing to have the test. It is the resident's responsibility to explain the risks of both the anesthetic and the radiation exposure to both the patient and a possible fetus. If the patient remains adamant about refusing the test, the discussion should be fully documented, and a release from liability should be signed by the patient.

Work with health care professionals, including those from other disciplines, to provide patient-focused care.

If the anesthesia resident is unsure of the radiation risks to the patient, a colleague from the radiology department should be consulted.

Provide health care services aimed at preventing health problems or maintaining health.

The patient states that she has been compliant with her oral phenobarbital regimen, but her blood level (drawn 2 days previously) is slightly subtherapeutic. Given the absence of further seizure activity, it is advisable to proceed with the case. Premedication with a benzodiazepine will further raise her seizure threshold. Her neurology or neurosurgical team should be made aware of the lab values.

Medical knowledge

Residents must demonstrate knowledge about established and evolving biomedical, clinical, and cognate sciences and the application of this knowledge to patient care.

Demonstrate an investigatory and analytic thinking approach to clinical situations.

Prior to the anesthetic, the resident must consider the following:

- What do I need to know about this patient's pathology? AVMs can be fragile structures that are exquisitely dependent on the patient's blood pressure parameters. Even a transient spike of hypertension during induction or laryngoscopy could result in rupture and subarachnoid hemorrhage.
- What do I need to know about the surgical and anesthetic management of AVMs (endovascular therapy vs. clipping via open craniotomy)? Since this patient will receive endovascular treatment, a flow-directed microcatheter will be used to access the lesion. During the portion of the procedure in which the neuroradiologist gains access to the AVM, the patient's blood pressure should be kept no lower than the preinduction value as hypotension will frustrate the effort to properly direct the catheter. During the embolization itself, the neuroradiologist will likely request that the blood pressure be reduced approximately 20%. This will slow flow through the AVM and give the liquid embolic material more time to harden within the target area. Owing to the small tortuous vessels that will be navigated, any patient movement could be catastrophic. Therefore adequate neuromuscular paralysis is mandated.
- What do I need to know about the neuroangiography suite? This may be an unfamiliar territory for the resident. He or she

should familiarize himself or herself with the area prior to the patient's arrival. The location of emergency equipment, such as a difficult airway cart and a malignant hyperthermia cart, should be ascertained (systems-based practice [SBP]: work effectively in various health care delivery settings and systems relevant to their clinical specialty). Because many neuroangiography cases are done without anesthesiologists' involvement, the resident may need to coordinate the anesthetic plan with the allied health care providers in the room. The nurse should be aware that continuous suction must be available, and the radiology technicians must confirm that the anesthesia machine and cart will not obstruct the mobile radiology equipment.

Interpersonal and communication skills

Residents must be able to demonstrate interpersonal and communication skills that result in effective information exchange and teaming with patients, their patients' families, and professional associates.

Create and sustain a therapeutic and ethically sound relationship with patients.

The patient is brought to the neuroangiography suite. She is alone and somewhat nervous. This is an ideal time to review the risks and benefits of the anesthetic plan with the patient and solicit any further questions or concerns. When this is complete, confirm with the nurse that all appropriate consents have been signed and witnessed and that a time-out has been performed. Quality patient care includes checking with the neuroradiologist before sedation is given to ascertain if he or she requires any further input from the patient or if a final neurological examination is warranted.

The patient is moved off the stretcher, positioned, and given a sedative dose of midazolam. Again, the benzodiazepine offers a dual advantage of sedation and elevation of the seizure threshold.

Show compassion, integrity, and respect for others.

The patient has calmed significantly, and you are ready to place monitors on the patient. Clearly the ASA standard monitors are required. Additionally, the patient will need an arterial line. Constant beat-to-beat blood pressure monitoring is essential during these procedures, and the arterial line will also facilitate the multiple blood draws necessary for following the ACT. However, because the patient is in good health, the arterial line can be placed after induction to spare her the distress. Central venous pressure monitoring is not standard in these cases unless clinically warranted by coexisting disease. It would not be indicated in this case. An anesthesia awareness monitor (e.g., BIS monitor) will be impossible to use as the strip placed on the forehead will preclude the proper radiographic imaging of the AVM. A neuromuscular twitch monitor is mandatory.

The patient has a 20-gauge intravenous catheter in her right hand. Is this adequate intravenous (IV) access? These cases do not involve large volume shifts or significant blood loss. In fact, it is advisable for us to limit our IV fluids as the patient will be receiving significant boluses of saline and contrast via the femoral catheter. It is not unusual for the neuroradiologist to flush the microcatheter with over 1 L of fluid and 200 cc of contrast per hour; these boluses provide a road map for the flow-directed catheter. That being said, many practitioners feel uncomfortable with only a 20-gauge IV. It would not be unreasonable to heparin lock this site and seek larger access elsewhere. A urinary catheter is mandatory, given the large amount of fluid that will be administered.

The patient is comfortable and ready for anesthetic induction. Baseline vital signs show a sinus rhythm of 72 bpm, a respiratory rate of 8, and a blood pressure of 118/62.

No drugs are specifically contraindicated during this patient's induction. Sodium thiopental or propofol would be good choices for an induction agent but must be titrated to avoid prolonged significant hypotension. Narcotics, if given, should be given sparingly; after the punctures of the arterial line insertion (by the anesthesiologist) and the femoral artery access (by the neuroradiologist), both of which will occur within the near future, there should be no further painful stimuli. A moderate- to long-acting muscle relaxant should be given and must be rebolused as needed (or given via a continuous infusion) until the conclusion of the case.

How should the ventilator settings be managed for this patient? Is the use of N_2O contraindicated? The patient should be maintained with an $ETCO_2$ in the range of 35–40 mmHg. Keeping the patient minimally hypercapnic may allow for dilatation of the intracerebral vasculature, thereby making it easier for the neu-

roradiologist to manipulate the microcatheter. N_2O is not contraindicated, and the small sympathetic boost it provides may help to counteract the hypotensive effects of isoflurane.

Systems-based practice

Residents must demonstrate an awareness of and responsiveness to the larger context and system of health care and the ability to effectively call on system resources to provide care that is of optimal value.

One hour later, the patient is doing well; she remains in sinus rhythm with a blood pressure of 124/60 and is adequately paralyzed. SpO_2 reads 100% on an FiO_2 of 0.3, FiN_2O is 0.7, and isoflurane is set at 1.3. The neuroradiologist informs you that he is preparing to embolize the first branch of the AVM and requests induced hypotension to a systolic of approximately 100 mmHg. How will you accomplish this?

Practice cost-effective health care and resource allocation that does not compromise quality of care.

Many agents can be used to induce controlled hypotension. The key in this case is that the period of hypotension will be transient; the neuroradiologist will inject that material, it will harden within the AVM within 30 seconds, and the blood pressure can then be brought back to its normal range. Therefore we want to choose an agent that is titratable and short acting. Once these criteria have been met, we would also prefer an agent that is easy to prepare and that is inexpensive. Labetolol works well, but the hypotension may last longer than desired. Sodium nitroprusside has a very short duration of action, but unless it is set up in advance, this may be a time-consuming chore. Small doses of nitroglycerine (50 mcg boluses) titrated to the desired blood pressure seem to work well and fulfill all the preceding requirements.

Work effectively with others as a member or leader of a health care team or other professional group.

Three minutes after the injection of the embolic solution, the patient experiences a rapid oxygen desaturation to 72%. The other vital signs remain stable. How do you proceed?

Your primary action should be to inform the neuroradiology team of this occurrence and ask them to temporarily halt the embolization until you can troubleshoot the problem. FiO$_2$ should be increased to 100%. As with any episode of desaturation, you must first investigate the most common culprits such as circuit disconnection, tube occlusion, endobronchial tube advancement, bronchoconstriction, and so on. Once these factors have been ruled out, it is reasonable to conclude that there may be a cause and effect relationship between the injection of the embolic particles and the desaturation, given their close temporal connection. Despite the induced hypotension, it is not uncommon for embolic particles to traverse the AVM and pass into the venous drainage system. From there, they may freely flow until they lodge in the pulmonary microcirculation. (If the patient has a patent foramen ovale or other intracardiac passage, they may enter the arterial circulation.) Depending on the volume and size of the particles that lodge in the pulmonary vasculature, there may be an immediate increase in dead space ventilation and a drop in the oxygen saturation. This is the likely scenario that occurred in this patient. Treatment is mostly supportive and rests on a cornerstone of positive end-expiratory pressure (PEEP). PEEP should be introduced starting at a level of 10 cm H$_2$O and gradually increased if the patient's saturation doesn't respond. Resolution of the desaturation typically occurs within 30 minutes. Although the exact mechanism of recovery is not known, it has been theorized that the increase in pressure proximal to the obstruction forces the opening of collateral circulation, thereby reducing the effect of the dead space ventilation. Large embolic pieces may need to be removed manually via the fluoroscopic introduction of an intraarterial basket or retrieval device.

Accountability to patients, society, and the profession.

Within 20 minutes, the patient's oxygen saturation has returned to 98% on an FiO$_2$ of 0.3 and a PEEP of +5. With your approval, the neuroradiologist continues the procedure and uneventfully embolizes two additional arterioles supplying the AVM. The neuroradiologist announces that he has a meeting to attend and decides to stop the case, despite the fact that the patient still has four arterial feeding vessels that will require embolization. He states that the patient will be rescheduled for a second-phase embolization in 4 weeks. Because the patient is hemodynamically stable and her desaturation has resolved, you question the decision not to complete the entire embolization now. How do you proceed?

It is important that we be advocates for our patients, and at no time is that sponsorship more important than when the patient is under general anesthesia and unable to represent his or her own interests. In this case, it may seem easier not to challenge the neuroradiologist and allow the case to end. Human nature may encourage us to let the patient return in 4 weeks to have the procedure finished; at that time, the case may be someone else's concern. However, good patient care demands that the neuroradiologist be questioned as to whether the best course of action is being pursued. In this case, the decision to abandon the procedure was in fact made on medical grounds and not out of convenience. It is dangerous to embolize a large number of vessels feeding a single AVM during a single session. As each arteriole is embolized, the blood supply that it used to carry to the AVM is rerouted to the remaining feeding vessels. Each feeder that is embolized therefore increases the pressure and volume in its remaining brethren. Embolization of too many arterioles may therefore result in rupture of one of the residual vessels feeding the AVM. Therefore the embolization is done in stages to allow the remaining arterial feeders time to adjust to their increased blood flow and pressure.

The procedure is complete, and the patient is ready for emergence. Are there any special considerations for this patient? The primary factor to consider during emergence is the maintenance of normotension. An infusion of an antihypertensive drug may be necessary for a short period following emergence. As with any neurosurgical procedure, it is valuable if the patient can be relatively alert following emergence so that a neurological evaluation can be performed.

You are called to the neurosurgical intensive care unit 2 hours later to see the patient. She is awake and crying hysterically. She states that she has not been able to see anything at all since she awoke from surgery. Her family is also present, and they are also justifiably concerned about the patient's new-onset blindness.

Participate in identifying system errors and implementing potential systems solutions.

Postoperative blindness is one of the scariest scenarios an anesthesiologist can face. One of the leading causes, retinal artery ischemia, is typically caused by faulty head positioning or continuous pressure on the eyes. In this case, during which the patient was supine and had no pressure applied to the globes, this seems unlikely. We must therefore proceed with a three-way approach. First, we must talk with the patient and her family and assure them that all measures will be taken to solve the problem and restore the patient's sight. Next, we must alert the neuroradiology team and immediately involve them in the resolution. It is also a good time to decide if input from any other specialists would be valuable. Finally, we must review the record to ascertain if this might be an anesthetic complication.

The neuroradiology team is called, and they order a stat computed tomograhy (CT) scan of the head without contrast to rule out a bleed in the occipital cortex. They will meet the patient in the CT suite to evaluate her. A stat ophthalmology consult is also ordered. In the interim, you are called back to the operating room to proceed with your next case. You update the patient and the family and return to the operating room.

After your next case is finished, you return to the intensive care unit to visit the patient. She is now 5 hours postop and still has no vision. You review the results of her CT scan, which reveal no evidence of ischemia or hemorrhage. The ophthalmology team has visited and left the following note in the chart:

1. Pupils 5 mm bilaterally, reactive to light and accommodation
2. Fundoscopic exam normal
3. No nystagmus in response to optokinetic drum rules out hysterical response
4. Suspect idiosyncratic (anaphylactoid) reaction to Optiray 300
5. Recommend methylprednisolone 30 mg/kg IV, then 5.4 mg/kg/hour, as well as increased hydration
6. We will follow up

Know how to partner with health care managers and health care providers to assess, coordinate, and improve health care and know how these activities can affect system performance.

You're not sure you understand their suspicion of an anaphylactoid reaction, so you page the team to discuss it with them. In the meantime, how can you proceed?

Anaphylactoid-mediated blindness to intravenous iodinated contrast is a rare but not unheard of complication. A literature search should be performed, and this would reveal several published case reports describing this phenomenon (PBLI: locate, appraise, and assimilate evidence from scientific studies related to their patients' health problems; use information technology to optimize learning). This condition is caused by the entry of high-osmolality contrast into the occipital cortex, resulting in localized swelling. Although it will correct itself with time, the administration of intravenous steroids and continued hydration will reduce the duration of the complication. Vision should begin to return within 72 hours, starting with the peripheral fields and moving medially.

The patient begins to regain her vision by postoperative day 3 and has a complete resolution of her blindness by postoperative day 5. She is discharged from the hospital the next day.

Participate in the education of patients, families, students, residents, and other health professionals.

Job well done. Owing to the interesting set of complications you faced, you should consider presenting this case at a morbidity and mortality conference.

Additional reading

1. Harris EA. Pre-anesthetic assessment of the patient for endovascular coiling. Anesthesiology News 2005 May; 31(5): 39–42.

2. Barr JD, Lemley TJ. "Interventional neuroradiology" in *Alternate Site Anesthesia: Clinical Practice Outside the Operating Room*. Russell GB, ed. Butterworth-Heinemann, Boston, 1997, p 171–194.

3. Blackburn T, Taekman J, Cronin A, Russell G. "Anesthesia considerations for interventional neuroradiology" in *Alternate Site Anesthesia: Clinical Practice Outside the Operating Room*. Russell GB, ed. Butterworth- Heinemann, Boston, 1997, p 195-223.

Contributions from the University of Miami Miller School of Medicine under Michael C. Lewis

47 Cardiac catheterization laboratory to cardiac operating room

Lebron Cooper and Adam Sewell

The case

An 87-year-old female with severe and symptomatic aortic stenosis was to undergo a percutaneous aortic valve replacement in the cath lab under general anesthesia. Workup included a "tight" AS by transthoracic echo, with an aortic valve area of 0.4 cm^2 and a transvalvular gradient of 85 mmHg. She had a history of HTN, on metoprolol, and NIDDM, controlled with Glucophage, although she had forgotten to refill her prescription after her last doctor's appointment. She was short of breath and had episodes of syncope. Her EKG showed NSR with a HR of 68 bpm. Her labs were all within normal limits, with a HCT of 30 g/dL and a glucose level of 283.

General anesthesia was induced with etomidate and fentanyl. Muscle relaxation was achieved with rocuronium. Anesthesia was maintained with sevoflurane in oxygen. Twenty units of intravenous (IV) insulin were given to treat the elevated glucose level.

Two hours into the procedure, just prior to deployment of the valve, a wire passed across the valve inadvertently transected the wall of the proximal aorta. The patient rapidly decompensated and the blood pressure dropped to 70 mmHg systolic, with a pulsus paradoxus noted with each ventilator breath. Rapid administration of crystalloid solution was initiated, and the blood bank was notified to send 4 units of packed red blood cells.

Cardiac surgeons responded, and the sternum was rapidly opened. In spite of rapid fluid administration, blood pressure continued to fall. Epinephrine was given in 10-mcg boluses to no avail. Open cardiac massage was done by the surgeons, and the patient was transported to the operating room (OR) to control the bleeding, repair the proximal aorta, and complete the AVR.

On arrival to the OR, heparin was administered and the groin was cannulated for cardiopulmonary bypass. The blood bank was called again, but the supervisor stated that the cross-match had "expired," so he

needed another sample of blood. Simultaneously, an ABG previously sent came back with a hemoglobin of 5 g/dL. Rapid infusion of crystalloid was slowed, but blood pressure could not be sustained.

The blood bank was called again, and emergency-release, type O negative blood was requested. The blood bank supervisor refused to release the blood, stating that he needed a cross-match. The anesthesiologist spoke with the supervisor and reiterated the need for immediate release of the emergency type O negative blood. The supervisor was upset and stated that he would only send a form that needed to be completed as a written request for him to release any emergency blood product. The anesthesiologist yelled into the phone, "Don't you know what emergency means?" The blood bank supervisor hung up the phone.

The blood bank was called again, and the supervisor was told to send the type O negative blood immediately. Five minutes later, a blood bank technician came into the OR with a form in hand, but no blood. The anesthesiologist completed the form, and the blood bank tech returned to the blood bank.

The surgeons succeeded in groin cannulation, but the CPB pump had been primed with crystalloid. A repeat ABG showed a hemoglobin of 3 g/dL. The anesthesiologist, in conjunction with the surgeon, decided to delay initiating CPB until blood arrived to prime the pump.

Fifteen minutes later, 4 units of O negative blood arrived, and 2 units were rapidly infused into the patient, while 2 units were added to the CPB prime (crystalloid solution was removed simultaneously). CPB was then initiated, and the case proceeded uneventfully.

On weaning from CPB, epinephrine infusion at 0.5 mcg/kg/minute was administered. An IABP was inserted via the remaining groin, and separation from CPB was successful. Bleeding was controlled following protamine administration, and the chest was closed.

The patient was transported to the intensive care unit.

Patient care

Residents must be able to provide patient care that is compassionate, appropriate, and effective for the treatment of health problems and the promotion of health.

Communicate effectively and demonstrate caring and respectful behaviors when interacting with patients and their families.

This case doesn't actually provide the opportunity to meet and discuss risks and benefits with the patient, but obviously, that would have been necessary prior to inducing general anesthesia. Understanding and explaining the risks of valve replacement and the possibility of failure in the cath lab requiring emergency surgery in an 87-year-old patient is paramount to good clinical practice.

Gather an accurate information about their patients.

The history obtained from this patient was essential in determining the risk the patient would undergo if she decided to and consented to the procedure. A history of hypertension, although not uncommon, was treated effectively with metoprolol, and the heart rate seemed to be well controlled, thus, it was hoped, reducing the risk of myocardial ischemia during general anesthesia. Her diabetes did not appear well controlled, and it was appropriate to obtain the glucose level to determine if there was an opportunity to decrease her risk of neurologic and other organ damage, which may result from high glucose levels. It also provides the opportunity for the physicians to find out *why* she didn't refill her prescriptions. Although she may have told the doctors that she "forgot," in fact, she may not have had the finances, or possibly may not have had transportation, to have her prescriptions refilled. Seldom do patients who have diabetes simply "forget" to refill their prescriptions. This is an example of how you may be able to identify social issues that may be better addressed (at a later time, of course) by involving a social worker.

Finding out about the severity of the aortic stenosis via transthoracic echo findings, aortic valve area, and gradient across the valve allowed the anesthesiologist to make an informed decision concerning induction agents. The choice of etomidate in this case may have prevented a drop in systemic vascular resistance, which could have been catastrophic, as a decrease in SVR in critical AS can lead to acute cardiac arrest secondary to decreased coronary artery perfusion during diastole.

Knowing your patient's medical history can prevent a catastrophic or deadly mistake!

Make informed decisions about diagnostic and therapeutic interventions based on patient information and preferences, up-to-date scientific evidence, and clinical judgment.

The choice to administer insulin to treat an acutely elevated glucose is an example of this. Another example is the reaction in the face of sheer crisis – once the wire transected the aortic root, close observation of decreased blood pressure and a concomitant pulsus paradoxus suggested pericardial tamponade and impending cardiovascular collapse. The decision to call the cardiac surgeons was an example of good clinical judgment, as was the decision to rapidly infuse volume. Evidenced-based literature suggests treatment of tamponade for supporting circulating volume and calling for help in a crisis situation.

Develop and carry out patient management plans.

There is no real time for the development of a plan – you just need to act. Emergency chest compressions and ACLS protocol had to be initiated immediately. Organization to get ready for transport to the OR, with CPR in progress, and ventilation via Ambu-bag were critical. During transport, the plan to eventually go on CPB includes thinking ahead about what you will need as you're going down the hallway. That includes heparin.

Counsel and educate patients and their families.

Prior to the initial procedure, during your preop assessment, would have been the only time to speak to the patient and family because you planned general anesthesia up front. The question is, how much do you tell them? There is always a risk of crisis and surgical intervention, but detailed possibilities frequently frighten patients. Simply informing them of the possibility of a need to go to surgery is usually sufficient.

Use information technology to support patient care decisions and patient education.

Electronic medical and anesthesia records are available and in use in many hospitals. Other textbooks address specifics as well as the advantages and disadvantages of these systems, but suffice it to say here that automated alerts that remind you of critical incidents (such as antibiotic timing or low blood pressure) are a feature that can help you improve patient care.

Perform competently all medical and invasive procedures considered essential for the area of practice.

Obviously, intubation is critical. Bagging the "goose" gets you nowhere, really, really fast! Whether you considered invasive central line monitoring or access was of paramount importance, even if the case had gone smoothly. You can't expect to rapidly infuse large amounts of volume through standard peripheral IV catheters, especially in a crisis situation. Absolutely making *sure* your line is in the central vein is critical. Either transducing the catheter prior to placing a wire or checking placement with ultrasound is mandatory. Had you failed to know the line was in the right place, you would have been in a heap of trouble!

Provide health care services aimed at preventing health problems or maintaining health.

Well, this isn't really a case that meets this part of the competency, huh? Your decision to proceed with general anesthesia was the best example of how you did this. Providing immediate volume and chest compressions, while planning ahead on your trip to the OR to give heparin prior to instituting CPB, also meets this.

Work with health care professionals, including those from other disciplines, to provide patient-focused care.

This is *exactly* what we do in every single case. While the surgeon is the patient's primary doctor, we are the consultant physicians. Surgeons and anesthesiologists are typically the only specialists working so that the primary physician takes care of the patient *simultaneously* with the consultant physician. Also included in the mix are the nurses and techs in the cath lab, followed by the nursing and tech team in the OR. Add in the perfusionists and the transporters, and you have a whole slew of people you work with, all in an interdisciplinary manner.

Medical knowledge

Residents must demonstrate knowledge about established and evolving biomedical, clinical, and cognate (e.g., epidemiological and social-behavioral) sciences and the application of this knowledge to patient care.

Demonstrate an investigatory and analytic thinking approach to clinical situations.

In this case, we have to think fast – everything was going well until the wire "slipped" past the valve and transected the aorta. The rapid decompensation and the pulsus paradoxus are clinical signs that you can use to determine the severity of the injury and plan your next steps.

We know that a wire transected the proximal aorta – what we need to determine is the amount of damage that it caused. So we look at our patient – a sudden rapid decrease in blood pressure and the presence of pulsus paradoxus – what did that pesky wire do? We know that the hemodynamic change and the development of pulsus paradoxus were very rapid – too rapid for just plain bleeding from the aorta.

So now we think back to what pulsus paradoxus is: an exaggeration of the normal change in pulse when the patient inspires. What kind of injury could be caused by a small wire that would give us such rapid development of pulsus paradoxus? If the bleeding were inside the pericardium, then that would cause decreased expansion of the entire heart (because the heart is competing for space with the blood).

We would then see pulsus paradoxus from the LV being able to fill less during inspiration, due to decreased space available inside the pericardium. Neither the right ventricle nor the left ventricle can fill. Our stream of thinking points us toward the conclusion that the patient has a cardiac tamponade.

Rapid developments call for rapid diagnoses. Waiting to get imaging or validation will only delay treatment and may result in patient death.

Know and apply the basic and clinically supportive sciences that are appropriate to their discipline.

For us to be good physicians and treat patients correctly, we need to understand the basic cardiac physiology and be able to detect common physical findings that might be important. In this case, we would need to draw on our knowledge of the following:

- cardiac physiology
- respiratory physiology
- how breathing affects pressures inside the chest
- how respirations affect blood flow
- normal clinical findings (e.g., pulsus paradoxus with SBP change less than 10 mmHg)
- what clinical findings would correlate to which illness

Practice-based learning and improvement

Residents must be able to investigate and evaluate their patient care practices, appraise and assimilate scientific evidence, and improve their patient care practices.

Analyze practice experience and perform practice-based improvement activities using a systematic methodology.

In this case, analysis of your practice experience tells you that you will need three things:

- a CT surgeon to open the chest
- an OR that will have the necessary setup, including cardiopulmonary bypass, for you to perform open heart surgery
- an OR nursing/tech staff, and perfusionists, who can handle an open heart surgery
- a lot of blood and pressors to resuscitate the patient

Unfortunately, this is not the time to work on practice-based improvement activities as you have a serious emergency. However, after this case, it will be important to go over the major issues that occurred in the case and ensure that if something similar to this case happens again, your practice will have all the resources to deal with the situation:

- When performing percutaneous heart procedures, is a CT surgeon available in such an emergency?
- Make sure the necessary equipment is available for crashing on CPB.
- Ensure that a good communication system is in place to allow for quick communication between teams and resources.
- Make sure that when a type and cross is completed, it is valid and the patient has blood readily available.

- Ensure that staff of the blood center understand what emergency release means and perform their functions appropriately.
- Eliminate barriers to patient care in emergency situations such as bureaucratic processes, unnecessary forms, and personnel who cannot perform efficiently during times of emergency.

Locate, appraise, and assimilate evidence from scientific studies related to their patients' health problems.

Ideally, before this procedure, we would need to develop our skills at being able to analyze what literature is good and what literature is flawed and invalid. Before starting the case, it would be good to read about (if there *is* anything to read about)

- anesthesia treatment goals for the patient with AS
- outcome of patients with AS and percutaneous replacement versus open replacement
- common complications that occur during percutaneous repair
- intraoperative monitoring of patients undergoing such procedures
- standard of care for patients who are undergoing such a procedure

Obtain and use information about their own population of patients and the larger population from which their patients are drawn.

When reading through the literature, it's always a good idea to see if it is applicable to the types of patients you deal with. Who are the patients you usually treat? Is the population with which you work different from the population of the literature? Are your patients more likely to have certain issues, and should you take steps to be prepared for such issues? Are the studies you read applicable to your population of patients?

Apply knowledge of study designs and statistical methods to the appraisal of clinical studies and other information on diagnostic and therapeutic effectiveness. As we have gone over before, we should always make sure that the studies we read are performed correctly and have valid significance before we start putting them into practice.

Use information technology to manage information, access online medical information, and support their own education.

With all the available technology, we quickly, and sometimes easily, access a vast amount of resources very quickly. Before the case, we could have done a search to review the literature. Perhaps, if we weren't confident in the physician who was performing the percutaneous valve repair, we could have reviewed the common complications of such procedures and the best ways to manage them.

During this crisis period, we could have an electronic OR record system that would be recording the various vital signs so that when things slow down again later in the case, we can accurately document what occurred as well as what steps we took, and when, to correct these issues.

Professionalism

Residents must demonstrate a commitment to carrying out professional responsibilities, adherence to ethical principles, and sensitivity to a diverse patient population.

Demonstrate respect, compassion, and integrity; a responsiveness to the needs of patients and society that supersedes self-interest; accountability to patients, society, and the profession; and a commitment to excellence and ongoing professional development.

So, in this case, respect and compassion can be demonstrated to the patient in the preoperative holding area. Integrity can be demonstrated by being honest to the patient about risks and benefits of the procedure and the anesthetic. Being mentally alert and ready, having all necessary equipment, and ensuring that all labs and studies are correctly done and ready are just as important. For example, the type and cross could have been confirmed prior to proceeding.

The interaction between the anesthesiologist and the blood bank director could definitely be classified as unprofessional. A better approach would be to keep your cool and speak calmly, even if at that very moment, you don't agree with what you are being told. Listening to the concerns of other health care professionals may help you understand their points of view, and they may help prevent you from making an error that could cause harm to a patient.

Demonstrate a commitment to ethical principles pertaining to provision or withholding of clinical care, confidentiality of patient information, informed consent, and business practice.

We can make sure that the patient is properly consented and that everyone on the team is aware of the details of the patient and is prepared. Making sure that the patient's information is confidential and not left open for anyone to see is not only a HIPAA requirement, it's the right thing to do to protect the patient's privacy. Perhaps most commonly, make sure that our conversations regarding patients and their care are confidential and not conducted in front of people who are not members of the health care team.

Demonstrate sensitivity and responsiveness to patients' culture, age, gender, and disabilities.

Cultural issues come into play more often than most of us notice. Being sensitive doesn't mean that you need to pretend as if you're one of the characters from a Lifetime miniseries; just take note, and take the proper steps. Is the patient from a culture in which they don't discuss medical matters with their family? Perhaps the patient is from a culture in which they don't have choices in medical care, and they don't understand that now, they have options.

The patient's age, gender, and disabilities are very important as well; will the patient have a different set of risks or be unable to perform or understand important tasks that the procedure requires?

Consider putting yourself in your patient's shoes to see what he or she sees: an unfamiliar environment; myriad people interacting with the patient, using words with which the patient may not be familiar, or perhaps in a language that could be the patient's second or third language. It doesn't take a leap of the imagination to see how this could be overwhelming for many people.

Interpersonal and communication skills

Residents must be able to demonstrate interpersonal and communication skills that result in effective information exchange and teaming with patients, their patients' families, and professional associates.

Create and sustain a therapeutic and ethically sound relationship with patients.

Just like you've heard a gazillion times before, wash your hands *before* you see a patient. It not only sets a professional tone, but it's also the right thing to do! Health care workers are notorious for spreading contamination around the hospital, and hospital-acquired infections can increase morbidity and mortality.

During your preop assessment, don't just "pop in" and stay for a second or two, and don't sit in front of the patient with your nose in the chart or writing on a piece of paper at the expense of talking *and listening* to the patient. Make her feel like you care.

Use effective listening skills and elicit and provide information using effective nonverbal, explanatory, questioning, and writing skills.

Listening, as stated earlier, is one of the most important parts of your preop assessment. Writing everything down you see in a medical record, although important for documentation purposes, doesn't give you any information, except what someone else has already obtained. If you listen to the patient, you will frequently learn more from the patient personally, which will make a *major* difference in the patient's care.

Work effectively with others as a member or leader of a health care team or other professional group.

Working with others was addressed earlier, under the "Patient Care" competency section. Teamwork is of utmost importance, and all members of the team should feel equally welcome to raise questions or point out potential hazards or errors that are about to occur. Intimidation by any team member, whether surgeon, cardiologist, anesthesiologist, nurse, or perfusionist, is simply unacceptable, and studies have shown an increase in morbidity and mortality directly related to intimidation in critical settings such as an OR.

Of course, someone has to be in charge in a crisis, just like an airplane pilot is in charge of an airplane, but any team member should feel welcome to bring up concerns with any step in patient care. Arrogance has no place in the OR or any other setting.

In this case, once the crisis in the OR happened, discussions among the cardiologist, surgeons, and anesthesiologist took on a new meaning of "quick consult." Everyone had to be on his or her toes, rapidly acting to stabilize the patient, while consulting the surgeons emergently, giving report of the situation, and communicating effectively the need to urgently move the patient to the OR. Without effective and pointed communication, disaster could just as easily have happened.

Once in the OR, though, communication fell apart. Attempts to obtain O negative, emergency-release blood were unsuccessful, and while the patient circled the drain, the anesthesiologist quickly lost his cool, with a less than appropriate response to the blood bank director, who, although being somewhat obstructionist in this crisis situation, did not deserve to be yelled at over the phone. The upset anesthesiologist, who became condescending and yelled into the phone, only caused a further delay in receiving the blood. The blood bank director should *not* have hung up the phone; an alternative solution should have been sought. However, the anesthesiologist did not know the specifics of the blood bank policies for emergency release of blood and assumed that the blood bank director was an imbecile.

These interactions show specifically how *not* to behave. The delay caused by the personal interactions between the anesthesiologist and blood bank director only put the patient at further risk. It is imperative that although you may not understand or know all the details about an interdepartmental policy or reasoning, you *listen* and state your concerns in a calm, cohesive fashion. Never lose your cool and stoop to denigration of anyone else on the team. Doing so has the potential to cause extreme patient harm, or even death.

Systems-based practice

Residents must demonstrate an awareness of and responsiveness to the larger context and system of health care and the ability to effectively call on system resources to provide care that is of optimal value.

Understand how their patient care and other professional practices affect other health care professionals, the health care organization, and the larger society and how these elements of the system affect their own practice.

There are several examples in this case concerning systems-based practice. The simple fact that general anesthesia was chosen allowed the procedure in the cath lab to proceed without patient movement. That decision further made it easier to immediately respond to the inadvertent placement of the wire through the wall of the aorta by concentrating on crisis management in conjunction with the cardiologist, prompting immediate volume resuscitation and chest compressions as well as activation of the cardiac surgeons.

The challenge incurred with the blood bank offers a great example of how systems in a health care facility can be improved. The form that was required to release O negative, emergency-release blood was an obstacle to receiving the blood. An electronic approach, or a different system implemented to allow release of the blood in such a crisis situation, is begging to be found.

The communication between the anesthesiologist and the blood bank director is an example of how patient care was hindered by their interaction. This suggests that a system solution is needed to address how physicians and other health care professionals approach problems, speak to each other, and learn to manage their emotions in a crisis.

Can a system be sought that doesn't require telephone communication or paper forms that may delay care? These are perfect examples of how to improve interactions, health care delivery, and patient care.

Know how types of medical practice and delivery systems differ from one another, including methods of controlling health care costs and allocating resources.

This case is a great example for showing how medical practices and delivery systems differ from each other. Working within the cath lab, frequently, vigilance may be lacking, but things can quickly go awry without much warning. Seldom in an OR environment are things out of control.

Practice cost-effective health care and resource allocation that does not compromise quality of care.

If you've ever worked in a cardiac catheterization or elecrophysiology laboratory environment, you've seen the loads and loads of catheters used to stent, dilate, ablate, or somehow treat a certain cardiovascular disease. Sometimes it may seem the catheters are used with no consideration of cost, while things in the OR are watched closely. The question from a financial perspective is this: does opening and using another costly catheter that allows successful treatment of the disease, yet prevents a further, more invasive procedure, such as open heart surgery, save money, or does it just add to the overall cost? You have to consider prolonged intensive care unit care, if surgery is your answer, when you make these types of decisions.

Is society better off by providing less invasive care, even at greater initial cost than if the definitive, more costly procedure were done? How can we justify spending so much money on staffing and equipment if we're only doing a nondefinitive treatment? Or by spending that money on staff and equipment, are we avoiding the increased costs in the long run?

Working within the health care system to determine the best approach, which is most cost-effective and has the best patient outcomes, is exactly what this competency is all about. Deciding the proper mix of types of practice allows for best use and allocation of limited and costly resources.

Advocate for quality patient care and assist patients in dealing with system complexities.

As stated earlier, the situation in this case with the blood bank begs for a solution. As the anesthesiologist, the patient's physician, it is your responsibility to follow up on this situation to see if you can come up with, within the scope of practice of the blood bank practitioners, a better system to get blood to the clinical areas much faster in a crisis. Setting up meetings with the blood bank director and/or supervising pathologist may be the first step in identifying challenges associated with release of un-cross-matched blood and offers the opportunity to create and write policies and procedures that meet the goals of the hospital, the requirements of the physicians, and the needs of the patient.

Know how to partner with health care managers and health care providers to assess, coordinate, and improve health care and know how these activities can affect system performance.

Following such a case, reviewing the challenges with other health care providers, such as the surgeons and cardiologists, is really important. Identifying problems encountered and coming to consensus solutions that may prevent those problems from recurring in the future is the goal.

Involving hospital administrators in your discussions with the blood bank and pathologist may reveal budgetary constraints or hospital administrative policies about blood transfusion unknown to you before the incident. Perhaps you find that the blood bank policies have been set to be able to meet demand, based on limited staffing due to budgetary constraints.

Meeting with these folks will give you the opportunity to identify issues that may be solved by updating policies or supporting the need with the financial guys to give greater funding to the blood bank.

Contributions from the University of Miami Miller School of Medicine under Michael C. Lewis

Lap choly in someone great with child

Amy Klash Pulido and Shawn Banks

The case

A 28-year-old female presents for a laparoscopic chole-cystectomy for acute cholecystitis. She is 18 weeks pregnant (G1P0). She has no other past medical history and no allergies. She had general anesthesia in the past for a tonsillectomy at age 7, with no anesthetic complications. The patient was symptomatic and a decision was made to do the operation as conservative treatment had failed. Her obstetrician was contacted regarding fetal monitoring. She recommended that fetal heart tones be monitored immediately prior to induction and then postoperatively as well.

Once the patient was in the operating room (OR), she was laid supine on the OR table with some lateral uterine displacement, and standard ASA monitors were applied. A labor and delivery nurse recorded the fetal heart rate at approximately 160 beats per minute. The fetal monitoring was then discontinued.

The patient received a nonparticulate antacid in the holding area preoperatively. A rapid-sequence induction was performed with propofol, and neuromuscular relaxation was achieved with succinylcholine. Once general anesthesia was attained, the surgery commenced.

At conclusion of the operation, the patient was extubated and taken to the postanesthesia recovery unit. The same labor and delivery nurse was available to monitor the fetal heart beat, and it was documented as being within normal limits. The patient did very well postoperatively and was discharged home from the hospital on postoperative day 2.

Patient care

Residents must be able to provide patient care that is compassionate, appropriate, and effective for the treatment of health problems and the promotion of health.

Gather essential and accurate information about their patients.

Besides the usual preoperative information, a history about the pregnancy was necessary, as well. Had the patient been receiving regular prenatal care? Were there any related complications? Has she been feeling the baby move regularly?

Develop and carry out patient management plans.

Management for a laparoscopic cholecystectomy is not a difficult management plan to formulate. However, adding a second unborn patient into the mix increases the stakes. We will err on the side of safety and avoid nitrous oxide and midazolam. This patient will be treated as a full stomach, and we will reduce the risk of aspiration by giving a nonparticulate antacid and performing a rapid sequence induction. Uterine displacement will be maintained and hypotension promptly treated.

Counsel and educate patients and their families.

The patient was nervous for obvious reasons. What effect will the surgery have on her and, more important to her, the baby? Sensing this, I gave her my routine spiel about what to expect when going back to the OR plus some extra information on anesthesia and pregnancy. The goal is to inform her without unnecessarily burdening her with scary details.

Use information technology to support patient care decisions and patient education.

Every time is the right time for a Google search! Don't forget UpToDate, MD Consult, and PubMed. We have such extensive resources literally at our fingertips; it would be a crime not to utilize these resources.

Perform competently all medical and invasive procedures considered essential for the area of practice.

Luckily, the procedure is a simple one, and the patient does not have any comorbidity that would require more invasive monitoring. For the fetal heart tones, we will have an expert come, just because we can.

> Work with health care professionals, including those from other disciplines, to provide patient-focused care.

This one is easy. We spoke with the patient's obstetrician to get current recommendations as well as to alert her to the fact that the patient was requiring surgery. We were fortunate to have a labor and delivery nurse present to record fetal heart tones immediately before and after surgery.

Medical knowledge

Residents must demonstrate knowledge about established and evolving biomedical, clinical, and cognate (e.g., epidemiological and social-behavioral) sciences and the application of this knowledge to patient care.

> Know and apply the basic and clinically supportive sciences that are appropriate to their discipline.

As inferred from the preceding verbiage, this competency is intimately linked to patient care. One must have core knowledge of the medical problems with which patients present to anticipate problems that may arise in the perioperative setting. Because we understand from embryology that organogenesis is primarily a first-trimester phenomenon, the surgery will be safer during this trimester. Pharmacology teaches us that midazolam is a category D drug, according to the U.S. Food and Drug Administration. This means that there is positive evidence of risk. Investigational or postmarketing data show risk to the fetus. We will avoid this drug. Most important, our medical knowledge tells us that anesthesia is safe. This is because of a Swedish study published in the 1980s. It showed that the risk of congenital anomalies and stillbirths is not increased in women requiring anesthesia versus those having procedures without general anesthesia.

Practice-based learning and improvement

Residents must be able to investigate and evaluate their patient care practices, appraise and assimilate scientific evidence, and improve their patient care practices.

> Use information technology to manage information, access online medical information, and support their own education.

Have there been further studies since the Barash chapter was written? Most likely so.

Clinicians can resort to looking at the current practice guidelines and recommendations. Many review articles will even grade these suggestions. Unfortunately, most are grade 2C recommendations. This means that it is a weak recommendation from moderate-quality evidence. Because few would want to do prospective, randomized, controlled trials on pregnant women, most of the data are retrospective or from animal studies. Case studies are another way to fill in the gaps lacking in the current literature.

The medical student is yearning to learn all about how hormonal changes during pregnancy increase the viscosity of bile and relax the gallbladder, leading to stasis. We also can take time to educate the OR nurse about pregnant women's increased risk for thromboembolism. This way, he or she can understand why we are so insistent about putting sequential compression devices on the patient.

Professionalism

Residents must demonstrate a commitment to carrying out professional responsibilities, adherence to ethical principles, and sensitivity to a diverse patient population.

> Demonstrate respect, compassion, and integrity; a responsiveness to the needs of patients and society that supersedes self-interest; accountability to patients, society, and the profession; and a commitment to excellence and ongoing professional development.

Was it mentioned that this procedure was just getting going at 11:00 P.M.? Your dinner has long since been eaten, and you have been doing cases nonstop since 7:00 A.M. Nonetheless, you down some performance-enhancing drugs, that is, caffeine, and get to work. This competency happens every time a resident makes the patient feel that the resident would much rather be taking care of her than sleeping.

> Demonstrate a commitment to ethical principles pertaining to provision or withholding of clinical

261

care, confidentiality of patient information, informed consent, and business practice.

We take care to interview the patient without family members in earshot for her own privacy as well as to enhance the potential for the whole truth and nothing but.

Interpersonal and communication skills

Residents must be able to demonstrate interpersonal and communication skills that result in effective information exchange and collaboration with patients, their patients' families, and other health professionals.

Use effective listening skills and elicit and provide information using effective nonverbal, explanatory, questioning, and writing skills.

For the anesthesiologist, the preoperative evaluation is where the money is. It is akin to speed dating, in which you have 5 minutes to make a good impression, but instead of getting someone's phone number, you get his or her life in your hands. There is such limited time in which to create this relationship that everything you say or don't say to the patient matters. This patient, in particular, had many questions about anesthetic implications to her baby, which deserved informative answers. The word *doctor* comes from the Latin term for "teacher," and it is especially during these preoperative conversations that we can perform this role.

Systems-based practice

Residents must demonstrate an awareness of and responsiveness to the larger context and system of health care and the ability to effectively call on system resources to provide care that is of optimal value.

Understand how their patient care and other professional practices affect other health care professionals, the health care organization, and the larger society and how these elements of the system affect their own practice.

In this case, with an unborn child hanging in the balance, it is easy to see how this would affect future resources. A child born with a birth defect or severely premature will incur an enormous cost to society at large.

Practice cost-effective health care and resource allocation that does not compromise quality of care.

We reuse whatever items we can, such as the blood pressure cuff, pulse oximeter, and electrocardiogram electrodes, and send her to the recovery room with those, as well. We only set up what we expect to use during the case. This includes not opening five differently sized endotracheal tubes or setting up more than one intravenous bag. Only essential drugs will be drawn up. These small efforts can add up to save hundreds of dollars.

Contributions from the University of Miami Miller School of Medicine under Michael C. Lewis

Renal transplant

Carlos M. Mijares and Sana Nini

The case

A 54-year-old African-American female with a long history of renal failure presents for a kidney transplant. The patient has been undergoing peritoneal dialysis for the last 10 years. Hemodialysis had been attempted in the past but she had problems with infection and thrombosis in the fistulae. On admission laboratory investigations revealed a BUN 80, creatinine 5.0, and potassium 4.0 mEq/L. An admission electrocardiogram revealed normal sinus rhythm with left bundle branch block and left ventricular hypertrophy. Physical examination was unremarkable. She was accompanied to the hospital by other family members.

Anesthesia management of renal transplants requires a thorough understanding of the metabolic and systemic abnormalities in end-stage renal disease (ESRD). Knowledge concerning transplant medicine and expertise in managing and optimizing these patients produce the best possible outcome. The related co-morbid conditions increase the complexity of anesthesia and perioperative morbidity and mortality. Hence, optimal anesthesia management of these patients includes a multidisciplinary approach with well-designed strategies.

Patient care

Residents must be able to provide patient care that is compassionate, appropriate, and effective for the treatment of health problems and the promotion of health.

Following an initial history and physical, the patient was confirmed for renal transplant. All investigations were reviewed. In the preoperative holding area the patient was interviewed with her family members. Risks, benefits, and options concerning anesthesia technique were outlined to both the patient and the family. Having considered all the presented issues, an anesthetic plan was developed with the agreement of the patient. It was agreed to administer general anesthesia. Regional anesthesia for post operative pain control was refused as it was assumed that the risks (given her renal failure) were too high. All consent documentation was signed and witnessed.

In the holding area a peripheral IV was started and standard premedication (midazolam 2 mg and glycopyrrolate 0.3 mg) was administered. A nonparticulate antacid (bicitra) was administered to increase gastric pH and reduce the risk of acid aspiration on induction. Once an initial time-out was completed the patient was transferred to the operating room.

Standard ASA monitors were applied. Intraoperative monitoring included heart rate, noninvasive blood pressure, oxygen saturation, end tidal CO_2 and electrocardiogram in all patients. Peripheral intravenous access was secured in the hand opposite to the pre-existing fistula and induction of anesthesia was done with propofol (2 mg/kg-1). A modified rapid sequence technique used. Neuromuscular blockade was maintained with rocuronium (0.6 mg/kg). The patient was intubated and ventilated. Anesthesia was maintained with 40% N_2O in oxygen supplemented with 1–2% isoflurane with fresh gas flow of 2 l/min. Analgesia was maintained with fentanyl (2–5 mcg/kg) and at the end of the case morphine was administered for long-term pain control (0.1 mg/kg).

The patient was intubated easily using a glide scope. It was decided to use both continuous invasive arterial pressure and central venous line (CVP) monitoring. The CVP line was placed in the right internal jugular vein. Strict asepsis was maintained at all times. Normal saline was administered during the surgery. It wasn't necessary to give colloid or blood.

Immunosuppressant therapy was given. Surgery lasted approximately 5 hours. Following reperfusion urine output and arterial blood gas values (ABG's) were within acceptable values. The patient was extubated to the intensive care unit.

The patient had no complications. A chest x-ray was normal. The patient was discharged after 5 days.

Medical knowledge

Residents must demonstrate knowledge about established and evolving biomedical, clinical, and cognate (e.g., epidemiological and social-behavioral) sciences and the application of this knowledge to patient care.

Every year in excess of 16,000 patients undergo kidney transplant in the United States. This number is expected to increase. Because the 1-year survival rate for the majority of transplant recipients is around 90%, an increasing number of transplant patients present like our patient in a semi-elective fashion for surgery. Transplantation provides an almost normal life and outstanding rehabilitation compared to dialysis and as in our case is the favored means of treatment for end-stage renal disease patients.

It would be expected that if the resident physician had not administered anesthesia for a renal transplant before they would read and review any institutional protocols for patients undergoing transplant surgery. Residents should also review biochemical sciences pertinent to the case.

Practice-based learning and improvement

Residents must be able to investigate and evaluate their patient care practices, appraise and assimilate scientific evidence, and improve their patient care practices.

The resident had done enough prior transplants to feel comfortable. **In our case** the resident had a strong understanding of immunosuppressants; sterility; whether to extubate at the end of surgery; using an ABG to monitor a patient's optimal physiology, particularly around the events of reperfusion; and being vigilant about urine output throughout the case.

In this transplant case, the resident physician had reviewed all scientific evidence and had simulated and planned for general anesthesia, keeping in mind sterility when placing invasive lines. The patient was aware of better outcomes with living related donors than cadaveric donors. The resident had reviewed outcomes of related procedures, rejections, and complications post transplant. The resident continued to monitor the patient postoperatively.

Professionalism

Residents must demonstrate a commitment to carrying out professional responsibilities, adherence to eth-

ical principles, and sensitivity to a diverse patient population.

Resident physicians should follow the guidelines below:

1. interact in a professional manner with other members of the health care team intensive care unit
2. wash hands before and after examining the patient
3. maintain patient confidentiality and respect patient privacy
4. demonstrate empathy and compassion for the patient
5. prior to seeing the patient review current management practices and research in transplant anesthesia
6. act in a professional manner when coming in contact with patients
7. have the patient's safety in mind at all times
8. develop ethically based relationships

Interpersonal and communication skills

Residents must be able to demonstrate interpersonal and communication skills that result in effective information exchange and teaming with patients, their patients' families, and professional associates.

Residents should do the following:

1. interact with the patient, family, and other members of the health care team
2. act in a professional manner when coming in contact with patients
3. have the patient's safety in mind at all times
4. explain all issues involved with surgery and anesthetic care
5. work effectively with transplant surgeons and medical staff before, during, and after procedures

If, after surgery, the resident sees the family in the hospital, and the family is requesting information, the resident should show empathy and explain to the family that the procedure went well from his or her point of view on the anesthetic care team, but further details on the surgery should be discussed with the surgical attending.

Systems-based practice

Residents must demonstrate an awareness of and responsiveness to the larger context and system of health care and the ability to effectively call on system resources to provide care that is of optimal value.

Residents should do the following:

1. remain focused on the care of the transplant patient, including preoperative visits and evidence-based knowledge of organ transplants – in this case, a kidney transplant due to ESRD, which can have different etiologies (e.g., polycystic kidney disease)

2. provide the most sterile environment possible

3. ensure safe positioning of patients, especially diabetic patients, who may already have preexisting neuropathies, to avoid deterioration of marginal nerve function

4. provide a safe environment so that the patient is not injured by anesthesia procedures (like line placement) by using an ultrasound device and airway devices, particularly for patients with a history of difficult airways

5. review previous anesthesia records and the patient's history of blood transfusions

6. recognize that this transplant will have an impact on the patient in both the short term and the long term

7. ensure that organs are preserved as well as possible, according to the resident's current level of training, and show perseverance in ensuring the patient's well-being

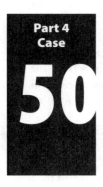

Contributions from the University of Miami Miller School of Medicine under Michael C. Lewis

50 Surprise! It's a liver and kidney transplant

Michael Rossi and Sujatha Pentakota

The case

A 16-month-old girl with end-stage renal disease due to primary hyperoxalosis is undergoing a combined liver and kidney transplant. The child's weight is 6.2 kg (less than the fifth percentile), and her overall state of health is poor. Her parents had traveled from Mexico for the surgery. They do not speak English, and their native language is Spanish. The family's religion is Judaism, and they are rigorously observant. The child is going to surgery late on Friday afternoon (the upcoming sabbath). The anesthesiology team had been unaware of this patient until the day of surgery.

Patient care

Residents must be able to provide patient care that is compassionate, appropriate, and effective for the treatment of health problems and the promotion of health.

Communicate effectively and demonstrate caring and respectful behaviors when interacting with patients and their families.

We conducted a thorough preoperative interview with the family, with the help of a Spanish-speaking colleague. Informed consent was obtained. We were honest with the parents and conveyed to them the major risks involved in the surgery, including the risk of death.

Gather essential and accurate information about their patients.

We reviewed the patient's medical record and obtained the results of the laboratory tests and various diagnostic imaging studies that had been performed. We noted that the preop blood chemistry was acceptable. We ascertained that the patient had undergone hemodialysis prior to surgery.

We performed a PubMed search to understand better the pathophysiology of primary oxalosis as it is a rare metabolic disorder. The girl had type I primary hyperoxalosis, for which the treatment of choice is combined liver and kidney transplant.

We discussed the plan with the surgeons, pediatric nephrologists, and other subspecialists involved.

Make informed decisions about diagnostic and therapeutic interventions based on patient information and preferences, up-to-date scientific evidence, and clinical judgment.

We were informed of this patient in the immediate preoperative period. We decided to proceed as the organs were immediately available, and given that we were at a major transplant center, we understood the difficulty of procuring a compatible organ for a small child (two, in this case).

During the intraop period, we performed regular arterial blood gas (ABG) analyses and acted on them. For example, peak inspiratory pressures were reduced to decrease tidal volume and increase $PaCO_2$, and calcium and PRBC were given to correct hypocalcemia and low hematocrit. Along with the initial ABG, a blood sample was drawn for thromboelastography.

Develop and carry out patient management plans.

After induction, we placed radial and femoral arterial lines. We decided to use the patient's hemodialysis catheter as a central line as a preop ultrasound had revealed thrombosis in the internal jugular veins. After the IVC clamp was on, the surgeons began pushing on the diaphragm, causing difficulty in effectively ventilating the patient, and we communicated to the surgeons the problem we were having. As the surgery progressed and the patient's hemodynamic status deteriorated, we called for help. Another pediatric anesthesiologist and CRNA came to the operating room. Intraop, the patient developed pulmonary edema and had a low hematocrit. We did an exchange transfusion with packed red blood cells to increase the hematocrit without increasing the blood volume. On reperfusion, the patient developed severe hyperkalemia, resulting in cardiac arrest. Defibrillation was ineffective. The surgeons attempted direct cardiac massage.

Counsel and educate patients and their families.

We impressed on the parents the risks involved with the surgery – the probable need for intensive care unit care, the prolonged rehab that would be involved, and the significant probability of death.

Use information technology to support patient care decisions and patient education.

Primary hyperoxalosis is a rare, autosomal, recessive genetic disorder. We did a literature search on PubMed and reviewed the Mayo Clinic hyperoxalosis registry to understand better the varied presentations of this disorder. We reviewed the patient's ultrasound imaging to establish the patency of the neck vessels because the patient would need an internal jugular central line for CVP monitoring, for blood product transfusion, and for resuscitation.

Perform competently all medical and invasive procedures considered essential for the area of practice.

In the operating room, the preop ASA standard monitors were placed. Postinduction, we established a radial and femoral arterial line for monitoring.

Provide health care services aimed at preventing health problems or maintaining health.

Postinduction, we gave the patient preop antibiotics. Preincision, we held a final time-out, per our hospital guidelines. We started immunosuppressive agents in a timely manner. We observed barrier precautions and asepsis in placing all lines.

Work with health care professionals, including those from other disciplines, to provide patient-focused care.

Preop, we tried to contact the nephrologists to discuss our concerns about two adult organs being transplanted into a 1-year-old girl and the necessity of having an intraop renal replacement strategy, if required. We contacted the postanesthesia care unit attending and ascertained that they had a bed for the patient for postop monitoring and care. Intraop, when the patient

developed refractory hyperkalemia, we attempted to contact the nephrologists again for CVVHD. Throughout the case, we were in constant communication with the surgeons.

Practice-based learning and improvement

Residents must be able to investigate and evaluate their patient care practices, appraise and assimilate scientific evidence, and improve their patient care practices.

Analyze practice experience and perform practice-based improvement activities using a systematic methodology.

Our experience with this patient made us realize the importance of preoperative planning and a multidisciplinary approach to optimize patient care. We realized the need to establish a better bereavement process, especially for families with diverse cultural and linguistic backgrounds.

Professionalism

Residents must demonstrate a commitment to carrying out professional responsibilities, adherence to ethical principles, and sensitivity to a diverse patient population.

Demonstrate respect, compassion, and integrity; a responsiveness to the needs of patients and society that supersedes self-interest; accountability to patients, society, and the profession; and a commitment to excellence and ongoing professional development.

We informed the parents in a nonjudgmental manner of the realistic probability of death involved in the case. We understood the significance of the linguistic and cultural barrier that existed in this situation. Hence we took advantage of the help of one of our Spanish-speaking colleagues in our discussions with the parents.

Interpersonal and communication skills

Residents must be able to demonstrate interpersonal and communication skills that result in effective information exchange and teaming with patients, their patients' families, and professional associates.

Create and sustain a therapeutic and ethically sound relationship with patients.

We need to understand the concerns of the family as a whole while taking care of pediatric patients. We need to appreciate the level of understanding and emotional involvement of the family. It is imperative that the family understand the probability of various risks involved in each case. In the present situation, we did our best to convey these to the parents. At the end of the case, we did our best to explain the outcome gently to the parents, with the help of a Spanish-speaking colleague. We honored their request to remove all the lines before transferring the patient to the mortuary. We accommodated their wishes for postmortem care and made arrangements to contact the Jewish chaplain.

Systems-based practice

Residents must demonstrate an awareness of and responsiveness to the larger context and system of health care and the ability to effectively call on system resources to provide care that is of optimal value.

Understand how their patient care and other professional practices affect other health care professionals, the health care organization, and the larger society and how these elements of the system affect their own practice.

An interdisciplinary case review was performed after this case. The transplant service held an intradepartmental case review. We had a departmental M&M so that we could share our experience with our colleagues and get their input in an attempt to improve the outcome of similar cases in the future.

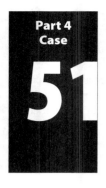

Contributions from the University of Miami Miller School of Medicine under Michael C. Lewis

Left lower extremity pain

Omair H. Toor and David A. Lindley

The case

The patient is an 81-year-old female with an onset of left lower extremity pain that began 1 month ago. The patient states that her pain radiates down to the toes on her left foot and describes the pain as sharp and full of pressure; she denies any burning qualities. The patient sustained a fall 3 months ago and suffered a pelvic fracture at that time. The primary care team ordered a magnetic resonance image (MRI) last night.

The patient had a CVA between 2 to 3 years ago, affecting left lower extremity motor powers. Her past history includes hypercholesterolemia, HTN, GERD, and a fall with pelvic fracture 3 months ago. Her past surgical history includes cholecystectomy and a cesarean section. Medications include ASA 81 mg po qd, Lipitor 40 mg po qd, Aciphex 20 po qd, and HCTZ 25 mg po qd. The patient has an allergy to codeine.

The patient denies a history of alcohol or drug abuse. She quit smoking 30 years ago, after 40 pack years. She lives with her daughter and grandchild. Previously, she was a housewife, but she has been widowed for 20 years.

Vital signs are as follows:

temperature, 97.0°C
pulse, 88 beats per minute
respiratory rate, 20 breaths per minute
blood pressure, 138/80
height, 5 feet 8 inches
weight, 79 kg

In general, the patient is alert, awake, and oriented. Her gait is antalgic on the right, and her stance shows postural landmarks aligned. Bilateral manual muscle testing reveals 5/5 in the L2, L3, L4, L5, and S1 muscle groups. Bilateral L2 to S1 dermatomes are intact to light touch. There is no rash or allodynia. Paresthesias are noted in the stocking distribution of the distal third of the leg and foot on the left. Negative straight leg raising tests bilateral lower extremities. There is no

tenderness, concordance, or reproduction of pain with palpation of the lower extremities.

A lumbar spine MRI dated this week shows multi-level degenerative disc disease and multilevel degenerative joint disease with mild multilevel central canal stenosis. Pelvic fractures are noted in computed tomography.

Patient care

Residents must be able to provide patient care that is compassionate, appropriate, and effective for the treatment of health problems and the promotion of health.

> Communicate effectively and demonstrate caring and respectful behaviors when interacting with patients and their families.

Interpreters should be used when indicated for effective communication. We would introduce ourselves to the patient and family members who are present before starting a careful history and physical exam. Eye contact and a handshake help to reassure the patient and family members that they have your complete attention and interest.

> Gather essential and accurate information about their patients.

Essential information here includes a careful history regarding when the pain started, the quality of the pain, the intensity of the pain, positional provocative factors, positional alleviating factors, associated symptoms, past treatment efficacy, failures, and side effects. History should also include circumstances around the fall. Was it a trip and fall, or a loss of consciousness and a fall? Was it a fall and then a loss of consciousness? On physical examination, essential information includes gross observation, stance, gait, palpation, range of motion, concordance, muscle strength testing, reflexes, sensory testing, and provocative maneuvers. Imaging studies should then be reviewed to help support the resident's impression from history and physical examination. In this case, pertinent imaging studies may include past brain imaging, plain films, and lumbar imaging.

Develop and carry out patient management plans.

Because, in the detailed history taking, the patient reported loss of consciousness and the subsequent fall 2 months ago, a portion of the workup will include metabolic, neurologic, and pharmacologic etiologic causes in coordination with primary care physicians and other specialists on the team. Further brain imaging may be indicated to evaluate for evolving cerebrovascular events that may contribute to a central pain state.

We reviewed past plain films of pelvic fractures for correlation with any palpatory concordance with our physical exam. In this case, there was no concordance with the previous fracture sites and palpatory findings.

We reviewed a recent lumbar spine MRI. In this case, MRI findings included multilevel degenerative disc disease and degenerative joint disease of the lumbar spine. No significant disc displacements were noted. Mild multilevel central canal stenosis was noted. No significant neuroforaminal stenosis was noted.

Because evidence from the history and physical examination suggests central pain syndrome, which often presents a few years after stroke, we will start central pain syndrome therapies. We will start low-dose gabapentin and plan for future dose optimization. We may consider a serotonin-norepinephrine reuptake inhibitor, which are used in central pain syndromes, among other pain syndromes. However, consideration must also be given to the patient's age and the side effects of such drugs in the elderly. The axiom "start low and go slow" is a good rule of thumb for titration and optimization of the dose.

Counsel and educate patients and their families.

In each case, level of education and cognition needs to be assessed and the terms used adjusted accordingly. Educating the patient and/or family in this case may sound something like this: "There are several possible causes of your pain, but we think the most likely cause is pain that occurs after damage to the brain after a stroke. This type of pain may start even several years later after the stroke, as we believe is your case. This is called *central pain syndrome*. The treatment is primar-

ily medications, in addition to physical therapy and cognitive therapies, which are therapies usually conducted with a psychologist who specializes in pain." Use of models and diagrams is also helpful, and drawings used in such discussions are suitably added to medical records.

Use information technology to support patient care decisions and patient education.

If the patient and/or family members have Web access, then we would provide Web addresses for treatment of central pain syndrome. A support group would also be helpful in designing the treatment plan along with the physician and would provide emotional support.

Perform competently all medical and invasive procedures considered essential for the area of practice.

Competence here is demonstrated by not performing an interventional modality that is not indicated for central pain syndrome. As far as demonstration of competence of medical modalities goes, this can be achieved by discussing the risks and benefits of opioid and adjuvant therapies.

Provide health care services aimed at preventing health problems or maintaining health.

As pain physicians, we would make certain that the patient is being followed by a primary care physician or neurologist for health maintenance and to help prevent a repeat stroke.

Work with health care professionals, including those from other disciplines, to provide patient-focused care.

The role of other health care professionals is essential to working as a team to provide care for the patient. This requires verbal and written communication with other physicians to form a complete and thorough treatment plan and preventative health plan.

Medical knowledge

Residents must demonstrate knowledge about established and evolving biomedical, clinical, and cognate (e.g., epidemiological and social-behavioral) sciences and the application of this knowledge to patient care.

Demonstrate an investigatory and analytic thinking approach to clinical situations.

The patient was referred for "pain status post-fracture." The investigatory and analytically thinking physician will examine the other possible causes of the patient's pain. After careful history and physical examination, the resident will identify the differential diagnoses and the most likely diagnosis, as supported by evidence.

Know and apply the basic and clinically supportive sciences that are appropriate to their discipline.

Understanding and recognizing the pattern of pain and the sequence of events is key to identifying the source of pain in this patient. Her previous pelvic fracture and degenerative disc disease can be red herrings. It is important to recognize the characteristics of shooting, burning, and electric pain associated with neuropathic pain so that the appropriate medications and therapies can be initiated.

Practice-based learning and improvement

Residents must be able to investigate and evaluate their patient care practices, appraise and assimilate scientific evidence, and improve their patient care practices.

Analyze practice experience and perform practice-based improvement activities using a systematic methodology.

Medical diagnostics and therapeutics are continuously changing. Residents need to implement and augment their lifelong learning behaviors. This includes continuous perusal of the literature, efficient knowledge and use of medical informatics, problem solving, and utilizing resources such as contacting and consulting colleagues. Applied to this case, recognition of the central pain state leads to further questions as to appropriate and inappropriate treatment modalities. With a quick look at review articles or consultation with an experienced colleague, one will find that appropriate therapy includes "polypharmacy involving combinations of physical and psychological therapies, antidepressants, anti-seizure medications, NMDA antagonists and opioids."

Locate, appraise, and assimilate evidence from scientific studies related to their patients' health problems.

As mentioned previously, a quick PubMed search will reveal a good review article on central pain, with a discussion of several medical modalities as well as potential motor cortex stimulation.

Obtain and use information about their own population of patients and the larger population from which their patients are drawn.

This patient is from the so-called elderly population. Consideration has to be given to obtain appropriate pain goals and to "start low, go slow" titration. Particular attention should be given to organ systems and systemic effects of medications. Comorbidities should be reviewed. In particular, many opioid and adjuvant pain medications can contribute to cognitive and somnolent effects much more in the elderly than in younger populations. Elderly patients are much more sensitive to the anticholinergic effects of cyclobenzaprine, tramadol, tricyclic antidepressants, and other serotonin-norepinephrine reuptake inhibitors.

Apply knowledge of study designs and statistical methods to the appraisal of clinical studies and other information on diagnostic and therapeutic effectiveness.

Analysis of study designs and statistical methods in the literature is needed to interpret their validity to implement this information into our practice management. A review of these studies and methods can guide our course of various therapies and modalities. A bit old but still helpful study of central pain compared a serotonin-norepinephrine reuptake inhibitor, amitriptyline, to both placebo and other active agents [1]. This was a double-blind, randomized cross-over study. One should take into account, however, that although statistical significance was achieved, this study involved only 15 patients. Also, titration was performed up to an amitriptyline dose of 75 mg. One should take such limiting factors into account when initiating and titrating in their own patients.

Use information technology to manage information, access online medical information, and support their own education.

The resident should be well versed in the use of medical informatics systems such as PubMed. Journal access is frequently granted through institutional library sources. This access information should be at the resident's fingertips for access to literature at all times, whether at home or work. For example, at the time of this writing, a PubMed search for "central pain" yields 35 items. A quick glance at these will show that some are pertinent, such as review articles titled "Efficacy and Safety of Motor Cortex Stimulation for Chronic Neuropathic Pain" [2] and "Lamotrigine in the Treatment of Pain Syndromes and Neuropathic Pain" [3], as well as some articles that are not pertinent, such as "Nerve Growth Factor of Red Nucleus Involvement in Pain Induced by Spared Nerve Injury of the Rat Sciatic Nerve" [4]. The latter is obviously not relevant due to its involvement of an animal model of *peripheral* nerve injury.

Professionalism

Residents must demonstrate a commitment to carrying out professional responsibilities, adherence to ethical principles, and sensitivity to a diverse patient population.

> Demonstrate respect, compassion, and integrity; a responsiveness to the needs of patients and society that supersedes self-interest; accountability to patients, society, and the profession; and a commitment to excellence and ongoing professional development.

We would wash our hands and then introduce ourselves to the patient and family members who are present before starting a careful history. Our main duties are to respectfully serve the patient and to help provide whatever needs are required. It is important to show empathy and to be easily accessible to the patient and staff. Accountability requires you to be up to date in your CME hours and licensing. Education is an ongoing process, which requires staying current with the literature and attending educational events and meetings.

> Demonstrate a commitment to ethical principles pertaining to provision or withholding of clinical care, confidentiality of patient information, informed consent, and business practice.

A selfish or unethical position may be to provide higher reimbursed services for a diagnosis that is typically not amenable to such therapy. In this case, if the impression is one of mainly central pain etiology, then neuraxial and/or peripheral nerve blocks would not be indicated. If there was a clinical suspicion of multifactorial etiology, then in that case, after discussion of risks and benefits with the patient and referring physicians, possible interventional techniques would be indicated.

> Demonstrate sensitivity and responsiveness to patients' culture, age, gender, and disabilities.

Enhanced communication can improve health outcomes, better patient compliance, reduce medicolegal risk, and improve satisfaction of clinicians and patients. Empathy is an important aspect of the physician-patient relationship. Empathy extends understanding of the patient beyond the history and symptoms to include values, ideas, and feelings, regardless of the patient's background.

Interpersonal and communication skills

Residents must be able to demonstrate interpersonal and communication skills that result in effective information exchange and teaming with patients, their patients' families, and professional associates.

> Create and sustain a therapeutic and ethically sound relationship with patients.

The chronic pain clinic is a good place to create and sustain this type of relationship. It is important to establish a good working rapport with the patient as well as family members and primary care and specialist physicians on the patient's team. This will ultimately lead to better gain of information and result in improved patient care. In some instances, communication with family members and physicians is more than just a good idea. When prescribing long-term chronic opioids, it is a medical and legal responsibility to obtain records to review for any suggestion of past compulsive use, abuse, or diversion activities. The chronic pain clinic is an excellent venue in which to utilize your longitudinal follow-up skills.

Use effective listening skills and elicit and provide information using effective nonverbal, explanatory, questioning, and writing skills.

One should dedicate sufficient and adequate time and attention to all patients. The history interview can be directed but should not be truncated prematurely. In the chronic pain population, however, one should not rely solely on patient history in some situations. For instance, cancer patients and geriatric patients tend to underreport their pain. In this case, this geriatric patient may underreport her pain. Reasons geriatric patients in general may underreport their pain are many and include the following:

1. When visiting with other specialists or primary care physicians regarding many issues, the pain issue per se becomes a side point.
2. Geriatric patients may accept pain as normal.
3. Patients may feel that an honest portrayal of their pain would lead to their being labeled as a "complainer."
4. Patients may feel anxiety regarding possible treatment for their pain.
5. Patients may feel scared that they will be forced into certain pain therapies that they do not want, be they medical, physical, cognitive, or interventional modalities.
6. Geriatric patients may have cognitive dysfunction resulting in poor history or poor communication. Family members sometimes help remind these patients of their actual complaint frequency.

Work effectively with others as a member or leader of a health care team or other professional group.

The pain physician should work in a multidisciplinary or interdisciplinary model. For instance, a pain physician who provides medical and interventional modalities should keep in mind, and refer, when appropriate, cognitive, physical, and complementary alternative modalities. A chronic pain physician should also be aware of clinical scenarios when communication and referral to other specialists is needed such as to rheumatology, gynecology, radiology, surgery, or oncology.

Systems-based practice

Residents must demonstrate an awareness of and responsiveness to the larger context and system of health care and the ability to effectively call on system resources to provide care that is of optimal value.

Understand how their patient care and other professional practices affect other health care professionals, the health care organization, and the larger society and how these elements of the system affect their own practice.

Health care spending comes from a number of sources, including Medicaid, Medicare, private insurance, and out-of-pocket expenditures, which include premiums and deductibles paid by those with insurance and full medical payments paid by those without insurance. The importance of using treatments that have a reasonable chance to help is essential to help keep the costs of health care down.

Know how types of medical practice and delivery systems differ from one another, including methods of controlling health care costs and allocating resources.

One option for slowing the increasing trend in health care spending is to increase the efficiency of health care delivery. In pain management, this can be achieved by adapting the use of new technologies. Increased efficiency can be achieved by training in ultrasound instead of fluoroscopy – this can lead to safer environments and reduced radiation exposure, allowing for an increased potential for bedside or office-based procedures that were previously done in the operating room. Another example of this is adapting e-prescribing practices. Evidence suggests that this reduces time spent by pharmacists and physicians in correcting errors and reduces the costs associated with uncorrected errors [5].

Practice cost-effective health care and resource allocation that does not compromise quality of care.

The "see one, do one" teaching model of the past is not optimal for patient care. In today's health care system and with today's resources, implementation of a simulation training program can be cost-effective [6]

273

by minimizing the suboptimal or harmful use of medical resources. Simulation training can lead to superior medical outcomes.

> Advocate for quality patient care and assist patients in dealing with system complexities.

Once a diagnosis is made, patients are often inundated with the complexities of the treatment plan and the logistics of obtaining services through third payer systems. The physician can help patients overcome these logistic barriers and be a patient advocate toward third-party payers. Directing patients toward disease and/or pain support groups can help them to become more active participants in their treatment. A little time and effort on the physician's part can relieve a great burden on the patient's part.

> Know how to partner with health care managers and health care providers to assess, coordinate, and improve health care and know how these activities can affect system performance.

Various members of the health care team participate to provide effective care for the patient. Communication and cooperation are keys to teamwork, which will ensure that the patient has his or her needs filled efficiently and safely.

Additional reading

1. Leijon G, Boivie J. Central post-stroke pain – a controlled trial of amitriptyline and carbamazepine. Pain 1989;36:27–36.

2. Fontaine D, Hamani C, Lozano A. Efficacy and safety of motor cortex stimulation for chronic neuropathic pain: critical review of the literature. J Neurosurg 2009;110:251–256.

3. Titlic M. Lamotrigine in the treatment of pain syndromes and neuropathic pain. Bratisl Lek Listy 2008;109:421–424.

4. Jing YY. Nerve growth factor of red nucleus involvement in pain induced by spared nerve injury of the rat sciatic nerve. Neurochem Res 2009;34:1612–1618.

5. Corley ST. Electronic prescribing: a review of costs and benefits. Topics Health Inf Manage 2003;24:29–38.

6. Wang EE. Addressing the systems-based practice core competency: a simulation-based curriculum. Acad Emerg Med 2005;12:1191–1194.

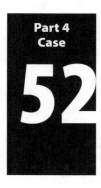

Contributions from the University of Miami Miller School of Medicine under Michael C. Lewis

Trauma

Edgar Pierre and Patricia Wawroski

The case

A 26-year-old male arrives via emergency transport at the trauma resuscitation bay after sustaining multiple gunshot injuries. Wounds are located in his chest, abdomen, and groin. On presentation, his blood pressure is noted to be 76/55, with a heart rate of 130 beats per minute. His body temperature is recorded at 35.2°C. He is noted to be pale, diaphoretic, and nonresponsive to verbal command.

The first step in the care of this patient is the primary survey. This is a coordinated effort between the trauma surgery and the anesthesia teams. The primary survey follows the A, B, C, D, E structure.

The first step is assessment of the patient's airway (A). The Glasgow coma scale is a helpful tool to determine the need for intubation. In general, patients with a score less than 9 will require intubation, in order to protect the airway. In this particular case, the patient is nonresponsive and will therefore need to have his airway protected. It is important to communicate with the surgeons that you plan to intubate. Tell them about any medications administered as these drugs may interfere with the remainder of the evaluation.

The second step is assessment of breathing (B). In this case, again, the patient is unresponsive and will get intubated, so breathing will be controlled with a ventilator. It is important to assess the adequacy of ventilation once the endotracheal tube is in place. Any thoracic injuries that may interfere with ventilation, including his gunshot wounds to the chest, should be addressed and corrected, if possible.

Third is circulation (C). The patient is currently maintaining a blood pressure, although his vital signs indicate that he is intravascularly depleted. Any source of bleeding should be assessed and addressed. Good intravascular access should be in place in the form of large-bore intravenous lines or central vascular access.

The fourth step is assessing the patient's disability (D). Initial assessment actually occurs before intubation because, as mentioned before, any medications that are given during intubation will affect the assessment. Any neurological defects should be noted during the primary survey.

The last step is complete body exposure (E) to assess occult injuries. The patient is log-rolled to assess spinal injuries.

The primary survey is typically completed as quickly as possible. Once the primary survey is completed, the secondary survey is initiated. This consists of a complete head-to-toe examination of the patient. Any remaining injuries are addressed and treatment is initiated. Laboratory values are evaluated and metabolic or electrolyte disturbances are treated.

Patient care

Residents must be able to provide patient care that is compassionate, appropriate, and effective for the treatment of health problems and the promotion of health.

Communicate effectively and demonstrate caring and respectful behaviors when interacting with patients and their families.

Trauma patients may present anywhere along a spectrum from unconscious to awake and agitated. It is important to explain procedures to any awake patient. Initial assessment focuses on stabilization of the patient. It is important to try to communicate with an awake patient and explain what is happening. When there are multiple people attempting to ask questions and assess for injuries, it can be very confusing to a patient. Technical terminology may also be confusing to a patient. Once the primary survey is complete and the patient is stable, additional information may be sought from the patient's family members or the patient himself, if he is awake. In this situation, the patient is usually not a good source of information.

Gather essential and accurate information about their patients.

Again, patients, as in this case, may not be able to give any information pertaining to their medical history or the type of injuries received. The greatest source of information can be the emergency medical transport team, who usually gather essential information at the scene of the injury. Although it is not appropriate to abandon the patient during the primary survey to speak to the family for information, it may be possible to delegate a nonessential member of the team to gather information from family and friends who may be present.

It is probably not appropriate to allow family members to be in the resuscitation bay during the initial treatment phase. This can be an emotional time, and family may become a distraction.

Make informed decisions about diagnostic and therapeutic interventions based on patient information and preferences, up-to-date scientific evidence, and clinical judgment.

The primary survey should be completed in a very efficient manner. On the basis of its results, it is important to make good clinical decisions regarding initial treatments. Although attempting to perform a literature search at the time of initial presentation is not appropriate, it is necessary to stay informed about current evidence-based treatment options. In this case, clinical decisions will be made in conjunction with the surgical trauma team. One of the first decisions to be made is whether the patient will need the operating room to address his injuries. This decision will be based on current literature and the experience of the team. Any injuries that can be addressed in the trauma bay should be treated. Other decisions may center on the choice of resuscitation fluids. Colloid and blood products are more expensive than crystalloids. In this particular patient, blood products and crystalloids will likely be most beneficial. The patient is apparently hypovolemic, as evidenced by his vital signs. He will need to have his intravascular volume deficit corrected.

Develop and carry out patient management plans.

Again, in a trauma situation, management of the patient is a team approach. Open communication should be occurring between surgical team members to determine treatment. Decisions regarding the airway typically are made by the anesthesia team, with input from surgical colleagues. The primary and secondary surveys should be completed jointly in a timely manner.

Counsel and educate patients and their families.

Discussions with the family and patient, if possible, are usually deferred until after the initial assessment is complete. In this emergency situation, the typical approach is treatment to preserve life, stabilization, then initiation of discussions. Any discussions with the patient's family should be realistic but hopeful. Family should be made aware of the extent of injury and the prognosis, but it should be made very clear that all efforts are being made to save the patient.

Use information technology to support patient care decisions and patient education.

Once the patient has been stabilized, it may be appropriate to perform a literature search to answer any remaining questions. Articles pertinent to the patient's care should be reviewed.

Perform competently all medical and invasive procedures considered essential for the area of practice.

Resuscitation of such a trauma patient is an emergency situation. This is not the time to have a medical student or even a junior resident attempt to intubate or place a central line for the first time. Personal limitations should also be recognized, and help from more experienced people should be immediately available. Techniques that are known to be safest for the patient should be employed.

Provide health care services aimed at preventing health problems or maintaining health.

The patient should be closely monitored to evaluate treatment outcomes. Sterile technique should be maintained at all times to prevent infection. Antibiotics should be administered in a timely fashion to prevent future infections.

Work with health care professionals, including those from other disciplines, to provide patient-focused care.

Communication is important among the whole trauma team, including the surgeons, anesthesiologists, and nursing staff. Future treatment plans should be conveyed among all care team members. This is especially important when care is being handed off from one care area to another, for example, from trauma to the intensive care unit.

Medical knowledge

Residents must demonstrate knowledge about established and evolving biomedical, clinical, and cognate (e.g., epidemiological and social-behavioral) sciences and the application of this knowledge to patient care.

Demonstrate an investigatory and analytic thinking approach to clinical situations.

In any trauma, it is important to evaluate and treat the whole patient. Attention should not be focused on one small detail. The overall clinical picture is more important. It is also important to adapt clinical treatments as necessary so that if one treatment does not seem to be helpful, a second modality should be sought and tried.

Know and apply the basic and clinically supportive sciences that are appropriate to their discipline.

The specific patient and clinical situation should be focused on when choosing treatments and medications. Pharmacologic principles should be recalled to anticipate any potential side effects or adverse outcomes from medication administration. Always be prepared to call for help when complications arise.

Practice-based learning and improvement

Residents must be able to investigate and evaluate their patient care practices, appraise and assimilate scientific evidence, and improve their patient care practices.

Analyze practice experience and perform practice-based improvement activities using a systematic methodology.

The initial trauma patient's evaluation should follow a systematic approach. This includes the primary and secondary surveys. Interventions should only be performed if they are deemed appropriate and clinically necessary.

Locate, appraise, and assimilate evidence from scientific studies related to their patients' health problems.

There is a great deal of information available for clinical practice. It is necessary to know the source of such information and be able to evaluate it objectively as not all articles are created equal. It is also necessary to understand whether clinical treatments are applicable to the current clinical situation.

Obtain and use information about their own population of patients and the larger population from which their patients are drawn.

Past experience is the most readily available information during an emergency situation. Patient populations can be unique in a hospital. Experience with the particular patients typically seen can be invaluable in the treatment of future patients. In addition, any knowledge gained from this patient can be used to better the treatment of future patients.

Apply knowledge of study designs and statistical methods to the appraisal of clinical studies and other information on diagnostic and therapeutic effectiveness.

As mentioned earlier, not all studies are designed equally. Each and every journal article read should be viewed in its entirety, and its limitations should be recognized. These limitations may come from the design itself or from the number of patients being studied. Overall, case reports, cohort studies, and randomized controlled trials each have their own strengths and weaknesses, which need to be recognized. It is also important to determine the validity and applicability of the results to clinical situations. An outcome that shows statistical significance may not necessarily be clinically significant.

Use information technology to manage information, access online medical information, and support their own education.

In this information age, there is a multitude of information available from several resources, including online journal articles, online textbooks, and lectures that are posted online by various educational institutions. These can be great sources of information on various injuries pertinent to patient care. All the information should be evaluated for validity. Online comprehensive literature searches should be employed to increase your knowledge base. Textbooks are also a great source for specific topics to support education.

Professionalism

Residents must demonstrate a commitment to carrying out professional responsibilities, adherence to ethical principles, and sensitivity to a diverse patient population.

> Demonstrate respect, compassion, and integrity; a responsiveness to the needs of patients and society that supersedes self-interest, accountability to patient, society, and the profession; and a commitment to excellence and ongoing professional development.

Trauma cases may present at any time of the day. Residents need to show equal dedication to the patient and case regardless of the time of arrival. Residents do have personal lives outside of the hospital, but separation between the two areas needs to occur. Personal issues should not interfere with patient care. Team members should be treated with respect. If a disagreement arises regarding patient care, other choices should be discussed in a calm manner.

> Demonstrate a commitment to ethical principles pertaining to provision or withholding of clinical care, confidentiality of patient information, informed consent, and business practice.

Patient confidentiality should be maintained throughout treatment and care. This includes being cognizant of areas of case discussion. Patient care discussions should not be held in the elevators or public areas. Family members should be taken to private areas for discussions. Informed consent should be obtained for procedures, unless it is an emergency situation and delay would be detrimental.

> Demonstrate sensitivity and responsiveness to patients' culture, age, gender, and disabilities.

All patients should be treated with equal respect. In this case, it is again important not to judge the cause of the injury or the situation in which it was obtained. Cultural background, age, or gender should not dictate treatment. In addition, personal preferences or religious beliefs should be recognized and respected when discussing treatment options (i.e., a Jehovah's Witness refusing a blood transfusion).

Interpersonal and communication skills

Residents must be able to demonstrate interpersonal and communication skills that result in effective information exchange and teaming with patients, their patients' families, and professional associates.

> Create and sustain a therapeutic and ethically sound relationship with patients.

Procedures should be described in detail. Results should be conveyed in a timely manner. All questions should be answered as best as possible. Patients should be given treatment options and alternatives.

> Use effective listening skills and elicit and provide information using effective nonverbal, explanatory, questioning, and writing skills.

Time should be taken to listen to patients and their families. Explanations should be given at a level appropriate to the patient's educational level. It is also important to realize that all notes become part of the medical record. Notes should be written in clear, concise language with good handwriting and no abbreviations. All notes should be legible to other members of the health care team.

> Work effectively with others as a member or leader of a health care team or other professional group.

Concerns should be communicated in a calm manner. We must stay calm at all times when dealing with patients and members of the medical staff.

Systems-based practice

Residents must demonstrate an awareness of and responsiveness to the larger context and system of health care and the ability to effectively call on system resources to provide care that is of optimal value.

279

Understand how their patient care and other professional practices affect other health care professionals, the health care organization, and the larger society and how these elements of the system affect their own practice.

In an ideal world, there would be unlimited resources available for every single patient. However, we do not live in an ideal world, and resources are limited. Patient care does not exist in a bubble, and it must be realized that resources (i.e., blood products) used on one particular patient may not be available for other patients.

Know how types of medical practice and delivery systems differ from one another, including methods of controlling health care costs and allocating resources.

It is necessary to triage appropriately operating room time and personnel as there may be only one operating room available for multiple patients. It is also important to realize that patient care and flow through the health care system may differ at various institutions, but the goals remain the same. Most residents will not remain at their training institution and must realize that different does not necessarily mean wrong.

Practice cost-effective health care and resource allocation that does not compromise quality of care.

Limitations to patient survival and futile care must be recognized. Trauma patients with a low likelihood of survival may be present. All efforts should be made for high-quality health care, but resources may need to be allocated in an efficient manner to provide for all patients.

Advocate for quality patient care and assist patients in dealing with system complexities.

Most residents do not understand how patients and their families should navigate through the health care system. A social worker should be contacted to help with the complexities of the health care system. Cost issues can be addressed as well as placement after acute, life-threatening issues are appropriately addressed. Provisions may also need to be made for home health care and rehabilitation, if needed, on discharge from the hospital.

Know how to partner with health care managers and health care providers to assess, coordinate, and improve health care and know how these activities can affect system performance.

Multidisciplinary meetings should be held to discuss ongoing issues in patient care. Each member of the team may have a specific area of interest regarding the health care of patients. These can seemingly interfere with other members' interests. Understanding must be reached to address the most life-threatening issues first. Discussions should also be held to critique performance and identify areas for improvement.

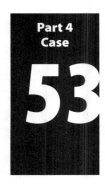

**Part 4
Case**

Contributions from the University of Miami Miller School of Medicine under Michael C. Lewis

53 Whack-an-eye

Steven Gayer and Shafeena Nurani

The case

A 15-year-old female presents to the emergency department with her father following an unusual gardening accident. The patient was helping her father with lawn work and was using a weed whacker to trim the area around a chain link fence separating their property from the neighbor's. A small barb of fence wire was whacked directly into her right eye. She complained of decreased visual acuity and pain in the right eye. There was no loss of consciousness, and she sustained no other injuries. While the lesion was outwardly apparent, nonetheless, a computed tomography scan of the eye was obtained, confirming the presence of a foreign body in the right eye. The ophthalmology service has determined that timely surgical repair of the open globe injury is warranted.

The patient ate a cheeseburger and fries for lunch approximately 3 hours ago. The patient has no past medical history. She had an appendectomy at age 8 under general anesthesia, without complications. She has no known drug allergies and is not on any medications.

Physical examination reveals the following:

temperature, 37°C
heart rate, 105 beats per minute
blood pressure, 118/78
respiratory rate, 20
pulse oximetry, 100% on room air
anxious, alert, and oriented to person, place, and time
Mallampati2, with full range of *motion* at the neck and with a thyromental distance greater than 6 cm
cardiac is S1, S2, regular rate and rhythm, with no murmurs
lungs are clear to auscultation bilaterally
abdomen is soft, *nontender*, and not distended
extremities are warm and well perfused

The ophthalmologists are concerned about the possibility of vision loss. The patient and her father are very anxious about the procedure.

Patient care

Residents must be able to provide patient care that is compassionate, appropriate, and effective for the treatment of health problems and the promotion of health. Residents are expected to:

Communicate effectively and demonstrate caring and respectful behaviors when interacting with patients and their families.

This is a very stressful situation for this family, given the potential for loss of vision. The patient and her family should be approached with kindness and consideration. While it is important to keep both the patient and the father feeling comfortable throughout the process, the patient is of foremost concern and it would be most effective to speak to her first and then address the concerns of her father. It would likely be best to speak to her in the absence of her father after an initial relationship has been established. This would allow addressing any questions or concerns that she has that she may not vocalize with her father present. It would assure her that she is your primary concern and allow for establishment of a relationship between the anesthesiologist and the patient. It would also facilitate determining if she is sexually active and if there is any possibility of her being pregnant. The need for a pregnancy test should be discussed with her, while proceeding with the workup, as this may have implications for her anesthestic management. It would be important to assure the patient that the results of this test would be kept confidential if she so wished.

Gather essential and accurate information about their patients.

As this is a case of traumatic eye injury, other injuries must be ruled out including skull or orbital fractures, intracranial trauma and trauma to any other part of the body. The patient should be interviewed and examined alone first to give her an opportunity to relay all relevant information including her reaction to her previous general anesthetic and to discuss the possibility of pregnancy as mentioned above. The father can then be present for the rest of the interview in order to obtain other relevant information about the patient including any childhood illnesses that the patient may not recall as well as a family history of adverse reactions to anesthesia.

Make informed decisions about diagnostic and therapeutic interventions based on patient information and preferences, up-to-date scientific evidence, and clinical judgment.

In this case, the decision to be made involves the ophthalmologist, the patient and the anesthesiologist in terms of whether to proceed to the operation room immediately. Given that this is an open globe injury, with the presence of a foreign body, the patient likely requires urgent intervention. There is increased incidence of visual loss and infection of the eye when surgery is delayed. The decision will ultimately be made by the ophthalmologist in regards to the timing of surgery based on current literature and outcome studies.

In regards to the type of anesthesia for the procedure, given that the patient has a full stomach and that the operation is an emergency the decision to choose general anesthesia or regional anesthesia needs to be made in consultation with the ophthalmologist (to determine the extent of surgery) as well as the patient. The risk of aspiration must be considered as well as the risk of blindness in the injured eye that could result from elevated intraocular pressure and extrusion of ocular contents.

Develop and carry out patient management plans.

Regional anesthesia is a useful alternative in trauma patients, however with an open globe injury, there is the risk of extrusion of ocular content by either the pressure generated by local anesthetics, the instrumentation of the orbit or the potential of orbital hemorrhage with performance of a regional technique. On the other hand, with a general anesthetic, there can be elevations in intraocular pressure from administra-

tion of succinylcholine of 1-8 mmHg, though this is transient. There is also the risk that the patient might cough or buck during intubation, and this can raise intra-ocular pressure by 35-40 mmHg. There have been recent studies that show that careful performance of regional anesthesia (including either retrobulbar, peribulbar or subtenon's administration of anesthetic) with direct visualization of the globe during anesthesia administration may be a safe alternative to general anesthesia in selected patients.

If a general anesthetic technique is used, preoperative treatment with a H2 blocker to reduce gastric acidity and volume as well as metoclopramide to enhance gastric emptying should be considered. The patient should also be given 30 ml sodium citrate before induction. A rapid sequence induction should be performed with the sellick maneuver. The use of succinylcholine in this situation is controversial, however due to its swift onset of action and short duration of action, if administered after pretreatment with a nondepolarizing neuromuscular blocker and an induction dose of thiopental, it results in only a small increase in intraocular pressure and therefore can be considered for this patient. Maintenance of anesthesia can be performed with a balanced technique using inhalational agents, opioids and neuromuscular blockers if necessary. The goals for anesthesia in this patient are patient safety (minimal fluctuations in intraocular pressure), no patient movement during the surgery as this can cause catastrophic complications, pain control and the avoidance of the oculocardiac reflex. Emergence should be smooth with minimal coughing and bucking, lidocaine 1.5–2 mg/kg should be considered prior to extubation. A prophylactic antiemetic should be considered as vomiting in the postoperative period can significantly elevate intraocular pressure.

Counsel and educate patients and their families.

In this situation the various risks and benefits of a regional technique versus a general technique should be discussed with both the patient and her father. Patient cooperation is essential for a regional technique and the choice should be presented to the patient with minimal use of technical terms and ensuring that she understands the options.

Use information technology to support patient care decisions and patient education.

As this is an emergent situation, there may not be enough time to perform a thorough literature search on the risks and benefits of general versus regional anesthesia or the use on succinylcholine in this situation, however a literature search should be performed at a later time to look for any recent articles that one is not aware of.

The patient should be counseled on the importance of not moving during the surgery should she opt for a regional technique. The patient and her family should be provided with reading material regarding the surgical procedure and recovery as well as on how the regional technique is done so that they have an idea about what to expect.

Perform competently all medical and invasive procedures considered essential for the area of practice.

Anesthesiologists and ophthalmologists are trained to perform regional anesthetic techniques of the eye. The individual experience and comfort with performing the block should be considered when deciding who is to perform the block, especially in this situation when one must closely observe the globe while administering the local anesthetic.

Provide health care services aimed at preventing health problems or maintaining health.

In this situation, the use of protective eyewear while performing any task where one might have flying debris should be emphasized as this measure could have prevented the current situation. Reading material on safe practices to protect the eyes should be provided to the patient and her family.

It is also very important to know the complications that can be caused by the various anesthetic techniques considered and be prepared to deal with them should they arise. All patients should be monitored with ASA standard monitoring when regional techniques are being performed. In addition, if any sedation is to be given, the patient should have supplemental oxygen delivered. In this case it is especially important to monitor for stimulation of the oculocardiac reflex, intra-arterial injection of local anesthetic and inadvertent brain-stem anesthesia among other possibilities. *It is important to have the resources to deal with the possible complications readily available.*

Work with health care professionals, including those from other disciplines, to provide patient-focused care

---

Communication is very important amongst the operating room team including the anesthesiologist, the ophthalmologist and the nursing staff. It is important to maintain good communication with all involved so that the operating room is a safe and efficient environment. It is especially important to communicate well with the ophthalmologists as this may change your anesthetic management and may alert you to potential problems early on giving you a chance to avoid them.

It is also very important to communicate with the patient, nursing staff and ophthalmologists in regards to any prophylactic antibiotics that may need to be administered prior to incision as well as to perform a time-out to protect the patient from wrong site surgeries.

Medical knowledge

Residents must demonstrate knowledge about established and evolving biomedical, clinical, and cognate (e.g. epidemiological and social-behavioral) sciences and the application of this knowledge to patient care. Residents are expected to:

Demonstrate an investigatory and analytic thinking approach to clinical situations.
Know and apply the basic and clinically supportive sciences which are appropriate to their discipline.

In order to understand the mechanisms that determine intraocular pressure and how different factors influence it, one must first understand the principles that go into its determination. Intraocular pressure normally varies between 10-21 mmHg. Three main factors influence intraocular pressure: 1) external pressure on the eye by the contraction of the obicularis oculi muscle and the tone of the extraocular muscles, venous congestion of ocular veins or conditions such as an ocular tumor; 2) scleral rigidity; and 3) changes in intraocular contents such as the lens, vitreous, blood and aqueous humor. Intraocular blood volume is determined primarily by venous fluctuations in pressure. If venous return from the eye is hindered, intraocular pressure can rise significantly. Straining, vomiting or coughing can increase venous pressure and therefore intraocular pressure by as much as 40 mmHg. While these changes in intraocular pressure dissipate rapidly, it can have disastrous consequences in the situation where the globe is open. Another factor to consider is that the maintenance of intraocular pressure is determined primarily by the rate of aqueous humor formation and its outflow. The most important factor in the formation of aqueous humor is the difference in osmotic pressure between aqueous humor and plasma. Therefore hypertonic solutions such as mannitol can be used to lower intraocular pressure as a change in the osmotic pressure of plasma can change the formation of aqueous humor and therefore influence intraocular pressure.

Practice-based learning and improvement

Residents must be able to investigate and evaluate their patient care practices, appraise and assimilate scientific evidence, and improve their patient care practices. Residents are expected to:

> Analyze practice experience and perform practice-based improvement activities using a systematic methodology.

One way in which analyzing practice experience can be performed is to follow up on all patients that the resident has any clinical interaction with to ensure that their outcomes are known and to find out about any complications that arose after the anesthetic was given. A more formal way to look at practice experience and to perform practice-based improvement activities would be to do a retrospective analysis of the patients undergoing a particular procedure and to look for events that occurred intraoperatively that resulted in different outcomes. For example, for this case, a review of the literature revealed that in one case series, there was no difference in outcome of the patients in terms of visual loss or eventual enucleation independent of the anesthetic technique used in a selected group of patients. This information supports the practice of either technique (general or regional) as long as the patients are carefully selected. However, if the resident were to do a retrospective analysis of the cases done at their institution and found that there was a difference in outcome, this would then lead to an attempt to determine if the technique used for regional anesthesia in their practice was different and, if so, could

lead to modification of the technique or the way in which patients were selected to receive general versus regional techniques for this procedure.

> Locate, appraise, and assimilate evidence from scientific studies related to their patients' health problems.

Residents should be able to perform literature searches on the issues relevant to the care of their patients and evaluate these studies for study technique, differences in patient populations, strength of the statistical analysis to evaluate the data that have been obtained as well as consistency in findings from different groups studying the same questions. There are often reports that suggest conflicting ideas in the literature and it is important to learn to read the primary literature and determine if the data being presented is valid to the patient in question. It is also important to determine possible sources of error in the studies performed. Randomized prospective controlled trials to evaluate the performance of regional versus general anesthesia in cases like a traumatic open globe injury would be difficult to perform and therefore in cases like this one must use the best available evidence, clinical judgment and confer with the ophthalmologist and the patient to determine what would be best for this patient in particular.

> Obtain and use information about their own population of patients and the larger population from which their patients are drawn.

It is very important to keep track of all the patients that are seen at the institution in which one works, so as to determine how best their needs might be served. For example, the growing number of elderly patients may be better served if more focus in the places treating them was to be placed on preventative interventions that this patient population is prone to. Residents should be aware of the population from which their patients are drawn to be more aware of the more prevalent problems in that population, such as in an elderly population, dementia, depression, Alzheimer's disease, systemic hypertension, and polypharmacy that may affect the anesthetic drugs that one would choose to use on the patients. There may also be regional differences in outcomes for various procedures related to the population of patients that one treats. For example, in the case of ophthalmologic surgery, a patient population that is not cooperative would likely benefit from general anesthesia so as to assure patient safety and patient akinesis during the procedure. A cooperative patient however, would likely benefit from a regional technique and be encouraged to stay still for the procedure, allowing for a quicker recovery time and less time spent in the hospital for the procedure. The anesthetic technique used for different procedures would vary significantly based on patient population seen at a particular institution.

> Apply knowledge of study designs and statistical methods to the appraisal of clinical studies and other information on diagnostic and therapeutic effectiveness.

As mentioned before, there are varying levels of confidence that can be placed in conclusions made by a particular study based on how it is designed, how large the study is, and what patient population is being studied. In general, to avoid bias in studies, they should be designed with a clear hypothesis, and specific outcome variables that are being looked at. The patients should ideally be randomized to the different treatment groups; there should be a control group and the evaluators of the outcomes should be ideally blinded to the treatment group. Systematic reviews and meta-analysis can be used to compile smaller studies, to make better inferences about the data collected. When reading clinical studies, it is important to keep in mind how the study was designed and what it was designed to assess so as not to make erroneous conclusions. It is important to determine if the patient population in which the study was performed related to your patient population. It is also important to determine if the hypothesis being studied has been studied by others and whether the results are similar.

> Use information technology to manage information, access on-line medical information; and support their own education.

Residents are increasingly able to access medical records online in a more legible format as well as use resources on the Internet such as Medline and online textbooks to quickly review information before proceeding with a particular procedure.

Professionalism

Residents must demonstrate a commitment to carrying out professional responsibilities, adherence to eth-

ical principles, and sensitivity to a diverse patient population. Residents are expected to:

> Demonstrate respect, compassion, and integrity; a responsiveness to the needs of patients and society that supercedes self-interest; accountability to patients, society, and the profession; and a commitment to excellence and on-going professional development.

It is important to treat all patients with respect and compassion. This is a very stressful time in the patient's life. The traumatic eye injury patient may present at any time of the day or night and should be treated with the same compassion and kindness regardless of the time or other circumstances in the resident's life. The first priority should always be to take care of the patient in the best way possible. It should be appreciated that this is a life-changing event should the patient lose their vision.

> Demonstrate a commitment to ethical principles pertaining to provision or withholding of clinical care, confidentiality of patient information, informed consent, and business practice.

In this case, informed consent with the patient understanding the risks and benefits of the various options is of utmost importance. Protecting the confidentiality of patient information is also an important principle in this case. In this case, it is very important to speak with the patient alone and offer a pregnancy test in a confidential setting so as to allow the patient to be given the opportunity to discuss any concerns that she might have, or to offer counseling regarding her health.

> Demonstrate sensitivity and responsiveness to patients' culture, age, gender, and disabilities.

It is important in this case to primarily address the patient when discussing options as she is a 15-year-old female and will soon be taking responsibility for her own health care decisions. It would empower her to make a choice that she would be comfortable with. It is also important as mentioned before to address any concerns that she might have in the absence of her parent in order to further establish a relationship with her and to allow her to disclose any further information. She would not be likely to foster a trusting relationship with an anesthesiologist that spoke only with her parents or primarily with her parents.

Interpersonal and communication skills

Residents must be able to demonstrate interpersonal and communication skills that result in effective information exchange and teaming with patients, their patients families, and professional associates. Residents are expected to:

Create and sustain a therapeutic and ethically sound relationship with patients.

It is important in the case of a teenage girl to create some rapport and trust with the patient, especially in this case, as it is a stressful situation with the possibility of vision loss. The patient is likely extremely anxious. Developing a good rapport with the patient and creating a trustful relationship are key elements in this case.

Use effective listening skills and elicit and provide information using effective nonverbal, explanatory, questioning, and writing skills.

In this case, listening to the concerns of both the patient and her father can help alleviate some of their anxiety. Explaining the process to the patient can be soothing as she may be less anxious if she knows what is going to happen next. Detailing the procedure of getting to the operating room, placement of monitors, and the people that will be present in the operating room may help to calm the patient down and to feel more in control of the situation. Providing some information about the things to expect postoperatively, such as an eye patch can also help to make the patient calmer in the postoperative recovery period.

Work effectively with others as a member or leader of a health care team or other professional group.

It is important to communicate effectively with the entire operating room team in order to provide the best care possible to the patient. Each member of the operating room team has a specific defined role to perform and the operating room works efficiently when there is good communication between all members of the team. It is important to address all members of the team in a calm and respectful manner.

Part 5

Contributions from Johns Hopkins Medical Institutions under Deborah A. Schwengel

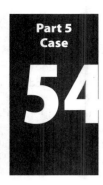

Contributions from Johns Hopkins Medical Institutions under Deborah A. Schwengel

Singin' the OSA blues

Jennifer K. Lee and Deborah A. Schwengel

The case

A 37-month-old boy with snoring and large tonsils is scheduled for an adenotonsillectomy and bilateral ear tubes. He was born 5 weeks early. His growth is on the 5th percentile for weight and the 10th percentile for length. His family says that he snores loudly and sleeps restlessly. He is an active child and his mother wonders if he has attention-deficit hyperactivity disorder (ADHD). He has some language delay. He has not had a sleep study. He has had many ear infections. He has a mild runny nose. All his other organ systems are healthy. He has never had an anesthetic. Family history is noncontributory. There is no history suggestive of coagulopathy.

On physical examination, he is 12 kg and thin. He is running around the room and comes over briefly to meet you but has to be held to listen to his chest. He has some crusted secretions around the nares and dark circles under his eyes. He breathes with his mouth open. He has kissing tonsils (they are touching in the midline). His chest sounds are clear and heart sounds normal. The abdomen is soft. Limbs appear normal.

Patient care

Residents must be able to provide patient care that is compassionate, appropriate, and effective for the treatment of health problems and the promotion of health.

> Communicate effectively and demonstrate caring and respectful behaviors when interacting with patients and their families.

This will be the first anesthetic for this child. The parents will have many questions and concerns about their child's care unless other children in the family have had similar operations. Even though the safety of anesthesia is established for most patients, many people come with preconceived ideas such as "Aunt Ethel *died* when she had an operation" or "Grandma's brother had surgery when he was 5 years old and never

woke up." Even though those events happened in 1922, you need to dispel myths and communicate your safety plans. If you talk about the course of events from induction, care during surgery, and common everyday side effects such as vomiting, emergence delirium, pain, and other postanesthesia care unit (PACU) events, it tells the family what to expect. It also demonstrates that you expect the patient to have a successful and safe anesthetic in the operating room, with normal recovery in the PACU. Spend enough time with the family to build trust and let them relinquish his care into your hands – hands that they think will handle him expertly, safely, and compassionately. If parents are allowed into the operating room for induction, prepare them for the expected crying, breath holding, and noisy breathing when the anesthetic mask is applied or crying when the intravenous (IV) line is started or propofol is injected.

> Gather essential and accurate information about their patients.

This child has snoring and presumably obstructive sleep apnea (OSA). It is essential to figure out how severe the OSA is. Without a sleep study, it is challenging to do so. It has been established that there are risks of postoperative morbidity and mortality in both adult and pediatric OSA patients. Although sufficiently sensitive and specific screening questionnaires for pediatric OSA to do not exist, a history of loud snoring, disrupted sleep, observed apneas, growth failure, and behavioral problems indicate severe disease. The challenge about observed apneas and disrupted sleep is that pediatric OSA is a REM-dominant event; REM sleep occurs in the dead of night, when most people are in bed, thus making it unlikely that the parents have fully observed the extent of the child's sleep abnormality. Comorbidities such as prematurity, hypotonia, or craniofacial anatomic disorders put children with OSA into a higher risk category. Unlike adult OSA, pediatric OSA does not have a gender predilection and is not usually associated with obesity, although obesity, when present, is a risk factor.

> Make informed decisions about diagnostic and therapeutic interventions based on patient information and preferences, up-to-date scientific evidence, and clinical judgment.

Would it be helpful to have sleep study information before proceeding with the case? Yes, but sleep studies are expensive and not always available to every patient, and they should be performed at a pediatric sleep study center. It is recommended that pediatric sleep studies use the apnea hypopnea index (AHI) rather than the respiratory disturbance index (RDI) because RDI scores measure central as well as obstructive events. Children normally have more central events than adults, so RDI should not be used in pediatric patients. Recent literature also recommends examining the oxygen saturation nadir. Patients experiencing desaturations to 80% or lower have more serious disease and may be at higher risk of perioperative morbidity [1]. Unfortunately, most pediatric patients presenting for adenotonsillectomy at most hospitals will not have had a sleep study. You and the surgeon will have to make a judgment about whether this patient will be admitted postoperatively or sent home the same day.

> Develop and carry out patient management plans.

Here's where the rubber meets the road. You have to make a plan with insufficient information. Much of clinical medicine is this way. You know you have matured as a clinician when you can say that you are comfortable with ambiguity and you can provide good medical care for complex patients using clinical experience. Several things about this child say to me "severe OSA": restless sleep, ADHD, thin body habitus, dark circles under his eyes, mouth breathing, kissing tonsils, and age. Therefore it is my gut feeling that this child should be assumed to have severe OSA; that means induction requirements are different, opioid sensitivity is likely, and postoperative admission is necessary. Premedicating should be done cautiously, if at all, because any pharmacologically induced decrease in airway tone could result in airway obstruction when the patient lies supine and during anesthesia induction. The plan is to place an IV while the child is breathing nitrous oxide and oxygen. Placing a local anesthetic cream like EMLA (eutectic mixture of local anesthetics, 2.5% lidocaine, and 2.5% prilocaine) for 1

hour preoperatively will provide additional analgesia. Once the IV is placed, an IV induction with lidocaine, propofol, and 0.5 mcg/kg fentanyl is performed. A short-acting paralytic can be considered if the patient is easy to mask ventilate, although some practitioners choose to avoid neuromuscular blocking agents due to the short duration of the case. Direct laryngoscopy and endotracheal intubation are accomplished. Care must be taken not to scrape or injure the enlarged, friable tonsils with the laryngoscope blade and endotracheal tube, or bleeding could occur.

It is not wrong to do an inhalational induction, but it might be fraught with problems. For instance, you might get an anesthetic level that is deep enough to obstruct the airway but not deep enough to instrument it. Remember that these patients are at significant risk of airway obstruction, and complications such as negative pressure pulmonary edema could occur if the patient makes respiratory efforts against an obstructed airway. It may be possible to relieve such airway obstruction with a jaw thrust, applying moderate continuous positive airway pressure (CPAP) of 10–15 cm H_2O or putting the patient in a lateral position. If an airway device is needed, an oral airway is safer than a nasal airway due to the risk of traumatizing the hypertrophied adenoids with blind placement of a nasal device.

During the case, volatile anesthetic is used to keep the patient deep enough to tolerate the surgery. The surgeon's rigid mouth gag can be quite stimulating, and the patient cannot gag or buck for risk of injuring the teeth, jaw, or cervical spine. Make sure the endotracheal tube (ETT) is still in good position after the gag is placed; placement of the gag can result in kinking or displacement of the ETT. The FiO_2 should be decreased to 0.21 by titrating in air as the patient's oxygen saturation tolerates. Although not as flammable as oxygen, nitrous oxide supports a flame in the presence of material that will burn, such as the ETT, so the concentrations of both should be minimized to lower the risk of an airway fire. No additional opioids should be used until the patient is extubated and fully awake. Postoperative emesis will also increase bleeding, so antiemetics should be administered and the surgeons should suction out the stomach under direct visualization of the oropharynx. Dexamethasone may decrease postoperative airway swelling and serve as an antiemetic.

The patient should be extubated fully awake to decrease the risk of postextubation airway obstruction.

If oropharyngeal suctioning is needed prior to extubation, it should be performed gently and only in the midline to avoid disrupting clot and initiating bleeding. Once the patient is awake and extubated, opiates can be carefully titrated to effect. Remember that patients with OSA have increased sensitivity to opiates [1]. Some surgeons use local anesthetics, and others do not. If local anesthetics are used by the surgeon the need for opiates will initially be reduced. Some surgeons allow the use of nonsteroidal anti-inflammatory drugs (NSAIDs) postoperatively, and others do not. Although aspirin is contraindicated perioperatively in tonsillectomy patients, there is the suggestion in the literature that postoperative ketorolac and ibuprofen may be safe [2,3]. In the PACU, the patient should be closely monitored. These patients are at high risk for hypoxia and airway obstruction due to residual anesthesia, airway edema, blood and secretions in the laryngopharynx, baseline anatomic and neuromuscular predisposition to airway obstruction, disordered sleep arousal mechanisms to hypercarbia and airway obstruction, and rarely, postobstruction pulmonary edema. There will be some postoperative discomfort; in addition to the above mentioned NSAIDs, pain can sometimes be managed with acetaminophen alone. Opiates should be avoided or given with caution in the patient with severe OSA [1].

Occult hemorrhage can go unnoticed as the patient may swallow most of the blood. Tachycardia, even with normal or elevated blood pressure, may signal hypovolemia from hemorrhage. If bleeding is suspected, the surgeons should be immediately contacted, IV access must be obtained for volume resuscitation, and red blood cell transfusion may be indicated. Ideally, check a hematocrit prior to transfusing blood. Airway management should be jointly coordinated between experienced practitioners in anesthesia and surgery. Because the stomach will likely be full of blood, rapid-sequence induction is necessary. The airway may be visually obscured with blood, and the uvula may be as big as your thumb if a hot tonsillectomy (with Bovie) was done, so everyone must be prepared to institute the difficult airway algorithm if the initial intubation attempt is unsuccessful. Listen up because tonsillectomies are bread and butter cases, and the case of the bleeding tonsil is a classic oral board scenario. The most common time for tonsillectomies to bleed is 7–10 days postop.

Fortunately, complications after adenotonsillectomy are not daily events. So after a successful recovery in the PACU, the patient is admitted overnight for observation with a continuous pulse oximeter on a nursing unit with adequate ability to observe the patient and respond to monitor alarms. Patients who used noninvasive ventilation (CPAP or BiPAP) prior to surgery should be permitted either to continue their PAP or to have continuous pulse oximetry if they are to sleep without PAP.

Counsel and educate patients and their families.

The family must be told that tonsillectomy patients all awaken with some discomfort and that it will be our goal to titrate the pain medication to balance pain management against respiratory depression. Patients with OSA are more sensitive to the respiratory effects of opioids [1,4]. Families also need to know that tonsillectomy isn't always an instant cure. There is perioperative edema, and the pharyngeal structures need time to recover, but pediatric OSA does improve in many patients following tonsillectomy [5].

Perform competently all medical and invasive procedures considered essential for the area of practice.

Procedures essential to this case are the pediatric IV, mask ventilation, and endotracheal intubation.

Provide health care services aimed at preventing health problems or maintaining health.

This is a case in which devastating complications can occur, but they are usually avoidable with preparation and knowledge of the pathophysiology, anatomy, effects of surgery, and pharmacodynamics.

Work with health care professionals, including those from other disciplines, to provide patient-focused care.

It is essential to discuss the plan for disposition with the surgeon. Both the surgeon and anesthesiologist must be comfortable with plans for either discharge or admission and the level of monitoring on admission.

Medical knowledge

Residents must demonstrate knowledge about established and evolving biomedical, clinical, and cognate (e.g., epidemiological and social-behavioral) sciences and the application of this knowledge to patient care.

Demonstrate an investigatory and analytic thinking approach to clinical situations.

The most important component of the knowledge base competency is to recognize that pediatric OSA exists and must be considered when screening patients for anesthesia. The prevalence is 1% to 3% [6]. The resident must know how most pediatric OSA differs from adult OSA. Some children are obese, with features of the disorder that are more like adult OSA, but most children are thin with large tonsils, and many have a narrow craniofacial construction. There is undoubtedly overlap between bony, soft tissue and genetic causes. Those with more than one cause may have severe disease or a higher likelihood of OSA that is not cured by tonsillectomy. An appropriate first screening question is, "Does your child snore?" If the answer is yes, proceed to ask more probing questions about the severity of sleep disruption. Most children with OSA do snore, with the exception of hypotonic children, who might not generate the noise but still have obstructive episodes. Down's syndrome patients are at risk for OSA and may not snore.

Know and apply the basic and clinically supportive sciences that are appropriate to their discipline.

The following topics are relevant to the discussion of OSA in children:

- basic and clinical science related to the study of Mu receptors and responses of patients with OSA to opioids
- effects of OSA on the heart, respiratory, and sympathetic nervous systems
- sleep medicine, REM sleep, sleep studies, and the perioperative use of CPAP
- bleeding risk associated with the use of NSAIDs in tonsillectomy patients

Practice-based learning and improvement

Residents must be able to investigate and evaluate their patient care practices, appraise and assimilate scientific evidence, and improve their patient care practices.

Analyze practice experience and perform practice-based improvement activities using a systematic methodology.

There is a range of practice that is sometimes based on evidence and sometimes not. When there is insufficient evidence in the literature to dictate practice, individuals determine their own judgment based on previous or similar cases. Pediatric OSA is one of those conditions for which judgment and experience have been the foundation for much of the management of patients. However, there is some compelling information to guide us, which is summarized in the review article by Schwengel [7].

Locate, appraise, and assimilate evidence from scientific studies related to their patients' health problems.

Studies do show that both adult and pediatric patients are at risk of perioperative morbidity. Children, especially under the age of 36 months, have a high risk of postoperative respiratory events and should be admitted overnight following adenotonsillectomy. Children with severe OSA are high risk and need to be observed, especially if given opioids. Children with comorbidities have increased risk, as well.

Obtain and use information about their own population of patients and the larger population from which their patients are drawn.

This patient is just barely over the "must admit age," and he has features suggestive of severe disease, although a sleep study would really be needed to confirm that. Prudence suggests keeping this patient overnight for respiratory monitoring.

Professionalism

Residents must demonstrate a commitment to carrying out professional responsibilities, adherence to ethical principles, and sensitivity to a diverse patient population.

Demonstrate respect, compassion, and integrity; a responsiveness to the needs of patients and society that supersedes self-interest; accountability to patients, society, and the profession; and a commitment to excellence and ongoing professional development.

The family might be prepared to stay overnight. For some families, an overnight stay is reassuring, and for others, it is distressing. It is important to respect the family's concerns, while explaining the reason for admission. Listen to them, while giving some structure to the conversation. Reiterate that every decision we make is primarily for the safety of the patient.

Professionalism must also be maintained in the discussion with the surgeons about patient disposition. Express your opinion about admission based on objective information. Be prepared to defend your decision rationally. Ideally, try to build relationships with the surgeons so that you can grow to mutually trust each other's decisions.

Interpersonal and communication skills

Residents must be able to demonstrate interpersonal and communication skills that result in effective information exchange and teaming with patients, their patients' families, and professional associates.

> Create and sustain a therapeutic and ethically sound relationship with patients.

Be supportive of the parents, who might be nervous about their child's surgery. Discuss possible effects of the anesthetic so that they can be prepared for the postoperative course.

> Work effectively with others as a member or leader of a health care team or other professional group.

Discuss the plans for induction, emergence, and postop care with the surgical team. The briefing and debriefing can help, but in this case, the discussion about admission must take place before going to the operating room.

Systems-based practice

Residents must demonstrate an awareness of and responsiveness to the larger context and system of health care and the ability to effectively call on system resources to provide care that is of optimal value.

> Practice cost-effective health care and resource allocation that does not compromise quality of care.

Sleep studies are considered the gold standard for determining the diagnosis of OSA, yet they are expensive and time-consuming tests, for which third-party payers might refuse to pay. The alternative options for patients with OSA of uncertain severity, but clearly more than mild, is to admit them overnight, discharge them home after a longer PACU stay, or avoid the use of postoperative opioids.

References

1. Brown KA, Laferriere A, Lakheeram I, Moss IR. Recurrent hypoxemia in children is associated with increased analgesic sensitivity to opiates. Anesthesiology 2006;105:665–669.

2. Dsida R, Cote CJ. Nonsteroidal antiinflammatory drugs and hemorrhage following tonsillectomy: do we have the data? Anesthesiology 2004;100:749–751; author reply, 751–752.

3. Jeyakumar A, Brickman TM, Williamson ME, et al. Nonsteroidal anti-inflammatory drugs and postoperative bleeding following adenotonsillectomy in pediatric patients. Arch Otolaryngol Head Neck Surg 2008;134:24–27.

4. Brown KA, Laferriere A, Moss IR. Recurrent hypoxemia in young children with obstructive sleep apnea is associated with reduced opioid requirement for analgesia. Anesthesiology 2004;100:806–810; discussion, 5A.

5. Nixon GM, Kermack AS, McGregor CD, et al. Sleep and breathing on the first night after adenotonsillectomy for obstructive sleep apnea. Pediatr Pulmonol 2005;39:332–338.

6. Anuntaseree W, Rookkapan K, Kuasirikul S, Thongsuksai P. Snoring and obstructive sleep apnea in Thai school-age children: prevalence and predisposing factors. Pediatr Pulmonol 2001;32:222–227.

7. Schwengel DA, Sterni LM, Tunkel DE, Heitmiller ES. Perioperative management of children with obstructive sleep apnea: a review. Anesth Analg, 2009;109:60–75.

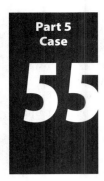

Contributions from Johns Hopkins Medical Institutions under Deborah A. Schwengel

55 Oxygen

Justin Lockman and Deborah A. Schwengel

Love is like oxygen. You get too much, you get too high. Not enough and you're gonna die.
– Andrew Scott and Trevor Griffen

The case

A 2-day-old, 26-week, 740-g male infant was admitted for repair of tracheoesophageal fistula (TEF).

The pregnancy was the product of a rape and was complicated by polyhydramnios, herpes simplex virus infection, preeclampsia, and ultrasound suggestion of fetal esophageal atresia and absence of the corpus callosum. The infant was delivered by cesarean section due to maternal preeclampsia. The infant was limp and required bag-mask ventilation, then endotracheal intubation and a brief period of chest compressions for bradycardia. Apgars were 1, 1, 5. Chest X-ray showed an enteric tube at the level of the clavicles, air in the stomach and intestines, and bilateral diffuse granularity of the lung fields. An echocardiogram showed patent foramen ovale (PFO), a small pulmonary artery and pulmonary artery hypertension, good left and right ventricular function, and otherwise normal cardiac structure. The child also had hypospadias and hydronephrosis.

The infant developed worsening lung compliance and was given surfactant and placed on an oscillator. You are consulted to take this child to the operating room for thoracotomy, ligation of TEF, and possible repair of the esophageal atresia; the team feels that the child is getting worse and that repair of the TEF might help improve oxygenation and ventilation. You think to yourself, "Yeah, if the baby survives the operation!" To make matters worse, it is 10 o'clock at night.

Patient care

Residents must be able to provide patient care that is compassionate, appropriate, and effective for the treatment of health problems and the promotion of health.

> Communicate effectively and demonstrate caring and respectful behaviors when interacting with patients and their families.

This is not an elective case, but you have enough time to answer questions for the mother. Not knowing how she might feel about the pregnancy, the baby, and now the baby's health problems, it is easy to understand feeling uncomfortable with the discussion. This is not the time to explore all those issues, so you give the same information to this mother as you would to any other mother faced with a premature newborn about to undergo major surgery. The mother should be counseled that the child could suffer cardiovascular or respiratory problems and neurologic complications of the anesthetic and surgical procedure.

> Gather essential and accurate information about their patients.

This child has a number of serious problems on which you need to focus tonight:

- prematurity: this baby is very premature and has a significant mortality based on the gestational age alone
- lung disease: the child needs ventilatory support with an oscillator
- tracheoesophageal fistula: the child is at risk of respiratory insufficiency and aspiration

> Make informed decisions about diagnostic and therapeutic interventions based on patient information and preferences, up-to-date scientific evidence, and clinical judgment.

Any child with a TEF needs to be evaluated for the components of VACTERL association. Key investigations prior to surgery include echocardiogram and renal ultrasound:

- vertebral anomalies
- anal atresia
- cardiovascular structural abnormalities (so an echocardiogram is essential prior to beginning an anesthetic)
- tracheoesophageal fistula
- esophageal atresia
- renal abnormalities
- limb anomalies

Develop and carry out patient management plans.

The diagnostic tests in this patient revealed evidence of TEF, PFO, pulmonary hypertension, and good bilateral ventricular function. The TEF is treated with an operation. The heart is treated by maintaining oxygenation and ventilation in an effort to avoid increasing pulmonary vascular pressures related to hypoxemia, hypercarbia, and acidosis. The child is ventilated with an oscillator. We must find out if the baby can tolerate coming off of the oscillator for the transport to the operating room, plus our surgeon does not want to operate on the oscillator, so a trial of conventional ventilation is done to make sure the baby doesn't crash and burn en route to the operating room. I hate it when my patient turns blue in the elevator! Seriously, transport is often the most hazardous part of any intensive care unit (ICU) case.

The child tolerated conventional ventilation and was transported without desaturation. The neonatal ICU staff had placed both umbilical arterial and venous catheters and a peripheral intravenous line. We had the lines we needed, blood was available, and our operating room was warm and set up. Temperature control is of particular importance in these very tiny patients. Their extremely high body surface area and lack of subcutaneous tissue puts them at very high risk for hypothermia. The operating room must be maximally warmed. As you pant and perspire, and the surgeons and nurses in the room complain, you take pride in the fact that your patient is warm. Heat loss in the operating room is primarily due to radiation and convection. Babies also have higher evaporative losses than older patients, both from skin and the respiratory tree. Conductive losses are the least. It has been shown that cold babies are at risk of higher morbidity and mortality from thermal stress [1]. Temperatures below

35°C can produce coagulopathy due to impaired von Willebrand factor – platelet interactions, clot instability, and slowed initiation of clot formation [2,3].

Most premature infants are treated with antibiotics, so giving additional doses in the operating room might not be advised. Their clearance mechanisms are not mature, and therefore dosing intervals are much longer than for older patients.

In most cases of TEF, the anesthetic induction and endotracheal intubation are accomplished in very specific ways. This patient was already intubated, but in the case of one who is not, the classic teaching is to keep the patient breathing spontaneously. Why do we do this? This is core anesthesiology teaching, analogous to the situation of a bronchopleural fistula. The patient has an abnormal connection from the trachea to the stomach. If you use positive pressure ventilation, in the worst case scenario, the stomach is a low-pressure sink. Air preferentially goes where the pressure is lowest, and so the stomach becomes a balloon that gets bigger with each breath, and you end up with aspiration of gastric contents or abdominal compartment syndrome, elevated hemidiaphragms, compressed lung tissue, massive atelectasis, severe loss of FRC, and therefore profound hypoxemia, complete failure of ventilation, cardiovascular compromise, and death. To avoid death, we let the baby keep breathing until the fistula is ligated, even if there is hypoxemia. And so we proceeded, letting the baby breathe spontaneously with a volatile anesthetic. With this, we accomplish unconsciousness, pain relief, and some degree of muscle relaxation. If we use too much opioid, we might burn bridges and end up with apnea, so we hold off on that.

For this baby, we started with 100% oxygen. When conditions allow us to mix in some air, we do. This patient and all severely premature infants are at risk for chronic lung disease and retinopathy of prematurity (ROP). This is the "get too much" part of the song. Both conditions are linked to high arterial oxygen tension and, possibly, swings in oxygenation that include periods of hypoxemia, all affecting retinal angiogenesis and pulmonary oxygen toxicity [4]. It is the standard of care to keep oxygen saturations in the low to mid-90s, rather than the high 90s, in premature babies less than 34 weeks' gestation.

The tricky part of the anesthetic beyond induction is maintaining oxygenation and ventilation during the thoracotomy. After all, the surgeon's hands are bigger than the kid's entire chest! Yet somehow they must find the fistula and ligate it. This is done by gently retracting the right lung (it is a right thoracotomy). You can bet that you will see oxygenation plummet in this tiny baby with respiratory distress syndrome, so hand ventilation is usually necessary to assist the baby's own respiratory efforts, positive end expiratory pressure (PEEP) can be used, and of course, 100% oxygen – this is the "not enough and you're gonna die" part. Our patient had episodes of desaturation and complete lack of ventilation noticeable by loss of end-tidal carbon dioxide (ETCO$_2$) and no perceptible lung movement. Possible explanations include kinking of the trachea, abutting of the endotracheal tube (ETT) against the mucosa of the airway, obstruction of the ETT by blood or mucus, or loss of all ventilation through the fistula. Assessment of compliance might help establish the diagnosis, but there isn't time for much diagnostic maneuvering, so you ask the surgeons to get their hands out of the chest to see if ventilation resumes, which, in this case, it did. Nevertheless, the ligation needs to get done, so brace yourself for multiple episodes of desaturation and loss of ETCO$_2$ – you will just have to work with the surgeons; allow them as much time as possible to get a ligature around the fistula, and then you can use positive pressure ventilation.

The fistula gets ligated, but you aren't done yet – now the esophageal anastomosis needs to get done. Finally, the case is completed; the patient did OK despite all the respiratory instability, but there was not much bleeding or hemodynamic instability.

Perform competently all medical and invasive procedures considered essential for the area of practice.

In this case, the technical procedures were done in the neonatal ICU, before you ever met the child. The umbilical catheters are a gift, providing reliable central venous access and arterial access. These catheters are not without complication but are much easier to place than peripheral, percutaneous catheters, especially in the artery. A backup plan would be to ask the surgeons to do a radial or posterior tibial cutdown. Femoral arterial lines in this size of a patient can cause the loss of a leg and so are avoided, unless there are absolutely no other options.

Provide health care services aimed at preventing health problems or maintaining health.

This case is all about keeping the child alive in the operating room and maintaining temperature, oxygenation, ventilation, blood pressure, and intravascular volume. We try to avoid some of the complications of prematurity: barotrauma, patent ductus arteriosus, hypothermia, hypoglycemia, intraventricular hemorrhage, and retinopathy of prematurity.

Medical knowledge

Residents must demonstrate knowledge about established and evolving biomedical, clinical, and cognate (e.g., epidemiological and social-behavioral) sciences and the application of this knowledge to patient care.

Demonstrate an investigatory and analytic thinking approach to clinical situations.

Prematurity is fraught with multiple possible serious medical consequences. Medical science has just not figured out how to duplicate the intrauterine environment. Additionally, prematurity is more common in babies with congenital anomalies, maternal infection, other maternal illness, and placental insufficiency, and neonates respond differently to physiologic stressors than mature humans do. Be prepared for all possibilities.

Know and apply the basic and clinically supportive sciences that are appropriate to their discipline.

Know the possible configurations of esophageal atresia or fistula. There are six possible variants (this is also something commonly found on the written board exam):

- proximal esophageal atresia and distal tracheoesophageal fistula – this accounts for 85% to 90% of defects
- proximal and distal esophageal atresia with no TEF
- proximal TEF and distal esophageal atresia
- proximal and distal TEF
- H-type TEF, no esophageal atresia
- esophageal stenosis, no TEF

Recent research has raised the question of the long-term safety of anesthesia for these patients. Laboratory experiments in rodents have suggested that apoptosis is common in the young and old and that learning deficits can also be demonstrated [5,6].

Practice-based learning and improvement

Residents must be able to investigate and evaluate their patient care practices, appraise and assimilate scientific evidence, and improve their patient care practices.

Analyze practice experience and perform practice-based improvement activities using a systematic methodology.

For most residents, a case like this is way beyond their comfort level. The patient is small enough to be completely lost under the drapes, medications are measured in tenths of milliliters, and the neonate's physiology is different from a more mature human's. So, unless the resident is very experienced with pediatric patients and babies, this case requires attending presence and constant vigilance. It is important to discuss the case afterward and to reflect on how it felt to care for this tiny baby, but the resident probably will not have enough experience with such small babies to have an internal barometer by which to evaluate the case.

Locate, appraise, and assimilate evidence from scientific studies related to their patients' health problems.

There is the need to learn about an infant's physiology and the complications of prematurity.

Obtain and use information about their own population of patients and the larger population from which their patients are drawn.

Residents can draw something from their experiences doing thoracotomies in adult patients and in caring for newborns having other types of surgeries. Some commonalities are generalizable, such as trying to avoid hypoxemia and hypotension, but the babies, especially premies, are really totally different. There is no such thing as a double lumen endotracheal tube for this case; indeed, the single lumen endotracheal tube is far smaller than the lumens of any of the double lumen tubes available. Consequently, life-threatening obstruction of the tiny (2.5 or 3.0) endotracheal tubes can easily happen due to mucus or blood.

Professionalism

Residents must demonstrate a commitment to carrying out professional responsibilities, adherence to ethical principles, and sensitivity to a diverse patient population.

Demonstrate respect, compassion, and integrity; a responsiveness to the needs of patients and society that supersedes self-interest; accountability to patients, society, and the profession; and a commitment to excellence and ongoing professional development.

Be prepared to put everything you have into this case: superb vigilance, constant communication with the surgeons, caring honesty with the mother, and strict attention to medication dosing and fluid administration.

Interpersonal and communication skills

Residents must be able to demonstrate interpersonal and communication skills that result in effective information exchange and teaming with patients, their patients' families, and professional associates.

Create and sustain a therapeutic and ethically sound relationship with patients.

The patient's family needs full disclosure of your plans for anesthetic management and real appraisal of risk for morbidity and mortality.

Use effective listening skills and elicit and provide information using effective nonverbal, explanatory, questioning, and writing skills.

Give the mother enough time to ask questions, knowing that she may be emotionally labile; she is postpartum, the pregnancy was the result of a rape, and the infant is ill.

Work effectively with others as a member or leader of a health care team or other professional group.

Team cooperation and communication is key, first with the neonatal ICU team, and next with the operating room team. As described, periods of patient instability are to be expected, and close communication with the surgeons is paramount. Additionally, the anesthesia team must closely communicate with the surgeons about where they rest their hands or equipment once the surgical drapes cover the patient; it is our job to protect the patient from inadvertent pressure injuries or difficulty with ventilation because of external forces.

Systems-based practice

Residents must demonstrate an awareness of and responsiveness to the larger context and system of health care and the ability to effectively call on system resources to provide care that is of optimal value.

> Practice cost-effective health care and resource allocation that does not compromise quality of care.

The most important way to practice cost-effective health care in this situation is to do things as safely as possible and try to avoid complications that might extend the patient's hospital course. All the complications of prematurity are possible for this extremely premature infant with congenital anomalies; they are also personally and economically costly.

References

1. Costeloe K, Hennessy E, Gibson AT, Marlow N, Wilkinson AR. The EPICure study: outcomes to discharge from hospital for infants born at the threshold of viability. Pediatrics 2000;106:659–671.

2. Kermode J, Zheng Q, Milner EP. Marked temperature dependence of the platelet calcium signal induced by human von Willebrand factor. Blood 1999;94:199–207.

3. Dirkmann D, Hanke AA, Görlinger K, Peters J. Hypothermia and acidosis synergistically impair coagulation in human whole blood. Anesth Analg 2008;106:1627–1632.

4. Sola A, Rogido MR, Deulofeut R. Oxygen as a neonatal health hazard: call for détente in clinical practice. Acta Paediatr 2007;96:801–812.

5. Jevtovic-Todorovic V, Hartman RE, Izumi Y, et al. Early exposure to common anesthetic agents causes widespread neurodegeneration in the developing rat brain and persistent learning deficits. J Neurosci 2003;23:876–878.

6. Wilder RT, Flick RP, Sprung J, et al. Early exposure to anesthesia and learning disabilities in a population-based birth cohort. Anesthesiology 2009;110:796–804.

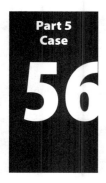

Contributions from Johns Hopkins Medical Institutions under Deborah A. Schwengel

"My patient's an airhead!"

Management of air embolism during sitting craniotomy

The case
Alexander Papangelou

A 52-year-old man presents to the preop area for a craniotomy for tumor. You reviewed the patient's records the prior day and noted that he was previously healthy but has recently developed severe headaches. Imaging of the head revealed a sizable mass compressing the brain stem, with some cerebral edema involving the pons.

Your attending for the day doesn't usually do neuro cases, especially craniotomies. The surgeon wants maximal operative exposure and really wants this to be an "awake crani" so that the patient can be quickly assessed for new neuro deficits. He strongly requests an awake crani in the sitting position. Your attending says, "Sure, whatever you want." You remember from your studies that these procedures are dangerous, but you can't really remember why. You convince your attending to put in both a central line and an arterial line. These are placed, with some sedation, into the right internal jugular vein and left radial artery, respectively.

The patient is positioned and sedated to a zombielike state with a dexmedetomidine drip. You've given the patient 1 g/kg of mannitol, 10 mg of dexamethasone, and 750 cc of normal saline. Incision goes well, partly due to your superb bilateral scalp block. You notice that the surgical field is rather dry, once the skull flap is removed. You're now smiling and excited. Things are going well! Thirty minutes later, the surgeon tells you that he got into the venous sinus but that he thinks he can control things quickly. As you go to text page your attending with the update, you notice that the patient just gasped. He then starts to get tachypneic, with shallow, irregular breathing. The ETCO$_2$ (end-tidal carbon dioxide) reading decreases rapidly, as does the pulse oximeter. You start playing with the connections to make sure the monitors aren't malfunctioning. You tell the surgeon what's going on, and he curses loudly, asking for your attending's presence stat.

Patient care

Residents must be able to provide patient care that is compassionate, appropriate, and effective for the treatment of health problems and the promotion of health.

Communicate effectively and demonstrate caring and respectful behaviors when interacting with patients and their families.

This is a must. In this case, you can very quickly let the patient know that everything is going to be OK. He probably won't hear you, but if he does, he'll later appreciate your calming words. Remember, however, that THIS IS A DIRE EMERGENCY requiring quick action, and not a moment should be wasted.

Gather essential and accurate information about their patients.

This case requires a tremendous amount of preparation and, quite frankly, some prayer. You should have looked at the surgical posting carefully, especially at the position preference. Cases done in the sitting position are particularly prone to air embolism; the patient spontaneously breathing just adds to this risk [1].

Your preop history and physical should have also included an assessment of intracranial pressure (ICP). This could be done by obtaining a history from the patient (headache worse in the lying position, headache worse in the morning, holocephalic unrelenting headache, nausea and vomiting, double vision, blurry vision) and physical examination (change in consciousness, bilateral sixth nerve palsies, papilledema, hyperreflexia). You should also question the surgeon about the scan and his or her assessment of ICP.

Make informed decisions about diagnostic and therapeutic interventions based on patient information and preferences, up-to-date scientific evidence, and clinical judgment.

Recognizing that the sitting position is dangerous should trigger the resident to read a book chapter or review article about this particular position or, even better, about venous air embolism.

Develop and carry out patient management plans.

All craniotomies should get an arterial line. You were right to want a central line. However, the line should have been of the longer variety – a Bunegin-Albin catheter of 30 cm length. This should have been positioned 2 cm below the superior vena cava–atrial junction [1]. You should have also obtained a precordial ultrasound Doppler to assist with early detection of venous air embolism. Along with a TEE, this is the most sensitive tool available to detect venous air embolism. You should be able to detect air before it becomes clinically apparent [2]!

You or your attending should have argued against the sitting position, especially with an awake patient. Positive pressure ventilation with PEEP (positive end-expiratory pressure) is somewhat protective against air embolism. The difference in venous pressure from the cranial veins to the right atrium drives shunting of air and subsequent embolism. An intubated patient in the prone position on 10 mmHg of PEEP, having brain-stem auditory evoked responses (BAERs) and somatosensory evoked potentials (SSEPs) performed as electrophysiological monitoring, would have been far safer.

Your plan should have included tight blood pressure control – not too high from baseline (increases risk of bleeding) and not too far below baseline (decreased cerebral perfusion). Low cerebral perfusion pressure (CPP) should be a substantial concern, especially in the seated position, with the head so far above the heart [2]. You should have aggressively volume loaded the patient, especially with the impending diuresis from a 1 gm/kg load of mannitol. A dry patient will further reduce right atrial pressure.

Counsel and educate patients and their families.

Your informed consent should have included the high probability of air embolism and all the possible sequelae. This includes right heart failure, arrhythmia, coma, and death. This is in addition to your routine preoperative discussion.

Use information technology to support patient care decisions and patient education.

The Internet and PubMed are wonderful resources. You must use them.

Perform competently all medical and invasive procedures considered essential for the area of practice.

It is hoped that you've become proficient at intubating, arterial lines, and perhaps central lines. The longer 30-cm central venous catheter needs positioning confirmed via chest x-ray (CXR). Proper positioning in the right atrium would be essential to treat air embolism.

Provide health care services aimed at preventing health problems or maintaining health.

Keeping this patient alive is now going to be a substantial challenge.

Work with health care professionals, including those from other disciplines, to provide patient-focused care.

Your preoperative discussion should definitely have included a chat with the neurosurgeon with regard to patient positioning and the lack of general anesthesia with mechanical ventilation. At this point, you can't turn back the clock, so working swiftly as a team is a must to save this patient's life.

Medical knowledge

Residents must demonstrate knowledge about established and evolving biomedical, clinical, and cognate (e.g., epidemiological and social-behavioral) sciences and the application of this knowledge to patient care.

Demonstrate an investigatory and analytic thinking approach to clinical situations.

Proper preparation for this case would have quickly helped you make the diagnosis. Even before the gasp, you should have been ready to act when the surgeons got into the venous sinus. Slow entrapment of air affecting 10% of the pulmonary circulation would produce a gasp reflex [1]. This, unfortunately, reduces intrathoracic pressure and right atrial pressure further.

This could cause a rapid entrainment of air and quick circulatory collapse.

> Know and apply the basic and clinically supportive sciences that are appropriate to their discipline.

You know you are in trouble but, what can you do now? The first thing would be to rapidly but safely secure the airway. Flatten the patient, and even put him in Trendelenburg, if possible. Ventilate and oxygenate with 100% FiO_2. *Avoid nitrous oxide* as this can expand air bubbles! Using high levels of PEEP may help prevent further air embolism. Be mindful, however, that PEEP can adversely affect performance of the right ventricle [3], which will already be strained pumping against high pulmonary artery pressures. It may be better to avoid it in cases in which there is impending circulatory collapse. Have an assistant start an inotropic pressor such as epinephrine or norepinephrine. With a longer central venous catheter, you could also manually remove air bubbles! The most air you can retrieve is about 50% of that entrained [1], but this may be the difference between life and death.

The surgeons should first flood the field with sterile saline. They should also get quick control of the venous bleeding. They should then assist the anesthesia team with patient positioning. It is hoped that the surgeons can help limit the danger to the patient during subsequent intubation.

Practice-based learning and improvement

Residents must be able to investigate and evaluate their patient care practices, appraise and assimilate scientific evidence, and improve their patient care practices.

> Analyze practice experience and perform practice-based improvement activities using a systematic methodology.

The first and biggest error in this case is the resident's lack of proper preparedness. Never get caught flat-footed like this again! Of course, your attending didn't help in this situation. You also had an insistent surgeon, who, for whatever reason, really wanted this patient awake in the sitting position. Certainly you will never forget this case during your entire career. Your points of improvement would be as follows:

1. Improve preparedness. Pay attention to positioning and the surgical plan. In neuro cases, be cognizant of elevated ICP, airway issues, and blood pressure control.
2. Read about topics you don't know well. This will allow you to have an intelligent conversation with your surgical colleagues and your patients.
3. Improve your history taking and physical exam skills.
4. Place the proper lines. You should understand whether central access is needed on the basis of potential infusion of vasoactive substances, blood loss (proximity to vascular structures), or in this case, treatment of venous air embolism.
5. Gather the proper equipment. You should have had a precordial Doppler.
6. Do not allow the neuro patient to get dry. This may exacerbate a dysautonomia, cause hypotension, and decrease cerebral perfusion pressure. In this case, a low CVP was clearly detrimental.
7. You should always anticipate the worst. Knowing the signs of venous air embolism, with the proper detection, may have limited the damage in this case.
8. Always simultaneously diagnose and treat a life-threatening problem.
9. Get help when you need it!

> Locate, appraise, and assimilate evidence from scientific studies related to their patients' health problems.

There have been several reviews of venous air embolism. The sitting craniotomy has gone out of favor due to the particularly high incidence of venous air embolism (VAE) (upward of 80% with sensitive detection) [1,2]. Experiments have been performed on different animals to understand what volume of air would be fatal and to follow physiologic changes as they occur. The lethal volume of air in dogs is 7.5 mL/kg injected rapidly. The number in humans is unknown, but injection of as little as 100 cc of air accidentally has led to death [1].

> Apply knowledge of study designs and statistical methods to the appraisal of clinical studies and other information on diagnostic and therapeutic effectiveness.

This is a no-brainer. When evaluating clinical studies, be aware of statistical tricks. In this case, a randomized, double-blinded study would never be performed for VAE. However, studies have been done evaluating the sensitivity of different methods of detection [2].

Professionalism

Residents must demonstrate a commitment to carrying out professional responsibilities, adherence to ethical principles, and sensitivity to a diverse patient population.

> Demonstrate respect, compassion, and integrity; a responsiveness to the needs of patients and society that supersedes self-interest; accountability to patients, society, and the profession; and a commitment to excellence and ongoing professional development.

You may get some Monday-morning quarterback chatter after this case. They may not even wait for Monday morning. Just be humble, respectful, and accept constructive criticism. You'll be a better doctor after your mistakes.

> Demonstrate a commitment to ethical principles pertaining to provision or withholding of clinical care, confidentiality of patient information, informed consent, and business practice.

I'm sure you did your best during informed consent. Sometimes it's tough to give informed consent if you don't know all the risks. If you understand the procedure, then you'll know the risks.

Interpersonal and communication skills

Residents must be able to demonstrate interpersonal and communication skills that result in effective information exchange and teaming with patients, their patients' families, and professional associates.

> Create and sustain a therapeutic and ethically sound relationship with patients.

This is a patient you should follow-up daily, until clinical resolution. Be honest with family members – they will always appreciate this.

> Use effective listening skills and elicit and provide information using effective nonverbal, explanatory, questioning, and writing skills.

Communication is very important, especially when charting a case such as this. This transcends every part of our profession.

> Work effectively with others as a member or leader of a health care team or other professional group.

Don't forget that everyone in the operating room is there to provide care to the patient. You are all there for the same purpose. There is no reason for conflict or anger.

Systems-based practice

Residents must demonstrate an awareness of and responsiveness to the larger context and system of health care and the ability to effectively call on system resources to provide care that is of optimal value.

> Understand how their patient care and other professional practices affect other health care professionals, the health care organization, and the larger society and how these elements of the system affect their own practice.

The outcome in this case is unclear but certainly could have led to intraoperative death or poor functional outcome. This would be even more likely if the patient suffered paroxysmal embolism (increased right-sided pressures, leading to shunting through pulmonary or cardiac channels, i.e., patent foramen ovale [PFO] leading to systemic arterial embolism). This could lead to central nervous system deficits or even death.

In case of death, the greater good of society should be considered. If the patient becomes brain-dead, attempt to maintain adequate organ perfusion. The patient may be a candidate for organ transplant.

> Practice cost-effective health care and resource allocation that does not compromise quality of care.

This was certainly a high-risk surgery, even avoiding the sitting position. Surgically, the tumor was in a terrible location. The possibility of postop deficit is relatively high. One may argue whether surgery should be performed in the first place. Once a decision has been made to proceed with surgery, we have an obligation to provide whatever care is necessary, in the best interests of the patient and society. This may lead to better outcomes, with less morbidity and savings to society.

> Advocate for quality patient care and assist patients in dealing with system complexities.

You are the patient's guardian and advocate, first and foremost. That probably best defines our role in anesthesia. You should always be willing to argue for the patient's best interests, whether with your hospital administrator or with an insurance company.

> Know how to partner with health care managers and health care providers to assess, coordinate, and improve health care and know how these activities can affect system performance.

Not everybody is interested in politics; however, your input from this case may lead to quality improvement at your institution. Presenting this case at morbidity and mortality (M&M) for neurosurgery or anesthesia may lead to helpful discussion. Again, providing excellent patient care should be first and foremost.

References

1. Palmon SC, Moore LE, Lundberg J, Toung T. Venous air embolism: a review. J Clin Anesthes 1997;9: 251–257.

2. Porter JM, Pidgeon C, Cunningham AJ. The sitting position in neurosurgery: a critical appraisal. Br J Anaesth 1999;82:117–128.

3. Neidhart PP, Suter PM. Changes of right ventricular function with positive end-expiratory pressure (PEEP) in man. Intensive Care Med 1988;14:471–473.

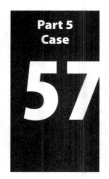

57 Fifty-one-year-old female with abdominal pain, diarrhea, flushing, and heart murmur for exploratory laparotomy

The case
Peter Lin and Ralph J. Fuchs

A 51-year-old, 59-kg woman was admitted to the hospital for elective exploratory laparotomy and resection of a pelvic mass, thought to be ovarian carcinoma. The patient gradually developed increasing abdominal and lower back pain, weight loss of 6 pounds, cough, nausea, and diarrhea over the course of 1 year. She also noted some facial flushing, described as redness of the central face that was persistent but would worsen from time to time, without any precipitating factor. Her medical history was significant for chronic anxiety disorder and mitral valve prolapse.

During the preoperative physical examination, the patient's heart rate was 120 beats per minute, and arterial blood pressure was 105/75 mmHg. There was redness of her central face, which was described as "facial rosacea" by the evaluating physician. A grade II/VI systolic ejection murmur was noted along the left sternal border, without radiation. She had increased bowel sounds. A firm, 18-week-sized uterus with a globular mass at the fundus was palpable. The remainder of her exam was unremarkable.

Laboratory investigations were unremarkable, with the exception of a hematocrit of 24.4 vol %. A colonoscopy to evaluate for chronic diarrhea was normal. An ultrasound of the abdomen and a computed tomographic scan showed bilateral ovarian masses within the pelvis, with ascites and a moderate right pleural effusion. The patient stated that a transthoracic two-dimensional echocardiography from 5 years ago (taken for her history of mitral valve prolapse) was normal, but these results were not available. A preoperative chest radiograph was not obtained. With the exception of a first-degree atrioventricular block, her electrocardiogram (ECG) was unremarkable.

Anesthesia was induced with thiopental sodium and fentanyl. Atracurium was given to facilitate endotracheal intubation. After induction, systolic blood pressure (SBP) decreased from 120 to 100 mmHg but was stable thereafter. Owing to the inability to obtain large-gauge peripheral intravenous access, a triple-lumen central venous catheter was placed in the patient's right internal jugular vein postinduction. Anesthesia was maintained with isoflurane supplemented with fentanyl and atracurium, as judged to be clinically appropriate.

The intraoperative course was hemodynamically uneventful; the heart rate varied from 70 to 100 beats per minute, and SBP varied from 85 to 110 mmHg. However, central venous pressure (CVP) was abnormally high, varying from 17 to 25 mmHg, despite the significant venous bleeding that occurred throughout the procedure. Small- and medium-sized veins in fibrotic tissue resulted in bleeding that was difficult to control surgically.

The CVP trace demonstrated large C-V waves, suggesting tricuspid regurgitation. A two-dimensional transesophageal echocardiographic (TEE) examination was performed, showing an enlarged right atrium and an abnormal tricuspid valve with tricuspid insufficiency. The tricuspid valve leaflets appeared thick, short, retracted, and hypomobile, resulting in incomplete coaptation. At this point, after discussions between the anesthesiologists and surgeons, a carcinoid tumor with cardiac involvement was considered.

Intraoperative surgical findings included amber-colored ascites, retroperitoneal fibrosis throughout the pelvis, and firm, irregular, bilateral ovarian masses. The appendix appeared normal and was left intact. A supracervical hysterectomy with bilateral salpingo-oophorectomy and omentectomy was performed. The patient was awakened and extubated uneventfully.

Postoperatively, the 24-hour urinary excretion of 5-hydroxyindoleacetic acid (5-HIAA) was elevated at 104 mg (normal is less than 6 mg per 24 hours). The final histopathological examination reported bilateral metastatic carcinoid ovarian tumors and omentum with metastatic carcinoid tumor. Both argentaffin and argyrophil stains were positive, suggesting the small bowel as the primary site.

Four months later, the patient underwent a second exploratory laparotomy for small bowel resection and appendectomy because there was evidence of carcinoid tumor involving the small bowel as well as metastatic carcinoid tumor of the appendix [1].

Patient care

Residents must be able to provide patient care that is compassionate, appropriate, and effective for the treatment of health problems and the promotion of health.

Communicate effectively and demonstrate caring and respectful behaviors when interacting with patients and their families.

In any case in which the suspected diagnosis is cancer, the anesthesiologist as well as any other health care provider must recognize the patient's potentially fragile state of mind. While most patients are already anxious prior to any major surgery, the patient in this case was also scared to discover the extent and pathology of her cancer. A patient's sense of self-identity often changes once they become labeled as a cancer patient (or survivor), and her anesthesiologist must recognize, respect, and react properly to these fears.

Gather essential and accurate information about their patients.

Every health care provider has wished, at least once, that his or her patients would carry copies of all their relevant medical studies. Until we have a uniform standard of medical record keeping, however, we must continue to fill in any blanks by taking a thorough history and physical.

For the patient in this case, a thorough preoperative history and physical suggested a possible complex underlying pathology. In retrospect, the presence of abdominal pain, diarrhea, facial flushing, and a heart murmur, together with the CT findings of bilateral ovarian masses, might have led the clinicians to include carcinoid syndrome in the preoperative differential diagnosis. In addition, the patient's earlier diagnosis of mitral valve prolapse may have been in error, and this finding may have actually represented a manifestation of her carcinoid cardiac disease.

The suspicion of carcinoid syndrome would have prompted the physician to request a urinary 5-HIAA level and might have led to an accurate preoperative diagnosis of carcinoid syndrome. The preoperative diagnosis of carcinoid syndrome would have permitted appropriate preoperative pharmacological preparation of the patient. Failure to offset the vasoactive substances that are produced by the carcinoid tumors may lead to profound hypotension or bronchospasm on induction of general anesthesia or during intraoperative manipulation of the tumor.

Develop and carry out patient management plans.

Medical decision making involves many factors, including patient preference, scientific evidence, clinician preference and experience, and clinical judgment. However, when a clinician is presented with a rare and unexpected disease, he or she is often forced to make decisions on the best available evidence.

In patients undergoing anesthesia, patient preference is often a moot issue (i.e., the patient agrees with whatever treatment the anesthetist deems necessary, with some exceptions such as blood transfusion). In a patient with a previously undiagnosed carcinoid tumor, clinical experience and preference are nonexistent and thus become nonissues. This means that whatever decisions are made in the operating room must be based on medical knowledge and on the best available scientific evidence. The scientific evidence and the details of managing a patient with carcinoid syndrome are discussed in more detail later.

Counsel and educate patients and their families.

The patient in this case was educated about carcinoid syndrome, which not only helped her to make informed medical decisions in the future, but also helped to allay some of the anxiety she felt about her new diagnosis. While discussing the implications of this disease with the patient, the health care providers were also vigilant to make sure that they provided an appropriate level of detail, balancing what the patient wanted to know with what she could understand.

It was explained to her that in approximately 2% to 5% of patients with carcinoid tumors, carcinoid syndrome develops. Normally, the release of vasoactive substances produces minimal, if any, symptoms, as the liver is able to rapidly inactivate these materials. Carcinoid tumors of neuroectodermal origin are slow growing and release at least 20 different humoral substances.

Manifestations of carcinoid syndrome usually occur in patients with liver metastasis, in situations in which tumors do not drain into the portal venous system such as ovarian or pulmonary tumors, or when the output of vasoactive substances overwhelms the ability of the liver to inactivate them. Classically, carcinoid syndrome is characterized by episodic flushing, bronchospasm, diarrhea, and right-sided valvular heart lesions. Carcinoid tumors in the appendix have never been reported to produce carcinoid syndrome.

Perform competently all medical and invasive procedures considered essential for the area of practice.

It was fortuitous that a central line was placed in the beginning of the case. This allowed the anesthesia providers to interpret the CVP tracing and recognize its implications. Subsequently, they also needed to perform a TEE and recognized that some of its findings were consistent with a carcinoid syndrome–related valvular lesion.

Indeed, carcinoid syndrome is a rare cause of acquired valvular heart disease. However, cardiac involvement has been recognized in more than half of patients with this syndrome [2], and it may be the cause of death in this condition [3]. Several authors have suggested that it is the exposure of the endocardium to elevated levels of serotonin that might lead to the development of heart lesions [3]. However, the exact etiology of the cardiac plaques that occur remains unknown. Despite treatment that resulted in significant reductions of urinary levels of 5-HIAA, Pellikka et al. [3] did not observe regression of the carcinoid heart lesions in any of the 74 patients in their study.

The definite diagnosis of carcinoid heart disease is difficult, and cardiac symptoms do not appear until the late stages of the disease [3]. In their large series, Pellikka et al. found that patients with cardiac involvement could not be distinguished on the basis of duration of carcinoid syndrome or histologic diagnosis. However, heart murmur and dyspnea were noted more frequently among those patients with carcinoid heart disease. Furthermore, the ECG and chest radiograph at presentation were nonspecific [3]. Changes showing evidence of cardiac enlargement may not occur until late in the course of cardiac involvement. Cardiac involvement in patients with carcinoid syndrome includes not only right-sided valvular heart lesions, but also left-sided involvement, myocardial metastases, and pericardial effusions [3]. Cardiac complications, including right ventricular failure secondary to tricuspid and pulmonic valvular disease, may be fatal. The typical right-sided valvular lesion appears to be one of combined tricuspid stenosis and regurgitation.

Medical knowledge

Residents must demonstrate knowledge about established and evolving biomedical, clinical, and cognate (e.g., epidemiological and social-behavioral) sciences and the application of this knowledge to patient care.

Know and apply the basic and clinically supportive sciences that are appropriate to their discipline.

Anesthetic management of patients with carcinoid syndrome has focused on blocking histamine and serotonin receptors and avoiding drugs that facilitate the release of mediators from tumor cells. Drugs that are considered to trigger mediator release include opioids, specifically meperidine and morphine; the histamine-releasing neuromuscular relaxants atracurium, mivacurium, and d-tubocurarine; and catecholamines. Drugs that are reported to provoke carcinoid crisis include epinephrine, norepinephrine, histamine, dopamine, and isoproterenol. The effect of thiopental has been controversial. Although in vitro studies have demonstrated dose-dependent histamine release from skin mast cells, thiopental sodium–triggered histamine release seems to be of minimal importance in this clinical setting. The use of succinylcholine has also been discouraged because the induced fasciculations can increase intra-abdominal pressure, which could potentially trigger mediator release. However, recent reviews have reported no adverse effects with the use of succinylcholine [4,5].

Carcinoid crisis can be precipitated by stress, physical stimulation, chemical stimulation, or tumor necrosis from chemotherapy or hepatic artery ligation or embolization [5]. Anesthetic premedication with benzodiazepines may be useful to alleviate anxiety. Furthermore, most reports of anesthetic management of carcinoid syndrome describe the use of one or more drugs that block the action of the various ectopic vasoactive substances. Methysergide, ketanserin, and cyproheptadine have been used as inhibitors of serotonin; however, they have not always prevented intraoperative crises. Steroids, to inhibit the action of bradykinin, and diphenhydramine and histamine blockers, such as ranitidine, have also been used.

More recently, anesthetic management of patients with carcinoid syndrome has focused on preventing mediator release from carcinoid tumor cells with the somatostatin analogue octreotide [5]. Octreotide appears to be the most efficacious treatment for carcinoid syndrome, reducing symptoms in more than 70% of patients.

Octreotide blocks hormonal release and inhibits the action of circulating peptides by the inhibition of either phosphatidylinositol or adenylate cyclase. It is a synthetic octapeptide somatostatin analogue, which retains the essential action of somatostatin, yet differs in its pharmacokinetic profile. In contrast to somatostatin, with a half-life of 1 to 3 minutes, octreotide resists degradation from serum peptidases, thus increasing its half-life to 1.5 hours and allowing it to be given by subcutaneous injection, instead of as a continuous infusion. A dose of 150 μg given by subcutaneous injection three times daily has been reported effective in relieving symptoms in patients with malignant carcinoid syndrome. Dosages of 50 and 200 μg given intravenously have been reported effective in rapidly reversing severe episodes of hypotension and bronchospasm. Recently, Claure et al. [5] reported the successful use of octreotide given prophylactically in the anesthetic management of liver transplantation for carcinoid tumor metastatic to the liver [5]. After anesthetic induction, an octreotide infusion was started at 50 μg/hour and was continued throughout the case. Adverse effects, which include pain at the injection site, nausea, vomiting, diarrhea, and abdominal discomfort, are uncommon and mild at dosages of 300 to 450 μg per day. Octreotide inhibits insulin secretion in response to hyperglycemia, and its use in combination with high-dose steroids in obese or non-insulin-dependent diabetic patients may complicate glucose management.

Practice-based learning and improvement

Residents must be able to investigate and evaluate their patient care practices, appraise and assimilate scientific evidence, and improve their patient care practices.

> Locate, appraise, and assimilate evidence from scientific studies related to their patients' health problems.

This is a case of a patient with an unusual diagnosis. That means it is unlikely that most anesthesiologists would be experts in the diagnosis or care of this patient. The literature is necessary to help determine treatment options and to better understand the pathophysiology involved. See the section on medical knowledge.

Interpersonal and communication skills

Residents must be able to demonstrate interpersonal and communication skills that result in effective information exchange and teaming with patients, their patients' families, and professional associates.

> Work effectively with others as a member or leader of a health care team or other professional group.

It is necessary to inform the surgeon of any hemodynamic or other physiologic derangements that become evident during the surgical procedure. Bringing in another diagnostic modality, the TEE helped to clarify the diagnosis and provide better care to the patient. When this was discussed with the surgeon, the diagnosis of carcinoid syndrome was considered.

Systems-based practice

Residents must demonstrate an awareness of and responsiveness to the larger context and system of health care and the ability to effectively call on system resources to provide care that is of optimal value.

> Understand how their patient care and other professional practices affect other health care professionals, the health care organization, and the larger society and how these elements of the system affect their own practice.

There is no mention that a frozen section of the tumor was submitted for pathology. Although carcinoid tumors are notoriously difficult to precisely diagnose by frozen section, consultation between the pathologist and the surgeon intraoperatively might have led to a more diligent search for the primary tumor. Additional diagnostic studies to help localize the primary tumor might have included a small bowel enteroclysis (small bowel enema), endoscopy, and an octreotide scan. If the diagnosis of carcinoid is suggested, but biochemical testing for vasoactive substances is not diagnostic, then provocative testing with a pentagastrin stimulation test can identify an occult carcinoid tumor [6].

Ultimately, effective treatment of a carcinoid tumor includes strong communication between all mem-bers of the treatment team. In addition to intraoperative discussions to find a primary tumor, the patient and the patient's family benefited from compassionate nursing and social work to better cope with her new diagnosis.

References

1. Botero M, Fuchs R, Paulus DA, Lind DS. Carcinoid heart disease: a case report and literature review. J Clin Anesth 2002;14:57–63. Adapted with permission.

2. Roberts WC, Sjoerdsma A. The cardiac disease associated with the carcinoid syndrome (carcinoid heart disease). Am J Med 1964;36:5–34.

3. Pellikka PA, Tajik AJ, Khandheria BK, et al. Carcinoid heart disease: clinical and echocardiographic spectrum in 74 patients. Circulation 1993;87:1188–1196.

4. Veall GR, Peacock JE, Bax ND, Reilly CS. Review of the anaesthetic management of 21 patients undergoing laparotomy for carcinoid syndrome. Br J Anaesth 1994;72:335–341.

5. Claure RE, Drover DD, Haddow GR, Esquivel CO, Angst MS. Orthotopic liver transplantation for carcinoid tumour metastatic to the liver: anaesthetic management. Can J Anaesth 2000;47:334–337.

6. Ahlman H, Nilsson O, Wangberg B, Dahlstrom A. Neuroendocrine insights from the laboratory to the clinic. Am J Surg 1996;172:61–67.

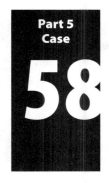

Contributions from Johns Hopkins Medical Institutions under Deborah A. Schwengel

58

DIC

Disseminated intravascular coagulation or devastating injury to the cervix?

The case

Sayeh Hamzehzadeh and Tina Tran

A 34-year-old female at 37 weeks' gestation with twins was admitted for induction of labor due to suspected preeclampsia. Successful delivery of two healthy baby boys was followed by concern for continuing postpartum hemorrhage. The initial diagnosis of cervical laceration was temporized with sutures and a Bakri balloon. The bleeding was resistant to the effects of oxytocin, Cytotec, Hemabate, and uterine massage. The patient had experienced 2 L of blood loss and counting. The decision to proceed to an emergent cesarean section required quick thinking and even quicker action. Of course, the blood that was contained in the abdomen came out to greet us quickly, in the form of a rapid gush. How quickly an oozing cervical injury transformed into disseminated intravascular coagulation.

Patient care

Residents must be able to provide patient care that is compassionate, appropriate, and effective for the treatment of health problems and the promotion of health.

> Communicate effectively and demonstrate caring and respectful behaviors when interacting with patients and their families.

The case originally began with an almost painless vaginal delivery. Result: happy parents, happy babies, happy doctors. So we let down our guard and wrap up the vaginal bleeding, reassuring the family that we are almost done. The nurses escort the father and babies to the recovery room, assuring him that we will be out to meet him in a few minutes.

> Gather essential and accurate information about their patients.

We ask our patient if she is comfortable and share in her joy. She is otherwise healthy and ready to intro-

duce the new twins to their big sister, who is anxiously waiting at home for their arrival. This pregnancy was surprisingly easy for her, compared to her first pregnancy, for which she was nauseated from the first month. She was surprised that a routine office visit would show elevated blood pressure, but if you take a car to the shop often enough, you will find something wrong. Otherwise, she is healthy and happy.

> Make informed decisions about diagnostic and therapeutic interventions based on patient information and preferences, up-to-date scientific evidence, and clinical judgment.

So then why is this healthy, happy mom continuing to bleed? Why can't the obstetrics (OB) team control her bleeding? So let's talk with patient about the possible need for blood transfusions. "You are continuing to bleed from the vagina. It is likely due to a cervical laceration during the delivery." The uterus is not contracting as it should, either due to the magnesium for treatment of preeclampsia [1] or the increase in size of the uterus needed to house the twins. "The OB team is attempting to repair the laceration quickly, but we will prepare to give you blood and monitor your blood pressure very closely. We will also keep talking to you continuously so that we know your head, heart, and lungs are ok." We know the risks and effects of low blood pressure and anemia and that administration of a lot of crystalloid can cause pulmonary edema.

> Develop and carry out patient management plans.

More oxygen, more fluids, call for blood. How do we know we're doing more good than harm? More monitors and more access. In come two more large-bore peripheral intravenous (IV) lines, fluids wide open. In pops the arterial catheter, which can monitor blood pressure on a continuous basis. A central line is in the horizon, but if we get a cordis introducer in the room, it might ward off evil spirits.

Counsel and educate patients and their families.

The patient's husband needs to come back because this is a family decision. We explain to the patient and her husband that we will likely need to place a breathing tube to protect the patient's lungs from pulmonary edema. We will put a big IV in her neck to give her fluids at a speed matched only by light. We will need to do this quickly because the blood pressure is quickly dropping and the patient is beginning to show signs of impaired oxygen delivery.

Use information technology to support patient care decisions and patient education.

We confirm that the uterus is still floppy by ultrasound and external palpation. We send a quick set of labs to rule out medical bleeding, that is, a coagulation profile, platelets, hemoglobin, fibrinogen, and fibrin split products. While we wait for results, let's put a small amount of blood in a test tube to see if it clots. All normal. Let's get to the source of this problem that can be solved by surgery: a floppy uterus that is expanding to hold more and more blood.

Perform competently all medical and invasive procedures considered essential for the area of practice.

Let's go down our checklist here. Large-bore peripheral IVs for rapid fluid resuscitation – check. Cordis introducer is ready to be introduced into the internal jugular for even faster fluid resuscitation – check. Large amounts of blood products are available in the room – check. Pressors made up and ready to go – check. Arterial line that allows for invasive blood pressure monitoring and frequent blood draws – check. Four surgeons on hand for rapid removal of the uterus – check.

Provide health care services aimed at preventing health problems or maintaining health.

We have administered antibiotics prior to vaginal delivery; however, in anticipation of a long surgery with potential for rapid blood loss, we need to have several doses available. We planned on repeating dosing of cefazolin every 4 hours or with estimated blood

loss of 1,500 mL. The last thing we would want to add to this woman's problems is a surgical wound infection.

Work with health care professionals, including those from other disciplines, to provide patient-focused care.

We want the OB team to be ready to work quickly under conditions in which they cannot see their target organ. The patient is at a great risk of rapid exsanguination, so they need to communicate with us about blood loss, and we with them about the patient's stability. At this point, their first estimation is about 700 mL, but it isn't that easy to estimate, so 700 ± 400 is probably a better guesstimate. That can't be good, especially since we know that the literature states that 1,000 mL is when things can get scary from a hemodynamic standpoint [2]. Do not open the abdomen until we have central access and a rapid infusing system. We all have to be focused on the care of this patient – not just the uterus, but the entire patient.

Medical knowledge

Residents must demonstrate knowledge about established and evolving biomedical, clinical, and cognate (e.g., epidemiological and social-behavioral) sciences and the application of this knowledge to patient care.

Know and apply the basic and clinically supportive sciences that are appropriate to their discipline.

Postpartum hemorrhage, or greater than 500 mL of blood loss after delivery, is estimated to occur in about 18% of births in developed countries [3]. Most often, the culprit is uterine atony, with the other potential causes being trauma to uterine structures, retained tissues, invasive placenta, or the coagulopathies. Our main concern now is to keep up with the blood loss to prevent hemorrhagic shock.

The first thing we think is that this woman's uterus is atonic and needs a little assistance from the keen physicians in the room. While the surgeons attempt to perform uterine massage to slow down the bleeding, our first approach is to use various uterotonics, including intravenous oxytocin (Pitocin), misoprostol (Cytotec), and carboprost (Hemabate). We start by giving oxytocin, which we know will help contract the upper portion of the myometrium and, it is hoped, constrict down on those darn spiral arteries that may be causing all this trouble [4]. When this does not work, then we turn to our prostaglandin options, misoprostol and carboprost.

The uterus is as toned as it can be at this point. The OBs have even placed a Bakri balloon inside the uterus to tamponade the bleeding, but this, too, was unsuccessful. The OBs tell us that based on their exam, there appear to be no obvious lacerations, and the placenta has been completely evacuated. Calculating blood loss has become even more difficult as we see clots and clots of blood being evacuated from the uterus. On the basis of our declining vital signs and the worried look on our surgeons' faces, we know that it's time for plan B – we are going to open the abdomen.

In the midst of all this alarm, we recall that although rare, coagulation disorders can be a cause of postpartum hemorrhage. The list of disorders include HELLP (hemolysis, elevated liver enzyme levels, and low platelet levels) syndrome, disseminated intravascular coagulation (DIC), idiopathic thrombocytopenic purpura, thrombotic thrombocytopenic purpura, von Willebrand's disease, and hemophilia. Preeclampsia, which our patient had, can, in 5% of cases, turn into HELLP syndrome. DIC was also high on our list as it can oftentimes occur with amniotic fluid embolism, preeclampsia, sepsis, and placental abruption [5]. In other words, once the arterial line was in, we immediately sent off a coagulation profile.

While we were investigating the cause of the bleeding, we were taking appropriate and clinically proven measures to stop the bleeding. We were also aggressively replacing the blood loss with crystalloid, colloid, and of course, packed red blood cells. To assist in coagulation, we also gave fresh frozen plasma (FFP), platelets, and cryoprecipitate.

Interpersonal and communication skills

Residents must be able to demonstrate interpersonal and communication skills that result in effective information exchange and teaming with patients, their patients' families, and professional associates.

Create and sustain a therapeutic and ethically sound relationship with patients.

While the patient is being resuscitated by skilled and adrenaline-filled anesthesiologists, a worried husband paces in the waiting room. In a brief moment of stability, an available member of the anesthesia team heads to the waiting room to talk with the husband. We explain to him that his wife has lost a lot of blood and continues to need it and will require a hysterectomy. Although he needs support, his wife is our first priority, and we turn all our attention to her.

Use effective listening skills and elicit and provide information using effective nonverbal, explanatory, questioning, and writing skills.

The husband is quiet, yet calm, which can sometimes be more concerning than a family member who is frantic, screaming, and crying. The important thing is that we recognize that everyone deals with stress differently. Our role is to listen, empathize, and let them grieve.

Work effectively with others as a member or leader of a health care team or other professional group.

Everyone in the operating room is working to save the life of this patient. As anesthesiologists, we can step back, away from the surgical field, and take in the big picture. The patient is continuing to bleed. We are running out of blood to transfuse. The patient's blood pressure is requiring high-dose epinephrine. She has high peak airway pressures indicative of pulmonary edema. The OBs cannot get the uterus out. Not a good picture. So speaking over the curtain, we suggest either occluding the aorta so they have a clear surgical field or calling for a trauma surgeon to help with the hysterectomy. A clamp goes on the aorta, and in comes the chief of gynecology and oncology. Now we are making progress.

Systems-based practice

Residents must demonstrate an awareness of and responsiveness to the larger context and system of health care and the ability to effectively call on system resources to provide care that is of optimal value.

Understand how their patient care and other professional practices affect other health care professionals, the health care organization, and the larger society and how these elements of the system affect their own practice.

We update the OBs on the progress of our resuscitation efforts and communicate our concerns for the patient's instability. We are all doctors and nurses caring for this patient, and we all need to respect each other's professional decision. Any moment of doubt, inconsistency, or hesitation can make a difference in this patient's life.

> Practice cost-effective health care and resource allocation that does not compromise quality of care.

In a patient with a presumed diagnosis of DIC, it is most important to find the cause and resuscitate quickly. It is easy to give cryoprecipitate to increase the fibrinogen levels and recombinant activated factor VII to stop the bleeding, but none are without risks to the patient. It is in the best interests of the patient and the health care system to work up a diagnosis before administering a therapeutic agent. Additionally, when you have found the problem and are faced with multiple options for treatment, do not just throw the entire kitchen sink at the patient. One has to balance the level of invasiveness, costs, and risks associated with a therapy before offering it to a patient. Recombinant factor VII, a treatment for patients with hemophilia A, has an off label-use in acute and uncontrolled hemorrhage. However, because a single 90-μg/kg dose for an 80-kg person can cost up to $4,500, it is almost never a first-line therapy for acute hemorrhage. Additionally, this agent is known to increase the risk of thromboembolic events. However, if, after giving FFP, platelets, and cryoprecipitate, one is unable to control intraoperative bleeding, then a discussion about giving factor VII is justified.

> Advocate for quality patient care and assist patients in dealing with system complexities.

While we are giving our undivided attention to the patient, we want to make sure the husband has support from the pastoral care and hospital staff. The charge nurse needs to keep the husband updated. A patient advocate should be at the husband's side should he have questions and should help him with minute-to-minute issues such as finding the nursery, finding water and the restroom, and locating an area in which to sit and rest. A pastor should be available to pray with the husband as this is a time to have support by someone who shares the same faith.

> Know how to partner with health care managers and health care providers to assess, coordinate, and improve health care and know how these activities can affect system performance.

After the successful surgery and resuscitation, the patient needs careful monitoring. The charge nurse calls for the intensive care unit (ICU) bed well before the end of the case in anticipation of immediate transfer to the ICU at the placement of the last staple. The ICU team needs to be ready with a ventilator, monitors, and pumps to deliver accurate doses of pressers. The ICU bed needs to have transport monitors and emergency medication and intubating equipment. The security guards need to have elevator doors open and waiting. The unstable patient on the move is a dangerous thing! We must anticipate all complications as we proceed in the shortest route possible from point A to point B. Do not stop at go, do not collect 200 dollars.

Did we mention that the labor and delivery suite is up and functional? That means that epidurals need to be placed and vaginal deliveries need to be performed on other patients. Call in the reserves: the anesthesia call team needs to have people available for elective epidural placement, and the OB team needs to call in another team to deliver babies on the labor and delivery floor. We need to make sure that the other operating room is available and set up in case we are lucky enough to have another stat cesarean section come through simultaneously. Our responsibilities extend to all the laboring patients, not just to our unstable patient in the operating room. All in a day's work.

References

1. Kantas E, Cetin A, Kaya T, Cetin M. Effect of magnesium sulfate, isradipine, and ritodrine on contractions of myometrium: pregnant human and rat. Acta Obstet Gynecol Scand 2002;81:825–830.

2. Bais JM, Eskes M, Pel M, Bonsel GJ, Bleker OP. Postpartum haemorrhage in nulliparous women: incidence and risk factors in low and high risk women. A Dutch population-based cohort study on standard (> or = 500 mL) and severe (> or = 1,000 mL) postpartum haemorrhage. Eur J Obstet Gynecol Reprod Biol 2004;115:166–172.

3. The prevention and management of postpartum hemorrhage: report of Technical Working Group, Geneva 3–6 July 1989. Geneva: World Health Organization; 1990.

4. Blanks AM, Thornton S. The role of oxytocin in parturition. BJOG 2003;110(Suppl 20):46–51.

5. Alamia V Jr, Meyer BA. Peripartum hemorrhage. Obstet Gynecol Clin North Am 1999;26:385–398.

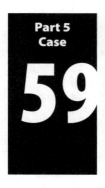

Contributions from Johns Hopkins Medical Institutions under Deborah A. Schwengel

All I had was a knee bursectomy; now do I have RSD (CRPS)?

Adam J. Carinci and Paul J. Christo

The case

Marcus is a 40-year-old dialysis technician who presents with severe, bilateral lower extremity pain following a right knee bursectomy in January 2006. His past medical history includes gastroesophageal reflux disease, coronary artery disease treated with a stent, hypertension, and a right knee bursectomy. He is married with no children. He has no history of substance or alcohol abuse; likewise, there is no family history of substance or alcohol abuse.

The patient's present pain began in January 2006, following a right knee bursectomy. The pain initiated in the right lower extremity and subsequently spread to the left lower extremity (contiguous and mirror image spread, respectively). He describes the pain as constant burning, aching, throbbing, shocking, stabbing, lacerating, wrenching, cruel, tearing, vicious, torturing, and unbearable. He is unable to wear pants due to allodynia and is unable to walk due to severe pain – he is wheelchair bound. His numeric rating pain score is 7 out of 10 at rest and 10 out of 10 with activity. Aggravating factors include cold, touch, walking, and standing, and alleviating factors include rest and sitting. The pain is associated with allodynia, vasomotor changes, sweating, swelling, and weakness, discoloration, and ulcers in lower extremities.

Marcus is angry and depressed secondary to pain. The pain has affected his relationship with his wife in the form of a decreased libido. Marcus is no longer able to socialize with friends or take annual vacations to the local state park. Previous treatments included physical therapy (water-based) and interventional therapy with lumbar sympathetic blocks. Previous medication trials included oxycodone/APAP, hydrocodone/APAP, gabapentin, morphine sulfate, pregabalin, methadone, duloxetine, and cyclobenzaprine.

The patient was eventually diagnosed with complex regional pain syndrome type I (CRPS type I). He subsequently underwent spinal cord stimulator (SCS) implantation, which has produced 70% relief of

bilateral lower extremity pain, and combined medical therapy (e.g., cyclobenzaprine, gabapentin, duloxetine, oxycodone/acetaminophen) relieves the remaining 30% of his pain. SCS therapy has permitted discontinuation of methadone (opioid sparing), increased mobility (out of wheelchair), elevated mood, 6-pound weight loss, and ulcer healing.

Patient care

Residents must be able to provide patient care that is compassionate, appropriate, and effective for the treatment of health problems and the promotion of health.

Communicate effectively and demonstrate caring and respectful behaviors when interacting with patients and their families.

Patients in chronic pain are desperately seeking relief. A compassionate, thorough history is indispensable in assessing the patient's complaints and crucial to establishing a diagnosis. Moreover, chronic pain patients may also have the additional burden of convincing the health care provider that their pain is, in fact, real because no objective signs or tests can confirm the diagnosis of pain. Caring and respect for patients are imperative.

Gather essential and accurate information about their patients.

Complex pain problems necessitate a thorough history and physical exam.

Make informed decisions about diagnostic and therapeutic interventions based on patient information and preferences, up-to-date scientific evidence, and clinical judgment.

CRPS is a debilitating neurologic syndrome characterized by pain and hypersensitivity, vasomotor skin changes, functional impairment, and various degrees of trophic change. No one treatment modality is the panacea; rather, a multimodal, combined pharmacologic and interventional approach is often necessary.

Develop and carry out patient management plans.

The goal of treatment in patients with CRPS is to improve function, relieve pain, and enhance quality of life. Current guidelines recommend interdisciplinary management, emphasizing three core treatment elements: pain management, rehabilitation, and psychological therapy.

Multimodal therapy is key to effective treatment of CRPS. A thorough algorithm for the treatment of CRPS can be found in the literature [1].

Counsel and educate patients and their families.

Psychosocial counseling in addition to medical and interventional treatments is important in patients with CRPS.

Use information technology to support patient care decisions and patient education.

Vascular studies, electromyogram/nerve conduction testing, magnetic resonance imaging, X-rays, and blood testing are warranted. These rule out possible causes of the patient's symptoms other than CRPS. Thermography, a three-phase bone scan, sudomotor testing, sympathetic blockade, and phentolamine infusion can help support the diagnosis of CRPS.

Perform competently all medical and invasive procedures considered essential for the area of practice.

Typical treatment incorporates medications (opioids, tricyclic antidepressants, antiepileptics, topical agents, bisphosphonates), interventions (sympathetic blocks, SCS, implantable drug delivery systems such as intrathecal pumps), and psychological counseling. No two patients will respond exactly alike, and oftentimes, a trial of therapy approach is necessary, and different combinations of interventions can be trialed to arrive at an acceptable regimen. All therapies assist in achieving the primary objective of functional restoration.

Provide health care services aimed at preventing health problems or maintaining health.

Ongoing patient education and follow-up are often needed to help patients deal with the chronic pain of CRPS. Once the patient is on a stable regimen and pain is well controlled, follow-up appointments can be made once every several months. Acute flares of CRPS will necessitate more frequent follow-up to reassess the patient's overall clinical presentation and any new changes that may have produced the acute exacerbation. CRPS is an extremely debilitating and disabling syndrome. Patients may experience months of adequate pain control, only to suffer repeated flares and setbacks.

Work with health care professionals, including those from other disciplines, to provide patient-focused care.

Referrals to pain psychologists and/or support groups often benefit patients dealing with pain and disability secondary to CRPS.

Medical knowledge

Residents must demonstrate knowledge about established and evolving biomedical, clinical, and cognate (e.g., epidemiological and social-behavioral) sciences and the application of this knowledge to patient care.

Demonstrate an investigatory and analytic thinking approach to clinical situations.

The diagnosis of CRPS can be challenging. Again, a thorough physical exam and history of the patient's complaints are essential to aid in diagnosis. Patients should report at least one *symptom* in each of the four categories and display one *sign* in two or more categories, according to the 1999 modified diagnostic criteria:

sensory: report hyperesthesia as increased sensitivity to a sensory stimulation; evidence of hyperalgesia or allodynia

vasomotor: temperature asymmetry or skin color changes

sudomotor/edema: edema or sweating changes

motor/trophic: decreased range of motion or weakness, tremor, dystonia or trophic changes (hair, nail, skin changes)

Once a presumptive diagnosis of CRPS is made based on physical exam and history, sympathetic blocks can then be utilized both to confirm the diagnosis of sympathetically maintained pain associated with CRPS and to treat the painful symptoms. Because

319

the pain in CRPS may be caused by the sympathetic nervous system, a sympathetic block (stellate ganglion block for upper extremities and ipsilateral face and lumbar sympathetic block for lower extremities) can interrupt the aberrant signaling and ameliorate the pain. Furthermore, the use of neuromodulation (spinal cord stimulation or intrathecal medications) may be required to facilitate treatment goals in patients who achieve limited benefit from more standard therapies.

Early recognition and diagnosis of CRPS is associated with better outcomes. It is essential for patients to continue using the affected limb to prevent atrophy and maintain function.

Know and apply the basic and clinically supportive sciences that are appropriate to their discipline.

Practitioners should be familiar with the typical presentation and physical exam findings as well as treatment modalities when caring for patients with CRPS. Refer to previous discussion for further details.

Practice-based learning and improvement

Residents must be able to investigate and evaluate their patient care practices, appraise and assimilate scientific evidence, and improve their patient care practices.

Analyze practice experience and perform practice-based improvement activities using a systematic methodology.

Proposed diagnostic and treatment algorithms for CRPS are available. Practitioners should avail themselves of such aides to help guide diagnostic and treatment decisions. PubMed is an excellent source for recent peer-reviewed research and investigations. In addition, secondary sources, such as UpToDate and MD Consult, provide review articles that synthesize the latest thinking and treatment approaches.

Locate, appraise, and assimilate evidence from scientific studies related to their patients' health problems.

Chronic pain literature [e.g., 2–7] is replete with case reports, case series, and investigational uses of medications and interventions that have shown benefit in treating patients with CRPS.

Obtain and use information about their own population of patients and the larger population from which their patients are drawn.

What benefits one patient may or may not benefit another. A broad exposure to a variety of patients will help expand the practitioner's knowledge base. Furthermore, seeking the opinion of more seasoned colleagues can be especially helpful in diagnosing and treating CRPS.

Apply knowledge of study designs and statistical methods to the appraisal of clinical studies and other information on diagnostic and therapeutic effectiveness.

References in the chronic pain literature are useful in diagnosing and treating CRPS [see 2–7].

Professionalism

Residents must demonstrate a commitment to carrying out professional responsibilities, adherence to ethical principles, and sensitivity to a diverse patient population.

Demonstrate respect, compassion, and integrity; a responsiveness to the needs of patients and society that supersedes self-interest; accountability to patients, society, and the profession; and a commitment to excellence and ongoing professional development.

Patients with CRPS have diverse pain needs. A compassionate, patient-focused, and comprehensive history and physical coupled with a multimodal treatment algorithm is essential in providing maximum benefit to patients.

Demonstrate a commitment to ethical principles pertaining to provision or withholding of clinical care, confidentiality of patient information, informed consent, and business practice.

Observe all HIPAA regulations (don't discuss the case where others can overhear the conversation; don't reveal any confidential patient information; provide the most relevant complications associated with specific nerve blocks, implantations, or pharmacotherapies).

Demonstrate sensitivity and responsiveness to patients' culture, age, gender, and disabilities.

A respect for culture, age, gender, and so on is important when diagnosing and treating patients with CRPS. No two patients are identical in their clinical presentation or psychosocial background; therefore practitioners must treat every patient as an individual with unique needs, requirements, and expectations.

Interpersonal and communication skills

Residents must be able to demonstrate interpersonal and communication skills that result in effective information exchange and teaming with patients, their patients' families, and professional associates.

Create and sustain a therapeutic and ethically sound relationship with patients.

Often patients with CRPS require intense support. This is an opportunity for practitioners to develop a firm physician-patient relationship with clear boundaries, expectations, and requirements. Patients with CRPS may often feel desperate or helpless, and this is a wonderful opportunity for physicians to establish compassionate avenues for communication and encouragement.

Practitioners should realize that CRPS is a syndrome that often waxes and wanes because patients may experience acute exacerbations that worsen their pain even after several months on a stable regimen. Patients may appear angry, exasperated, and dejected over these setbacks, and this may affect their personalities and ability to communication effectively with their providers. Residents need to be patient and kind with CRPS patients and maintain empathy.

Use effective listening skills and elicit and provide information using effective nonverbal, explanatory, questioning, and writing skills.

Thorough documentation of treatment successes and failures is ultimately necessary to ensure that failed treatments are not repeated and that patients are provided with procedural interventions and medications appropriate to their specific needs.

Work effectively with others as a member or leader of a health care team or other professional group.

Any treatment plan for CRPS must be multimodal. Interdisciplinary treatment is the mainstay of effective management of CRPS. Treatment plans will often involve physical therapists, pain medicine specialists, psychiatrists and/or psychologists, nurses, recreational therapists, and occupational therapists. Respect for each member of the team will ultimately improve patient care and patient outcomes.

Systems-based practice

Residents must demonstrate an awareness of and responsiveness to the larger context and system of health care and the ability to effectively call on system resources to provide care that is of optimal value.

Understand how their patient care and other professional practices affect other health care professionals, the health care organization, and the larger society and how these elements of the system affect their own practice.

CRPS is a challenging medical problem. Effective treatment will involve practitioners from multiple specialties over the course of several years. An understanding of a team approach to treating patients with CRPS within the greater context of the health care system will help ensure that patients receive appropriate treatment, follow-up, and monitoring.

Effective multidisciplinary teams may include a pain physician, psychiatrist, psychologist, physical therapist, nurse, physician assistants, and social workers. A treatment approach that encompasses physical and psychosocial needs is ideal.

Practice cost-effective health care and resource allocation that does not compromise quality of care.

An understanding of both effective and less successful medical and interventional treatments will prevent practitioners from repeating costly tests or therapies and will avoid patient disappointment from duplicating ineffective treatments.

Advocate for quality patient care and assist patients in dealing with system complexities.

In addition to the patient with CRPS, the patient's family members and social networks are also significantly affected. Engaging the family or social supports and educating them about the course of CRPS will help each group cope with the often protracted nature of the syndrome. It will further assist them with the substantial psychosocial impact of the disease.

Know how to partner with health care managers and health care providers to assess, coordinate, and improve health care and know how these activities can affect system performance.

The pain specialist should communicate regularly with the patient's primary care physician, physical therapist, and psychologist. Integrating available inputs will better help craft treatment and tailor interventions to the unique needs of the patient. Moreover, this allows for closer follow-up and greater patient satisfaction from knowing that the entire team is collaborating with the treatment plan.

References

1. Stanton-Hicks MD, Burton AW, Bruehl SP, et al. An updated interdisciplinary clinical pathway for CRPS: report of an expert panel. Pain Pract 2002;2:1.

2. Albazaz R, Wong YT, Homer-Vanniasinkam S. Complex regional pain syndrome: a review. Ann Vasc Surg 2008;22:297–306.

3. Grabow TS, Tella PK, Raja SN. Spinal cord stimulation for complex regional pain syndrome: an evidence-based medicine review of the literature. Clin J Pain 2003;19:371–383.

4. Harke H, Gretenkort P, Ladleif HU, et al. Spinal cord stimulation in sympathetically maintained complex regional pain syndrome type I with severe disability: a prospective clinical study. Eur J Pain 2005;9:363–373.

5. Stanton-Hicks M, Baron R, Boas R, et al. Complex regional pain syndromes: guidelines for therapy. Clin J Pain 1998;14:155–166.

6. Rowbotham MC. Pharmacologic management of complex regional pain syndrome. Clin J Pain 2006;22:425–429.

7. Van Hilten BJ, Van de Beek WJT, Hoff JI, et al. Intrathecal baclofen for the treatment of dystonia in patients with reflex sympathetic dystrophy. N Engl J Med 2000;343:625–630.

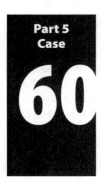

**Part 5
Case**

60

Contributions from Johns Hopkins Medical Institutions under Deborah A. Schwengel

Obstetricians cannot detect FH sounds, and Mom's cyanotic

What's an anesthesiologist to do?

Ramola Bhambhani and Lale Odekon

The case

During the early hours of the morning, you get a call to get yourself immediately to room 1 in the labor and delivery suite. On arrival, you find an apparently term, obese patient in bed. She looks blue and is foaming at the mouth. She is thrashing about and impeding attempts to keep a mask on her face and to secure intravenous access. For the same reasons, you have no way of getting a blood pressure or pulse oximeter reading, but heart rate on the electrocardiogram (ECG) tracing shows sinus tachycardia at 150–160 beats per minute. You are told that the patient ate dinner, got short of breath, her water broke, and she started having contractions at home. She came to the emergency department and was sent to labor and delivery right away, and now there are no detectable fetal heart tones. Your obstetrician colleague tells you that clinic notes on the patient indicate that she is at 40 weeks' gestation and has gestational diabetes mellitus, but there is no indication that she has preeclampsia. The patient's belly is tilted to the left while the obstetrics (OB) team is desperately looking for fetal heart motion.

Someone manages to get intravenous access and is told to guard it with her life. While the patient turns a darker shade of blue and is losing consciousness, despite oxygen being delivered by Ambu-bag, you attempt to suction whitish foam from the patient's mouth while she bites the Yankauer. Your assistant applies cricoid pressure while you are giving etomidate and succinylcholine. You do a direct laryngoscopy; suction the whitish, nonparticulate foamy stuff that is coming through the vocal cords; and quickly place an endotracheal tube. End-tidal carbon dioxide is positive, and there are bilateral breath sounds with crackles. Just as you are taking a sigh of relief, you hear the heart rate go from 160 to 60 beats per minute. You call out for atropine, and as you repeat your request, the heart rate goes to 40 and continues to drop. Atropine is given. You reach for the carotid and the bad news

is confirmed. Advanced cardiac life support (ACLS) is started.

Patient care

Residents must be able to provide patient care that is compassionate, appropriate, and effective for the treatment of health problems and the promotion of health.

> Communicate effectively and demonstrate caring and respectful behaviors when interacting with patients and their families.

The patient's significant other was in the room when she was hypoxic and combative and also heard the obstetrics team mention that they had no fetal heart tones. He just witnessed something that would be very stressful for anyone and is obviously anxious and concerned. At the moment, you would show the most respect by focusing on oxygenation, ventilation, and resuscitation of the mother and the child, so you ask the appropriate language interpreter and a nurse to kindly and respectfully escort the father of the baby to an adjacent room and stay with him to counsel him.

> Gather essential and accurate information about their patients.

Let us take a step back here. Neither the ambulance crew nor the emergency room staff spoke Spanish, and the patient and her partner did not speak English. On arrival to labor and delivery, a Spanish-speaking nurse finds out that in response to "Are you contracting?" the patient responded, "I can't breathe." Here is a crucial piece of information that was overlooked because of the language barrier. Other essential information would be the vital signs. None were available due to patient movement, except the ECG. The patient is obviously short of breath and cyanotic, and you can see secretions coming out of her mouth. As soon as you walk into the room and take one look at the patient, it is hard to miss the urgency of the situation even if no history and vitals are available. This is not the time to get a detailed history and physical exam, but you can keep your ears open to get as much information as you can from the nurse and the OB team while you are resuscitating. Prioritizing your actions and the appropriate use of time are critical in this situation.

Make informed decisions about diagnostic and therapeutic interventions based on patient information and preferences, up-to-date scientific evidence, and clinical judgment.

Clinical judgment directed you to ensure a patent and protected airway by rapid sequence induction as soon as possible to facilitate oxygenation and ventilation of the patient. This response is time-sensitive as the parturient can become hypoxic in a matter of seconds because of the physiological changes of pregnancy (decreased functional residual capacity [FRC] and increased oxygen utilization) and is also at a higher risk of aspiration. As you prepare for emergency intubation, keep in mind the possibility of an unanticipated difficult airway, given her pregnant state and obesity. Now you have cardiorespiratory arrest in a full-term patient and need to initiate ACLS protocol with attention to left uterine displacement and chest compressions at a somewhat higher point on the sternum than in the nonpregnant patient. Recall the differences between ACLS in pregnant and nonpregnant patients [1]. Also, you have not just the life of the mother at stake, but also that of the baby, and its survival depends on that of the mother while it is still in the uterus.

Develop and carry out patient management plans.

In developing a management plan, foresight would have directed the patient to the operating room rather than the labor and delivery suite. Also, the need to urgently call for help from other relevant teams is necessary. It is now clear that ACLS is in order, with special attention to the full-term status of the mother (the big uterus with the baby weighing on the inferior vena cava and decreasing the preload; the decreased FRC and increased oxygen utilization associated with pregnancy; and elevation of the diaphragm).

All medications listed in ACLS are to be given, even if some may decrease uterine perfusion: atropine, epinephrine, and vasopressin. You need to be aware that the patient should have at least 15° left uterine dis-

placement for cardiopulmonary resuscitation (CPR) to work. Chest compressions need to be two finger breadths above the accepted point because of changes during pregnancy. It goes without saying that volume resuscitation should also be ongoing. If, by 5 minutes into CPR, the mother has not recovered a perfusing rhythm, an urgent cesarean section is necessary for the success of the resuscitation of the mother and the best chance of recovery of a viable neonate.

Counsel and educate patients and their families.

This, of course, is no time to educate anyone, but we need to keep in mind that proper prenatal care has to be emphasized later on. Extending care to the uninsured and to illegal aliens (which was applicable in this case) and educating them on what they need to do in the case of an emergency is beneficial. Moreover, in populations where illiteracy is high, utilizing pamphlets with only pictures and instituting proper social policies may forestall the lifelong dependence of the mother and child on the system because of a preventable disability.

Fast-forwarding, the patient survives and is diagnosed with peripartum cardiomyopathy. She needs to be counseled as to the feasibility of a future pregnancy, her medical care, and the possibility of a heart transplant.

Use information technology to support patient care decisions and patient education.

Although ideally, one would use the clinical data management system of one's hospital prior to administering care to the patient, in this particular case, it will be used for the subsequent management of the patient. In the intensive care unit (ICU), where the patient is recovering, an ECG, serial echocardiograms, laboratory results, computer tomography of the chest, and an ultrasound of the lower extremities will be crucial to patient care. Also, the ready access to this information for sharing among professionals from various fields due to the development in technology will help in determining the etiology of the event that ended in the patient having a cardiopulmonary collapse.

Today, we are treating an increasingly older and sicker patient population (notwithstanding advanced maternal age, with its attendant comorbidities). The volume of medical information and the increasing complexity of the medical environment, and the requirement to abide by evidence-based medicine, have necessitated that each practicing physician acquaint himself or herself with the various information technology options available today. Devices such as PDAs can be used to carry information to the point of care.

Information found on the Internet may be helpful, but it is essential to verify the source. Library liaisons (librarians with special interests) help physicians discover information in a particular clinical setting. Additionally, the educational sites listed here are available to physicians looking to broaden their information base in a particular case:

1. http://www.theanswerspage.com
2. http://www.mypatient.com
3. http://www.nysora.com

The information gathered from the preceding sources will also help guide the patient's and her family's education and counseling about the etiology of the problem and help them make informed decisions in the future [2].

Perform competently all medical and invasive procedures considered essential for the area of practice.

In a pregnant, hypoxic, and cyanotic patient, a competent anesthesiologist would preoxygenate and perform a rapid sequence induction and intubation or an awake intubation to secure and protect the airway. He or she will also ensure that suction, all intubation equipment, medications, and an end-tidal carbon dioxide monitor are available and will induce via an available intravenous access (or place one in an upper extremity, if one is not available already) in a manner that is most likely to maintain cardiovascular stability (for left uterine displacement, a Cardiff wedge or at least 15° tilt included). Instituting effective CPR as per ACLS protocol, acting as a team leader for conducting the code, and eventually placing arterial and central lines when they are more feasible are also skills that one should possess.

Provide health care services aimed at preventing health problems or maintaining health.

Though not the domain of anesthesiology at that moment, this competency would involve attending to the patient's gestational diabetes and prenatal care and perhaps an astute observation that might lead to a suspicion of an impending cardiac failure. Additionally, one would follow up and treat the cardiomyopathy and counsel the patient as to the advisability of a future pregnancy. Antibiotic coverage during surgery and afterward (because the cesarean section was done in the labor and delivery suite, rather than the operating room) also becomes relevant once the patient is successfully resuscitated.

Work with health care professionals, including those from other disciplines, to provide patient-focused care.

A code is an excellent example of this interaction: the most qualified individual for coordinating care during the code in this case is the anesthesiologist, who should take charge and delegate firmly, clearly, and respectfully the necessary tasks to other members of the team (nursing, obstetrics, etc.). The others on their part need to repeat back to acknowledge the message and confirm that an action was taken (medications given, pulse checks done, compression cycles completed). If the obstetricians have not initiated an emergency cesarean section within 4 minutes of the code, then the anesthesiologist in charge will ask them to do an emergency cesarean section on the spot. If the request is met with any resistance due to the fear of delivering a neurologically affected baby, then you need to be persistent as it is a documented way of increasing the success of the parturient's resuscitation, as well. Also, the neonatologists and neonatal intensive care unit need to be made aware of an impending delivery in which a compromised neonate is a possibility.

Medical knowledge

Residents must demonstrate knowledge about established and evolving biomedical, clinical, and cognate (e.g., epidemiological and social-behavioral) sciences and the application of this knowledge to patient care.

Demonstrate an investigatory and analytic thinking approach to clinical situations.

You would think back to what could have caused this patient's respiratory distress. Was she sitting down in front of the TV for too long and a thrombus traveled to her lungs? She is reported to have ruptured membranes, so amniotic fluid embolism is also a consideration. She is obese, 40 weeks pregnant, and has gestational diabetes; could she also have preeclampsia that is presenting as pulmonary edema, or is she developing cardiac failure secondary to peripartum cardiomyopathy?

Or could it be aortic dissection? She had dinner some time back, so could it be "food in the wrong pipe"? But she should have a reason for the decreased mental status that led to aspiration in the first place (like seizures secondary to eclampsia). One also needs to draw on the physiologic changes during pregnancy that will hasten the development of hypoxia such as decreased FRC and increased oxygen utilization.

> Know and apply the basic and clinically supportive sciences that are appropriate to their discipline.

When working in labor and delivery, you will need to have a good understanding of changes in cardio-vascular, respiratory, airway, and full stomach status secondary to pregnancy (increased minute ventilation, decreased FRC, increased oxygen consumption, increased blood volume and the propensity for cardiac failure, increased possibility of difficult airway, and the risk of aspiration). In addition to these, she has changes related to obesity and gestational diabetes (not to forget a 10-pound baby resting on the inferior vena cava, which can cause all kinds of complications). The possibility of chronic hypoxemia secondary to obesity, leading to pulmonary hypertension, also exists. One should also realize the significance of left uterine displacement on facilitating venous return in the mother. Familiarity with the interpretation of fetal heart rate patterns is necessary, even though, in this case, none were detectable.

You need to focus urgently on the following:

1. The patient is tachypneic and cyanotic (she is in respiratory failure and decompensating fast, and you have less time than in a nonpregnant patient).

2. She has a full stomach in every sense of the word (she just had dinner, is obese, and is full-term pregnant and contracting). She might have already aspirated.

3. The patient is pregnant and has a large fetus due to gestational diabetes, which will impede preload and certainly not help with cardiac output. On top of that, she may be in cardiac failure (she had crackles all over the chest bilaterally on auscultation and had white froth coming out of her mouth even when she was awake and speaking earlier during transport).

4. She might be a difficult airway (combine obesity, pregnancy, and likely preeclampsia).

5. There are two lives at stake: mother and baby.

Practice-based learning and improvement

Residents must be able to investigate and evaluate their patient care practices, appraise and assimilate scientific evidence, and improve their patient care practices.

> Analyze practice experience and perform practice-based improvement activities using a systematic methodology.

The patient's oxygenation and ventilation are going down fast, and you need to act *now*. Not much of a chance to indulge in practice-based learning at that moment. After the case, you need to conduct a debriefing session with all involved parties, to be followed by a departmental morbidity and mortality (M&M) conference. There is always room for improvement, so discuss the good and the bad with intent to improve the system that is already in place. One of your colleagues showed up to help out of the goodness of his heart when he heard the overhead "rapid response team to labor and delivery" announcement. Other teams apart from the code and neonatal ICU team were called, and you had 20 people in the small room. The ones who were not participating in the resuscitation had to be escorted out by the nurse to decrease the noise level in the room. This is a place where the nursing team had not participated in a code or a code drill in years but did pretty well and, thankfully, the mother was revived without any evident neurological deficit (there were code drills conducted after this event to make the nursing team more familiar with such events). Should this patient have been taken directly to the operating room from the emergency department, rather than a crammed labor and delivery suite, in anticipation of badness? You had to overcome the reluctance of the obstetricians to perform the perimortem cesarean section due to the high probability of delivering a neurologically affected infant as they have not been able to detect any fetal heart tones or motion at all. Persist as the emergency cesarean section will improve the likelihood of saving the mother's life. Had the cesarean section and CPR not restored the mother's circulation, would you have been able to transport to a facility with extracorporeal membrane oxygenation? What about left ventricular assist device or intra-aortic balloon pump? Should someone – ambulance crew or emergency room staff – have placed an IV prior to transferring to labor and delivery or gotten vitals? Should the OB and rapid response team have been called to the emergency room instead? What would have happened if she had coded in the elevator during transport to labor and delivery? How do good communication, coordination, and foresight help in better transfer of care of patients between teams? There are a lot of questions to be considered and answered and changes to be made based on the lessons learned from this event.

Locate, appraise, and assimilate evidence from scientific studies related to their patients' health problems.

It is hoped that you would already have read and internalized the prevailing knowledge and guidelines on how to deal with a peripartum code. The literature will not have prospective, controlled, randomized, double-blind studies on peripartum codes. American Heart Association guidelines recommend left uterine displacement, all advanced cardiac life support (ACLS) medications irrespective of their potential effects on the fetus, and the delivery of the fetus within 5 minutes of the code (for the sake of both the neonate and the mother, if the fetus is alive, and for the success of the mother's resuscitation, if otherwise). However, there are several other issues that are relevant to this case that have controlled trial results available. You might want to brush up on these later: especially the effect of hyperglycemia on neurologic resuscitation and the effect of hypothermia on neurologic recovery post–cardiac arrest.

Obtain and use information about the population of patients and the larger population from which their patients are drawn.

Review published case reports on CPR/ACLS on parturients (when left uterine displacement [LUD] is necessary [more than 20 weeks], when the fetus is viable [more than 24–25 weeks], and there's the need and decision to perform an emergency perimortem cesarean section) and draw on the experiences of your colleagues. Fast-forward to a time after successful resuscitation of the patient; you need to review the differential diagnosis of the initiating event. It is now narrowed down to amniotic fluid embolism versus peri-

partum cardiomyopathy, so literature related to management of these conditions and the risks associated with future pregnancies are relevant.

Apply knowledge of study designs and statistical methods to the appraisal of clinical studies and other information on diagnostic and therapeutic effectiveness.

Statistics quantify uncertainty utilizing three methods: (1) data analysis, (2) probability, and (3) statistical inference. We need to be aware of the kind of data that are being collected and ascertain whether the analysis is appropriate for those data – this will provide the inference validity. "If we are to be role models of critical thinking, we need to evaluate claims based on evidence by adhering to the six essential elements for reasoning: falsifiability, logic, comprehensiveness, honesty, replicability, and sufficiency" [3, p. 730].

Use information technology to manage information, access online medical information, and support their own education.

The differential diagnosis for the patient was narrowed down to amniotic fluid embolism versus peripartum cardiomyopathy. We can use one of the search engines, such as PubMed, to search for information on these. Additionally, we can classify relevant literature by EndNote or RefWorks for future reference. Also, Web sites, such as http://F1000medicine.com, where experts in each field stratify the abundant literature under "must read" or "changes clinical practice," can be consulted.

Professionalism

Residents must demonstrate a commitment to carrying out professional responsibilities, adherence to ethical principles, and sensitivity to a diverse patient population.

Demonstrate respect, compassion, and integrity; a responsiveness to the needs of patients and society that supersedes self-interest; accountability to patients, society, and the profession; and a commitment to excellence and ongoing professional development.

Providing a Spanish interpreter, keeping the significant other informed about the condition of the mother and baby and their progress during and after resuscitation, and updating the mother and father about the baby's condition during the time when the baby is in another hospital are respectful and compassionate behaviors. Coming on time for work, well rested and under no influence of anything, and making sure that the code bag and the operating rooms are well stocked would be examples of integrity.

Although the parents are illegal aliens and do not have any insurance coverage, providing the care they need and assisting them in getting temporary insurance would be in line with responsiveness toward the patient and society.

Being up to date on ACLS and neonatal resuscitation with appropriate credentialing would be expected of an accountable professional.

Fellowship training in one's chosen subspecialty field would further professional development. Attending national and international meetings, grand rounds, and journal clubs would demonstrate a commitment to excellence.

> Demonstrate a commitment to ethical principles pertaining to provision or withholding of clinical care, confidentiality of patient information, informed consent, and business practice.

As this is an emergency, we do not have time to pause and get an informed consent. The same applies to the obstetrician performing the perimortem cesarean section. The requisite paper work will be completed after the case, dated, and timed to indicate that the notes were written after the patient's condition had stabilized.

During the case, keep meticulous detailed records of interventions and vital signs. Respect the confidentiality of the information discussed during the debriefing and the M&M. Ensure that the billing is appropriate for the type of anesthesia coverage the case received.

Even though our primary patient is the mother, we were also concerned about the survival and prognosis of the baby. Owing to undetectable fetal heart tones and low Apgars at delivery, the prognosis for the baby was guarded. Several management decisions were made by neonatal ICU staff in consultation with the parents. The possibility of hypoxic encephalopathy and need for withdrawal of care were considered, but luckily for this baby, her subsequent clinical improvement made this unnecessary.

> Demonstrate sensitivity and responsiveness to patients' culture, age, gender, and disabilities.

The parents were Spanish speaking only, illegal aliens in the United States, and with a much desired pregnancy now resulting in complications. They were embraced by the team as any other patient would be and were provided with care, support, and empathy.

Interpersonal and communication skills

Residents must be able to demonstrate interpersonal and communication skills that result in effective information exchange and teaming with patients, their patients' families, and professional associates.

> Create and sustain a therapeutic and ethically sound relationship with patients.

A person unable to breathe initially and who becomes unconscious later, and who is having her vital organs perfused by outside help, may not be receptive to a relationship initially! In this case, you might get a second chance by doing the right medical things first, and later visit her in the ICU. Inquiring about her health and that of her baby will be a good place to start the relationship during a postop visit. Not bringing her any bacterial gifts by remembering to wash your hands before the interaction will be much appreciated.

> Use effective listening skills and elicit and provide information using effective nonverbal, explanatory, questioning, and writing skills.

In this patient's case, the language barrier delayed getting crucial information. In the emergency room, the classical error of medical interviews, that is, incomplete and incorrect agenda setting, took place [4]. This is partly because of time pressure and partly because physicians usually err in assuming that the first thing about the patient that draws our attention is his or her most pressing need. In this case, her mentioning contractions and rupture of membranes (mostly in sign language, as no interpreter was available) distracted the emergency room physicians from her most urgent complaint, that is, her respiratory distress. This is one area of communication in which we all have to improve.

The time to practice perfect writing skills is when you are writing the postop note, which better be a detailed and exact text, without any blaming of other members of the care team, even if you are thinking that some things could have been done faster or better. We need just the facts, in the order in which they took place. If, later, you think of something you neglected to write down, you can always go back and write an addendum, clearly marking the time and date to complete the record.

Work effectively with others as a member or leader of a health care team or other professional group.

During the initial encounter with the patient, you are multitasking: assessing the patient (who is blue, thrashing about, and foaming at the mouth), acting on your initial assessment (she needs airway control, ventilation, and oxygenation), and also interacting with your OB colleagues to obtain available history (term pregnancy, gestational diabetes mellitus, not preeclamptic). You also note that the patient does not have IV access. You designate, perhaps, a nurse to this task (asking nicely) and emphasize how vital access is once it is obtained ("guard this with your life"). As the situation evolves, the trachea is successfully intubated, but as luck would have it, now the heart rate is decreasing rapidly, and your communication is directed to others in the room. You call one person by her name, asking her for atropine; it is hoped that she will call back the request and let you know when it is given. You note the nonperfusing rhythm on the monitor and check for a pulse (not there!). Now your communication effort is directed to another person, as you ask him to call the code team and your colleague upstairs (his name and number are given).

We have a term patient coding; designate one person to perform chest compressions, another to keep a record, and yet another to prepare and administer medications (atropine, epinephrine, vasopressin). Ensure that the patient has a CPR board underneath and is in LUD, and that compressions are high on the sternum. The next item on communication is a request to OB to deliver the neonate (they are reticent as they have not been able to obtain fetal heart tones), which, fortunately for all involved, happens quickly – and voilà! Mom gets her pulse back. The next step will involve an orderly and safe transport of the patient to the operating room. Take a minute to inform the father about the delivery of the baby and that the mom is doing better, check on the baby's status with the neonatal ICU team and then continue to designate tasks in the operating room, including central line and arterial line placement. Ask the obstetricians about their preference for antibiotic coverage as the surgery had started under less than sterile conditions.

After transfer to the ICU, there is another opportunity to interact as a member of the health care team. A detailed report to the nurse and physician in charge, a discussion of the pros and cons of hypothermia for this patient, and also, a discussion on optimal glycemic control should take place. Additionally, the patient's ventilator settings need to be reviewed to ensure that there will not be any additional insult to her lungs secondary to excessive volume.

Postoperative visits allowed the anesthesiologist to interact with the primary care team and to discuss the working diagnosis and treatment. In the ICU, the patient initially had an ejection fraction of 15%. Could this be attributed to "stunned myocardium" postcode, or to the natural progression of a peripartum cardiomyopathy? Did the patient develop respiratory distress secondary to amniotic fluid embolism (ruptured membranes, sudden onset of pulmonary edema)? A literature search on how fast the ejection fraction corrects itself in peripartum cardiomyopathy may answer some of these questions.

Systems-based practice

Residents must demonstrate an awareness of and responsiveness to the larger context and system of health care and the ability to effectively call on system resources to provide care that is of optimal value.

Understand how their patient care and other professional practices affect other health care professionals, the health care organization, and the larger society and how these elements of the system affect their own practice.

Encouraged by their training to be omniscient, physicians may find it difficult to ask for help. This may not always work in the best interests of their patients. For example, during the maternal code, we needed assistance from many members of the health care team. Our success in returning the patient to her family intact reinforced the high-quality image of our institution. If each element undertakes what it can, the whole may end up being more than the sum of its parts. The nursing, ICU, anesthesiology, OB, and neonatal

ICU teams worked together to save two lives. On the other hand, based on a judgment call, the failure of the ambulance and emergency department teams to get the patient's vital signs or an IV access negatively impacted the ability of subsequent health care givers to help the patient, albeit for a short time. It's all interdependent.

Know how types of medical practice and delivery systems differ from one another, including methods of controlling health care costs and allocating resources.

At times, the scarcity of resources, such as equipment, beds, time, or excessive numbers of patients, makes it difficult to provide all possible alternatives in health care. When these conditions of scarcity occur, we have to consider various factors to guide decisions for making difficult trade-offs in a fair and compassionate manner. At times, this can be alleviated by making the system more efficient or increasing investments (which may not always be an option), but in spite of this, a rationing decision must be made under certain unfortunate circumstances.

Hospital policies and protocols should clearly outline specific situations that call for activating the code or the rapid response team, and these should be adhered to as these teams involve different personnel and resources. Doing this will increase the efficient use of resources.

A question may arise as to whether a patient's quality of life seems so poor that use of extensive medical intervention appears unwarranted. During these moments, please consider who is making this quality of life judgment – is it the health care team, the patient, or the patient's family? For example, the neonatal ICU team was considering ECMO (extracorporeal membrane oxygenation) for the baby at one point, which is a scarce resource. They considered the absence of fetal heart tones in utero and low Apgar scores after birth, but the electroencephalogram and clinical assessment were better and more encouraging. Also, the wishes of the family should be respected. The allocation of resources (ICU beds and prolonged ICU care) would also have been relevant if the mother suffered significant neurological injury, although thankfully, that was not the case here, and she was neurologically intact.

Our hospital has a three-level system for operating room time allotment that classifies the cases into various levels, depending on the urgency of the surgery. This helps with prioritizing and proper allocation of operating room resources in an objective way.

What happens if a cesarean section is already being done by the night anesthesiology team? In such a situation, it is justified to call in the anesthesia backup team and an additional nursing team from another floor. Also, seeking help from the general operating room anesthesiology team if there is no emergency case in progress would be a good utilization of these resources.

Practice cost-effective health care and resource allocation that does not compromise quality of care.

In business circles, redundancy of staff is not cost-effective, and resources allocated to high-volume areas increase revenues. This approach has limited applicability to the medical setting. Keep in mind how this patient's fate might have changed if there were no 24/7 OB or anesthesiology team coverage available at labor and delivery. Would the code or rapid response teams be aware of the specific requirements of resuscitation in a term parturient? How is cost-effectiveness defined in this context?

Transporting this patient directly from the emergency department to the operating room would also have been a good way of optimally using our resources, as in this case it was obvious that a cesarean section was in order.

Advocate for quality patient care and assist patients in dealing with system complexities.

Quality patient care will involve timely airway intervention initially, a successful resuscitation, and an evidence-based management of ventilator support and invasive monitoring to avoid complications. Identify resources for the patient – medical coverage, legal access, and access to care and entitlement – and attend to their emotional and spiritual needs, and even offer transportation, as needed.

Know how to partner with health care managers and health care providers to assess, coordinate, and improve health care and know how these activities can affect system performance.

This patient was of Hispanic descent, which is a growing population in our society. There are often issues of language barriers and a certain misconception about medical interventions. For example, if this patient had presented in labor without respiratory distress, it is likely that she would have been reluctant to accept epidural analgesia for fear of paralysis. Work is already in progress at our institution (administrators, masters of public health trainees, nurses, physicians) to reach out to this population early in pregnancy and provide education. Administrative support is invaluable for outreach clinics, and distributing pictorial and written pamphlets in Spanish that provide patients with information about pregnancy and labor, the right time to seek medical help, and the pros and cons of epidural analgesia would be beneficial. Getting these endeavors operational paves the way for reducing complications in pregnancy, leading to healthier mothers and babies (due to a decrease in maternal mortality and morbidity and declining neonatal death rate) and, overall, a healthier society.

Additional reading

1. The 2005 International Consensus Conference on cardiopulmonary resuscitation and emergency cardiovascular science with treatment recommendations hosted by the American Heart Association in Dallas, Texas, January 23–30, 2005. Circulation 2005;112:IV-150-3.

2. Kurup V, Ruskin KJ. Information technology in anesthesia education, in Anesth Infs, Stonemetz, Ruskin eds. Springer-Verlag London 2008; pp397–407.

3. Shafer SL. Critical thinking in anesthesia. Anesthesiology 2009;110:729–737.

4. Baker LH. "What else?" Setting the agenda for the clinical interview. Ann Intern Med 2005;143:776–770.

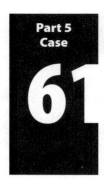

Contributions from Johns Hopkins Medical Institutions under Deborah A. Schwengel

A case of mistaken identity

Nishant Gandhi and Bradford D. Winters

The case

It is five o'clock in the morning, and you and your on-call team have been up all night pushing blood, scopolamine, and fluid (not necessarily in that order) into the parade of trauma patients and emergent cases that have come to your operating rooms (ORs). You have five people on your team (four residents and one attending), and two are in rooms already. A call comes out from the wilderness of the surgical intensive care unit (ICU) – a critically ill renal transplant patient with an open abdomen needs to come back to the OR emergently because he may be bleeding. You and the free members of your team hastily dispatch to the ICU to find the patient sedated, vented, and on pressors, with a pulmonary artery catheter in place that has been demonstrating worrisome values for the last few hours.

Many other patients in the unit are equally unhealthy, and the staff is in a surly and foul mood from a mixture of high patient acuity, a sick call-out, too much instant coffee, and some questionable salty snack foods. You and your team slunk through the unit seeking the fellow who provides a thumbnail sketch of the last eight-hour course and the general history of the patient. None of it sounds good. You attach your transport monitors – make sure you have your emergency drugs and airway equipment and undock from the mother ship, taking care not to rip any lines out of the patient or wires or tubing out of the wall. On the way out the door, a nurse comes running up to you with the patient's chart and squeezes it between the mattress and the bed frame, and you hurriedly race down the hall to the OR.

In the OR, you and your team get the patient transferred to the OR table and hooked up to the anesthesia machine monitors and breathing circuit and get the case under way. The patient is already anemic, and you and the surgeons agree to get some blood up to the room for the patient. While all of these preparations are going on, your pager goes off, informing you that there is a patient in the neuro critical care unit (NCCU)

who is not responding to maximal therapy for increasing intracranial pressure (ICP) and is therefore in need of an emergent decompressive craniectomy. You leave your very capable second year anesthesia resident in charge of the kidney transplant patient and rush off to the NCCU to start yet another case.

The craniotomy case does not start smoothly, and the acuity of the operation does not permit you to leave until well after 7:00 A.M. The anesthesiologist in charge of the room for the next day gets sign-out from you, and around 7:30, you finally get the opportunity to return to the room with the kidney patient. Your call resident has already signed out to the resident assigned to that room for the day and, like Elvis, has left the building to spend a well-deserved day communing with his pillow and studying the back of his eyelids. While in the process of signing off on this case, you note the bag of packed red blood cells hanging on the IV pole infusing into the patient, closely examine it, and to your horror, you realize that the blood has a different patient's name on it, and this is the second unit being transfused. What happened?

In a nutshell, the chart that the nurse shoved between the mattress and the bed frame had the wrong stamp card inserted in it. No check was performed. No time-out or briefing occurred. The process was rushed. The staff members involved were stressed and tired. The staff in the OR completely turned over shortly after the procedure began, except the surgeons, who were much distracted. The OR nurse, not realizing the card did not match the chart or the patient, stamped all the forms with the wrong card. You and your team knew who the patient was, but the new team taking over did not. You were occupied in another emergency. When the blood arrived in the OR for transfusion, the resident from your on-call team was already gone, and the new resident had no idea who the patient was and didn't recognize that the name on the blood did not match the patient. Multiple system failures occurred, leading to the patient, who was B positive, receiving

O positive blood. While this is not a dire situation (purely by dumb luck), the patient was also cytomegalovirus (CMV) negative and got CMV positive blood, which could have been a longer-term problem. As it turned out, the patient passed away a few days later, unrelated to this event.

"All systems are designed to give the exact results that they produce." This phrase is often heard and, at first glance, seems to be an example of pure circular logic. However, it is not. It simply underscores that you will only get good results from well-designed systems. The system described in the preceding vignette is poorly designed, and its breakdown, and the subsequent error, with or without patient harm, was predictable. Medical care is extremely risky, and the potential to cause harm, including death, is immense. It is incumbent on us as practitioners to strive to develop safer systems to reduce harm to our patients.

Patient care

Residents must be able to provide patient care that is compassionate, appropriate, and effective for the treatment of health problems and the promotion of health.

The primary failure in this case is that effective communication did not occur and the resident did not gather essential and accurate information about the patient. Obviously, one of the most important pieces of "essential and accurate information" is confirming that you have the right patient. The system in place to ensure that this information is correct, including ID bracelets, patient cards, and names on units of blood, failed. Why? Because they were not cross-checked with each other to ensure that they all matched. While the resident is partly responsible for this, so is everyone else participating in the patient's care. Blaming the resident or any one individual for the failure serves little purpose as systems need to be designed to protect against error, especially when the situation is stressful, hurried, and chaotic, much as it was during this situation. Such protections can include time-outs (not the kind your Mom did with you when you painted the cat orange when you were 4 years old) so all members of the team correctly identify the patients. Had a simple time-out been in place, by which the patient, the procedure, availability of blood, and other items on a time-out checklist are verified, the providers would likely have identified the problem and been able to correct it.

But you say, "This was an emergency; there was no time for a time-out!" While, yes, this was an urgent/emergent procedure, but there was time for a time-out. Even in very critical situations, a time-out can still be called out by a member of the team while the procedure is even getting under way. It takes only a few seconds to call out the patient's name (if known) and expected procedure and have everyone on the team communicate back his or her response. The airline industry does it all the time in emergencies, and analyses of airline disasters have frequently shown that failure to adhere to these checklists sealed the planes' fate. The mismatch between the card provided by the ICU nurse and the patient and his chart would have been recognized. While the theme for this particular competency is to take a professional responsibility to utilize the systems already in place to obtain essential information, it also underscores the physician's responsibility to participate in the design of systems to promote the accurate gathering of crucial patient information.

The current system of medical record keeping can provide for difficulties in this area. Due to the use of both computerized and paper charting for the many patients across institutions, and even within one institution, developing systems to protect against misidentification can be challenging. Until completely computerized systems are in place that take advantage of bar codes, radiofrequency tags, and other identification technology, we need to be vigilant to these risks and employ other strategies, such as the time-out and checklists, in safe care design.

Medical knowledge

Residents must demonstrate knowledge about established and evolving biomedical, clinical, and cognate (e.g., epidemiological and social-behavioral) sciences and the application of this knowledge to patient care.

The idea of analytical and investigatory thinking applies to this event, even though this may seem remote. How does this case of mistaken identity relate to medical knowledge? In the sense of knowing pharmacological, biochemical, or anatomical facts, it does not. However, the scientific method and process of asking and reasking questions is integral to the practice of the science of safe medical practice as much as it is in basic scientific, translational, and clinical research. When the resident took over the case from the night-call resident, a conversation probably occurred regarding issues such as physiological status and history.

What apparently was not discussed was patient identity and its confirmation, and the conversation was most likely only conducted between those two people. Unfortunately, because of lack of a time-out procedure, the signing out resident couldn't have known the problem that was coming. Perhaps the investigation inherent in transfer of care should have been expanded beyond that two-person process. Inquisitiveness and investigation by the new resident with the rest of the team, reidentifying the patient and any other issues from their perspective, rather than by the first anesthesiology resident, only would have uncovered the failure before the blood had been hung. While this is probably not the way most people go about their work, we would submit that perhaps we should expose those barriers and not work in isolation, either as individuals or as a specialty. Understanding and being cognizant of the science of safety and how it tells us how things can go wrong can offer additional opportunities to apply science beyond standard thinking. The science of safety should be part of medical knowledge, just as much as the Krebs cycle.

Practice-based learning and improvement

Residents must be able to investigate and evaluate their patient care practices, appraise and assimilate scientific evidence, and improve their patient care practices.

In the United States, an estimated 100,000 people die from health care errors, and many consider this to be a gross underestimate. Additionally, we provide inadequate care to many more based on our own definition of what people should receive. In terms of providing recommended quality of care for a range of conditions and diseases, a RAND Corporation study found that for only three conditions – low back pain, coronary artery disease, and hypertension – did the American medical system score above an F, and that grade was a D in the percentage of patients who actually received recommended treatment for their conditions. For other conditions, such as asthma, diabetes, and hip fracture, recommended care was provided less than 55% of the time. How can we harm patients in this fashion? How can we harm patients with medical errors such as the one described here?

It happens because we don't treat the delivery of health care as a science. We don't seek rigorous methods to analyze it, we don't standardize it, and we don't put broad and diverse input into the process. Read

through the five subcategories of this Core Clinical Competency. Very "disease"-oriented, isn't it? How much of your medical education has focused on disease and treatment evidence, but not on how the care for that disease and its treatment is delivered? While health care delivery and the science of safety may rarely be amenable to double-blinded, placebo-controlled, randomized trials, rigorous methodologies exist both inside and outside of medicine that may be appropriately applied to the delivery of health care. A full discussion of the science of safety is beyond the scope of this book, but while the science of safety is immature, to be sure, it deserves to be as much a part of practice as genetics, which itself was in its infancy only 30 years ago. All the elements of this Core Clinical Competency should be applied to this field with as much energy as they would be to the management of acute lung injury.

Professionalism

Residents must demonstrate a commitment to carrying out professional responsibilities, adherence to ethical principles, and sensitivity to a diverse patient population.

It is important for all health care providers to dedicate themselves to providing patient care in the most professional manner. There is little room for selfish or egotistical behavior, and one must always put the patient first. This becomes a difficult proposition in the reality of medical practice in the majority of hospitals, specifically those that are designated teaching institutions, with residents from various disciplines. House staff at times have seemingly unreasonable demands placed on them, which can be compounded with long work hours, frequent call, and lack of sleep. Despite these conditions, there must be a sense of accountability to the patient, and this is the element of this competency that most applies in this case. This accountability broke down at several levels and across disciplines – nursing, surgery, OR techs, and the anesthesiology team. Certainly there was never malice, simply error compounded by many factors, which have been previously discussed. How do we make ourselves and the system accountable under these circumstances? We do so not by blaming, accusing, criticizing, and denying, but rather, by making us accountable to safe practice and supporting the application of the science of safety. Whenever you witness others violating safe principles, such as not following checklists, procedures, standards, and policies, you demonstrate your accountability to your patients by speaking up and empowering others to speak up and correct the problem. We are accountable to educate ourselves and others and to participate in the development and application of safe practice principles. Our egos, self-interest, and professional autonomy take a backseat to these principles and the science behind them. You do not work in isolation. No individual can or should be asked to shoulder all the burden. You should not take it on yourself to do so, but nor should you assume it is for others to carry. We provide care in a complex system in which communication and cooperation are key elements. We must move away from the ABCDs of medicine (accuse, blame, criticize, and deny). If you are not willing to be dedicated to these ideals, perhaps you should consider another career.

Interpersonal and communication skills

Residents must be able to demonstrate interpersonal and communication skills that result in effective information exchange and teaming with patients, their patients' families, and professional associates.

Certainly the group taking care of this particular patient in the operating room thought, at the time, that they were performing this competency very well. The patient got transferred to the operating room from the ICU, incision was made, and the patient was kept alive. However, the irony of the situation is that this was the greatest failure: communication.

Several checkpoints are in place in most health care institutions to avoid such occurrences. Most nursing units have a checklist that must be completed before any patient goes to the operating room; this obviously includes checking the patient ID before he or she is whisked off to the OR, even in emergent situations. We should all be familiar with time-out procedures that should occur before every surgical case or procedure (central line placement, bronchoscopy, etc.). Unfortunately, at the time this case occurred, formal time-outs were not part of routine care where this happened. Even more unfortunate is the fact that where these are used routinely, they are often viewed with skepticism and may be performed in a haphazard fashion, where everyone in the room just agrees with what is said, name bands are not checked, and the paper work is signed blindly. A commitment to the culture of safety is essential. Would you want your airline pilot to just sign off on a checklist blindly, without going through it properly? The airline industry has a culture of safety that pervades everything they do. The number of accidents per flight takeoff is miniscule. Developing the same culture of safety in medicine can yield similar results.

An additional problem in this case was that there was a physician and nursing shift change during this case, and despite sign-out from the outgoing teams to fresh, well-rested teams, the grave error still went unnoticed. Perhaps such significant staff changes should require an additional time-out or some other formal mechanism to transfer the data. Clearly verbal sign-out was inadequate or was isolated between like practitioners (nurses vs. doctors) so that there was no cross-contact. Had a multidisciplinary conversation occurred, surely the error would have been quickly realized. Thus interpersonal skills and communication across disciplines are at the center of the culture of safety and safe practice and help ensure that mishaps, such as patient misidentification, don't occur.

Systems-based practice

Residents must demonstrate an awareness of and responsiveness to the larger context and system of health care and the ability to effectively call on system resources to provide care that is of optimal value.

This is what we've been talking about the whole time. Medical care is provided within a system, and you are part of that system. All the elements in this competency have been described earlier in this chapter because this is the core of what it means to practice safe medicine and prevent medical errors. While the elements of this competency may not have direct bearing on the immediate prevention of this patient misidentification at that moment, understanding and applying these elements is central to the science and practice of safety. Each one of these requires not only a knowledge of the side effects of ketamine or the potential complication of placing a central line catheter (safe technical work), but the understanding of safe design in teamwork (checklists, time-outs, standards, and protocols) and how diverse teams of people tend to make more wise decisions than individuals working in isolation. Had this group of people worked better as a team using safe design, the event would likely not have occurred.

(*First author's note:* Just like Case 39, we went straight to a discussion of the main ideas under each clinical competency. After 335 pages, you should be doing this automatically.

You'll also note, by now, how often we repeat the same things in discussions of systems-based practice, interpersonal and communication skills, and professionalism.)

Additional reading

1. Winters BD, Gurses AP, Lehmann H, Sexton JB, Rampersad CJ, Pronovost PJ. Checklists: translating evidence into practice. Crit Care 2009 Dec 31;13(6):210.

2. Clarke JR, Johnston J, Blanco M, Martindell DP. Wrong-site surgery: can we prevent it? Adv Surg 2008;42:13–31.

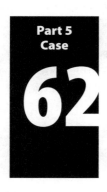
Contributions from Johns Hopkins Medical Institutions under Deborah A. Schwengel

62 "To block or not to block, that is the question"
Anticoagulation and epidural anesthesia

The case
Brandon M. Togioka and Christopher Wu

An 85-year-old gentleman with hypertension, known diffuse coronary artery disease with two stents to his left anterior descending artery, and now a recent diagnosis of prostate cancer is scheduled to have a radical retropubic prostatectomy in your room tomorrow. His stents are drug eluting and were placed just under 1 year ago, and thus the patient continues to be on clopidogrel. The good news is that he comes with a preoperative cardiac evaluation. In this evaluation, the patient is deemed safe for surgery "only under neuraxial anesthesia due to his many known stenotic lesions that were not stented open." Today, the patient presents with his family, angry because he is hungry and has been off clopidogrel for 5 days.

Patient care

Residents must be able to provide patient care that is compassionate, appropriate, and effective for the treatment of health problems and the promotion of health.

> Communicate effectively and demonstrate caring and respectful behaviors when interacting with patients and their families.

In this case, as in every case, the first order of business when greeting the family is to establish rapport, instill confidence, and act in a manner to relieve patient and family anxiety. State your name, your title, and what you will be doing. Starting off on a good note can pay big dividends later, when you have to talk about whether the surgery will be done.

> Gather essential and accurate information about their patients.

Check to make sure that the patient has in fact been off his clopidogrel for only 5 days. Verify all his medications, including whether he was on a beta-blocker or angiotensin receptor blocker and whether these were

continued. Complete the rest of that all important preoperative evaluation sheet, but before you begin, start with the most basic and often overlooked question: so this is you (pointing to the patient's bracelet), and we are taking your prostate out today, right?

> Make informed decisions about diagnostic and therapeutic interventions based on patient information and preferences, up-to-date scientific evidence, and clinical judgment.

In this case, patient management will involve a precise understanding of timing. This will include the time when the patient stopped taking his clopidogrel, the window of clopidogrel-free time required to put a needle in someone's back, and, if a catheter is put in his back, the time to wait before it can come out.

The incidence and risk of spinal hematoma after clopidogrel use in a patient who receives neuraxial anesthesia is unknown. As such, the American Society of Regional Anesthesia and Pain Medicine have relied on scientific data from the surgical, interventional radiology, and cardiology literature to come up with a consensus statement on this topic. In essence, a consensus statement is a compromise from a set of experts on how to answer a clinical question yet to be decisively answered by research. In this case, your best clinical judgment is likely their best clinical judgment, or the consensus statement. This statement recommends waiting 7 days from the time of last clopidogrel administration before a spinal or epidural is placed [1]. You best be waiting to take the patient back.

> Develop and carry out patient management plans.

> Talk to the patient, his family, the surgeon, and the nursing staff. This patient may be going home with a prostate.

> Counsel and educate patients and their families.

Now the family is a little upset. They say, "Isn't there another way? He must get his prostate out. He is going to die!"

At this point, some education is in order. Even if you did a great job of explaining why the patient could not get neuraxial anesthesia, the family may still be very confused. You are a doctor, and there is always more than one way to do something. Their thought is: use your education, be creative, and figure it out. Do not forget that they may not have been told by the cardiologist that the patient is only cleared for surgery if they get a spinal or epidural. Also, does the family know why neuraxial anesthesia is dangerous while being treated by an antiplatelet medication such as clopidogrel? Do they even know what clopidogrel is? Explain about the greater than average risk of bleeding from the procedure. Explain that this bleeding may lead to a blood clot (hematoma), and if this is in the wrong place, the patient can end up paralyzed. Discuss with the patient's family that although prostate cancer is technically "cancer," waiting an additional 2 days may lessen the risk of epidural hematoma (and thus paralysis), whereas waiting 2 days (although mentally difficult) will not affect the advancement of cancer in most cases. Such a discussion of risks and benefits can show the family that you are their advocate and that you are looking for the best possible outcome for their loved one. This can turn the conversation from competitive to collaborative and help to alleviate the family's fears, while helping them to accept that the surgery may not be performed today.

Use information technology to support patient care decisions and patient education.

The question here is whether there is some database of clinical information, such as an electronic medical record, to which you could get access that may help to explain why this patient's cardiologist felt so strongly against general anesthesia. This database may not include all the cardiologist's thoughts about the patient, but it may, at the very least, provide some data (echocardiogram results, stress tests, history of angina, etc.) that could help you support your decision not to allow the surgery and educate the patient and his family as to why you are doing this.

Perform competently all medical and invasive procedures considered essential for the area of practice.

Should this case have gone to the operating room (OR), you would have been responsible for putting in an intravenous line, bolusing the patient with fluid, and then placing either an epidural or spinal. An arterial line may have also been useful in this case, given the cardiac concerns related to this patient.

Provide health care services aimed at preventing health problems or maintaining health.

Again, going back to the scenario in which the patient goes to the OR for regional anesthesia, the block would have to be placed in a sterile fashion. This would include skin antisepsis, maximal use of barrier precautions, washing of one's hands before and after the procedure, and the opening of a new kit containing all new sterile equipment for each block.

Work with health care professionals, including those from other disciplines, to provide patient-focused care.

In essence, everything we do as anesthesiologists involves working with other physicians and health care professionals. In the OR, we collaborate closely with an OR nurse and a team of surgeons to provide care as a unit that would otherwise be impossible on our own. Preoperatively, as we prepare our anesthetic, we consult with radiologists, cardiologists, and primary care physicians, whether via written or verbal communication. Though it may be an oversimplification, anesthesiologists who have been tagged as lone rangers are, in fact, linked at all times to other health care disciplines by the simple fact that none of their clinical decisions can be made in a vacuum without information gained from other specialists.

Medical knowledge

Residents must demonstrate knowledge about established and evolving biomedical, clinical, and cognate (e.g., epidemiological and social-behavioral) sciences and the application of this knowledge to patient care.

Demonstrate an investigatory and analytic thinking approach to clinical situations.

Now back to the case: remember that comment by the family about there being other options? Quickly, in a matter of seconds, before giving your answer, you would have gone through the other options in your head, which, in this case, mainly involve general anesthesia. You would have thought about the options for a more hemodynamically stable cardiac induction, the drips that you may have gotten set up to help keep the patient's blood pressure within a well-defined range, and the types of monitors that you would have needed. You would have done this quickly and systematically because that is the way you do it every time, and in the end, that is what would keep you from missing anything. Having had this thought experiment, you would then be able to calmly, and in a logical manner, explain the other options to the patient's family.

> Know and apply the basic and clinically supportive sciences that are appropriate to their discipline.

You are now just about ready to address the family, but first, you feel that you should quickly refresh your memory about the patient's pathology and the physiology of anesthesia and a failing heart. After some review, you have narrowed it down to the following for easy discourse with the family:

- The patient has known limitations to blood and nutrient flow to his heart.
- Anesthesia in the surgical setting can bring out these limitations by increasing nutrient demand and potentially further limiting the body's ability to increase supply.
- If demand outweighs supply, the heart gets damaged, and if the extent of damage is large enough, the rest of the body can die.
- Published literature has not clearly shown a superiority of regional anesthesia over general anesthesia for patients with heart disease, though nonrandomized (or less than ideal) trials do seem to support lower incidences of heart attacks and death in high-risk patients with regional anesthesia [2].
- Given the fact that we do not know the extent of the patient's cardiac history and his cardiologist does, it may be the safest decision in this circumstance to follow the cardiologist's recommendation.

Practice-based learning and improvement

Residents must be able to investigate and evaluate their patient care practices, appraise and assimilate scientific evidence, and improve their patient care practices.

> Locate, appraise, and assimilate evidence from scientific studies related to their patients' health problems.

To help answer the patient's and your ultimate question as to whether the patient can still have neuraxial anesthesia, you will need to know if there were any good studies recently published on clopidogrel and the incidence of hematomas. In this case, no such studies have been published, but even knowing that there are no good studies can help you in making your decision.

> Obtain and use information about their own population of patients and the larger population from which their patients are drawn.

Let's say that there is a strong study out on the incidence of hematomas after stopping clopidogrel for 5 days. Does this study apply to your patient? Your patient is not on aspirin, but the majority of the patients in the study were. Does this affect the applicability of this study? Your patient is also elderly, but most of the patients in the study were under the age of 60. Can you still apply the incidence of morbidity and mortality to your patient, or is your patient more likely to have a poor outcome?

> Apply knowledge of study designs and statistical methods to the appraisal of clinical studies and other information on diagnostic and therapeutic effectiveness.

Similar to the preceding, let's say that in the study mentioned earlier, the patients off clopidogrel for only 5 days had a zero incidence of hematoma. Does this information help? Can you now safely place an epidural in this patient with full confidence that he will not get a hematoma? Before you can make such a bold prediction, look at the way the study was performed, and see if it is even a valid study. For instance, were inclusion criteria stated in the study? Were patients randomly allocated? How? Were the observers and those who carried out the study blinded? Were subgroups appropriately analyzed? Only if a study is deemed to be valid can it even begin to be considered as a new piece of information that may change how you manage patients. Changing patient care before appropriately appraising the source of information is unwise and potentially litigious.

Use information technology to manage information, access online medical information, and support their own education.

For most residents, this part of the practice-based learning and improvement competency is quite easy to meet. Online journals, metasearches, patient information databases, and, now ever more commonly, electronic charting are how we prefer to learn, accumulate data for research, and complete our daily clinical duties. Maybe they should change this part of the competency to include a statement that residents should make sure they still know how to use the Dewey Decimal System.

(*First author's note:* Egad! And to think we were told in a Stony Brook case that we were forever rid of the Dewey Decimal System.)

Professionalism

Residents must demonstrate a commitment to carrying out professional responsibilities, adherence to ethical principles, and sensitivity to a diverse patient population.

Demonstrate respect, compassion, and integrity; a responsiveness to the needs of patients and society that supersedes self-interest; accountability to patients, society, and the profession; and a commitment to excellence and ongoing professional development.

After weighing the potential gains and risks to pursing neuraxial anesthesia, we decided not to block this patient. Though it is a natural and necessary desire for a resident to want to get procedures under their belt, this should not by itself guide clinical decision making. Now, oftentimes, there can be many reasonable treatment plans for a patient with no one option being clearly superior to the others. In such cases, it could be reasonable to hope for the option that may expand your clinical experience, but even still, all options should be fairly presented with accompanying risks and benefits. Then, the patient should be given a chance to weigh in on the treatment options before an anesthetic plan is chosen.

Demonstrate a commitment to ethical principles pertaining to provision or withholding of clinical care, confidentiality of patient information, informed consent, and business practice.

As referred to earlier, for an informed consent to be valid, all options must be presented fairly and without bias. The patient must express a clear understanding of the facts, and he or she must have the mental capacity to understand the implications of the procedure about to be undertaken. In our case, it was assumed that our patient had the mental capacity to make his own decisions, but did he or his family have a clear understanding of the facts? The fact that the patient's family thought that he could die if he did not get his prostrate out right away points to the family not having a thorough understanding of the acuity of the situation. This is a problem that is often encountered in the hospital. Patients can grasp some understanding of the situation, but parts of the intended procedure or disease treatment will ultimately remain a mystery. In such instances, your commitment to the ethical principles of the fair allocation of health care resources, beneficence, nonmalficence, veracity, and fidelity is what your patients are counting on.

Demonstrate sensitivity and responsiveness to patients' culture, age, gender, and disabilities.

Revisiting our patient, I forgot to mention that in addition to his mentioned history, he has congenital sensorineural deafness, and as such, he is part of a unique subculture of deaf Americans who communicate through American Sign Language, or ASL. More times than I would like to count, I have done a preoperative assessment on a patient and seen notes from primary teams stating that a patient is "difficult," "non-cooperative," "unintelligent," "unable to follow commands," and "not oriented to person, time, or place." When I first read this, I think, wow, this patient has some anger management issues, or he or she has a mental disability or is delirious. I go into the room, and because I know ASL, I find a totally normal human being desperately waiting for someone who can communicate with him.

I understand that this example may be a little different than what people normally think of when they hear about cultural, age, gender, and disability sensitivity, but I mention it to make the strong point that sensitivity to a culture or characteristic requires both understanding and awareness of it. Without these things, we are helpless against stereotyping and inappropriately putting people into boxes of diagnoses that do not belong to them.

Interpersonal and communication skills

Residents must be able to demonstrate interpersonal and communication skills that result in effective information exchange and teaming with patients, their patients' families, and professional associates.

Create and sustain a therapeutic and ethically sound relationship with patients.

In our case, start by establishing a strong channel of communication, which means realizing what you are good at and what you are unable to do. If this patient happened to be Spanish speaking, I would have had to get a translator in the room, or at least on the phone. This would be a huge step toward establishing a good physician-patient relationship. Then, have patience; let the patient ask you all of his or her questions, ease his or her worries, and approach the dilemma of whether to get the patient's prostate out as a team – you and the patient working together toward a common goal.

Use effective listening skills and elicit and provide information using effective nonverbal, explanatory, questioning, and writing skills.

Again, this boils down to engaging with the patient and working with the patient, rather than at the patient. If you take the time to engage, you will be amazed at how easy this all becomes. These are simple communication skills that we developed over the years through our interactions with family and friends, only too often, because of time constraints, we fail to apply these extremely effective methods of communication to the perioperative time. Change this – you can! (You don't have to be Yoda to be successful. If you try, the force will be with you.)

Work effectively with others as a member or leader of a health care team or other professional group.

So, after excellent adherence to the communication principles described earlier, the patient and his family understand that waiting 2 days would be in the patient's best interest, and they go home. Two days later, they come back, and the patient has his prostate taken out with an epidural as the primary method of anesthesia. Now it is the postoperative period, and his catheter will need to be removed – at some time.

In this circumstance, in which timing for the removal of the patient's catheter will be extremely important, you will have to make sure that all those involved in the care of this patient understand the plan. Take time to explain the situation and plan for catheter removal with the nursing staff, the surgical team, and even the floor techs who will be cleaning the patient and may not understand that small tugs on that funny-looking wire coming out of the patient's back can lead to big problems. Furthermore, the surgical team should be cautioned about the use of drugs that can affect hemostasis, such as nonsteroidal anti-inflammatory drugs, platelet inhibitors, or other anticoagulants, while the catheter is still in place. Communication is the key here. Communication will lead to a safe discharge.

Systems-based practice

Residents must demonstrate an awareness of and responsiveness to the larger context and system of health care and the ability to effectively call on system resources to provide care that is of optimal value.

Understand how their patient care and other professional practices affect other health care professionals, the health care organization, and the larger society and how these elements of the system affect their own practice.

I'm not sure if you caught it, but you were just able to do something amazing in the last competency. You canceled an elective surgery and then brought the patient back in 2 days. No small feat, considering that the OR times and schedules are often set much further in advance, and the surgeon who was to take the patient's prostate out may only operate a few times a week. Congratulations! You did something difficult that ultimately led to a good outcome and high patient satisfaction. Undoubtedly, you did this knowing that it would require the surgical team to squeeze the patient into the OR schedule and the hospital to give up OR billing time, and that all this grief was back on your head. Wow, didn't realize you pulled off such a feat, did you?

Now don't just pat yourself on the back; after all, you still don't know why the patient ended up coming to the hospital for surgery after only having been off clopidogrel for 5 days. To be truly amazing, you would need to analyze the process and determine what chain in the link failed. Systematically follow all the preoperative instructions, from the receivers (the patient and family), to the primary surgical team, to the primary care physician who cleared the patient for surgery, to the cardiologist who was consulted by the primary care physician. Where did the message get messed up? Was there any problem with a lack of education with any of the physicians? Did communication get messed up? Was the appropriate information communicated at all?

Some have said that the next decade will be one in which the biggest strides in patient care will come in the area of refining hospital policies and protocols. In this case, our patient has encountered a problem that was entirely avoidable, could have been prevented without any extra charge, and that we already have the tools to eliminate; however, the simple fact is that such problems occur all the time in hospitals, and consequently, patients are not optimized for surgery. This kind of problem would not have happened if the patient had been seen at a preoperative evaluation clinic (PEC). In such clinics, providers with a keen awareness of anesthetic practice assimilate consultants' opinions into a perioperative and anesthetic plan. After all, consultants such as cardiologists are invaluable, but we as anesthesiologists do not always take their advice as they are not intimately involved in the formulation and implementation of the anesthetic plan. To help reduce day-of-surgery delays and cancellations, the use of established guidelines and clinical pathways are used in PECs to take the guesswork out of decision making and ensure a successful perioperative outcome [3].

Practice cost-effective health care and resource allocation that does not compromise quality of care.

In this case, you went with neuraxial anesthesia because it was safer, but evidence suggests that it was probably also cheaper. In a study done on patients undergoing radical retropubic prostatectomies, spinal anesthesia was found to be associated with less overall blood loss, less postoperative pain, less time to first flatus, and less time to ambulation, which ultimately led to a faster postoperative recovery – which has been linked to decreased hospital costs [4].

Advocate for quality patient care and assist patients in dealing with system complexities.

As described earlier, you pulled off a feat. You assisted your patient by maneuvering scheduling difficulties and hospital financial disincentives to get the best care possible.

Know how to partner with health care managers and health care providers to assess, coordinate, and improve health care and know how these activities can affect system performance.

Now that you pulled off this feat and got great patient satisfaction, share this success with hospital administration. Find out how these coordinated activities were able to be completed in such a short time span. Analyze what happened, congratulate those who made it happen, and make changes to help it happen again. Better yet, make changes so that the patient comes in at 7 days, rather than 5 days, so that jumping through the hoops isn't necessary. You are now thinking of the hospital as a system, and every system can be optimized. So, in the same way that research questions are systematically answered, systematically analyze your hospital system to get optimal performance.

References

1. Horlocker TT, Wedel DJ, Benzon H, et al. Regional anesthesia in the anticoagulated patient: defining the risks (the second ASRA Consensus Conference on Neuraxial Anesthesia and Anticoagulation). Regional Anesth Pain Med 2003;28:172–197.

2. Breen P, Park KW. General anesthesia versus regional anesthesia. Int Anesthesiol Clin 2002;40:61–71.

3. Fischer SP. Cost-effective preoperative evaluation and testing. Chest 1999;115:96S–100S.

4. Salonia A, Crescenti A, Suardi N, et al. General versus spinal anesthesia in patients undergoing radical retropubic prostatectomy: results of a prospective, randomized study. Urology 2004;64:95–100.

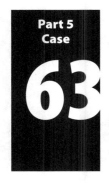

Contributions from Johns Hopkins Medical Institutions under
Deborah A. Schwengel

63 Anterior mediastinal mass with total occlusion of the superior vena cava and distal tracheal compression

The case

Andrew Goins and Daniel Nyhan

A 28-year-old female, with a medical history significant for mitral valve prolapse, has developed progressively worsening cough and orthopnea of 3 months' duration. A chest radiograph and computed tomograph (CT) revealed the presence of a large anterior mediastinal mass measuring 12 × 10 cm, with significant distal tracheal mass effect, but without occlusion. Chest CT also revealed dilated collateral venous involvement and a superior vena cava totally encased and occluded by the mass, which was suspicious for lymphoma.

Efforts to diagnose the mass via transbronchial biopsy and supraclavicular lymph node sampling were nondiagnostic, so the patient was referred to a thoracic surgeon for mediastinoscopy and biopsy. In the days leading up to her procedure, her symptoms worsened, and she required admission for further evaluation. Her chest radiograph featured a large right pleural effusion, and transthoracic echocardiogram revealed the presence of right ventricular compression, a depressed left ventricular ejection fraction of 35% with moderate diastolic dysfunction, and a large circumferential pericardial effusion. In the hours leading up to the scheduled operation, her oxygen requirement increased, and she required upright positioning with a nonrebreather mask to maintain adequate oxygenation.

Patient care

Residents must be able to provide patient care that is compassionate, appropriate, and effective for the treatment of health problems and the promotion of health.

Communicate effectively and demonstrate caring and respectful behaviors when interacting with patients and their families.

Informed anesthesia consent was obtained from the patient in the company of her mother for all aspects of her intraoperative and postoperative care. Owing to the significant intrathoracic mass effect, consent also included a detailed description of the potential for cardiopulmonary collapse in the operative theater, requiring mechanical support, and the possible need for prolonged postoperative intubation.

Gather essential and accurate information about their patients.

A comprehensive history and physical exam was performed, as was an extensive chart and imaging review. The thoracic CT was reviewed with the surgeon, who was also involved in the patient's anesthesia induction plan.

Make informed decisions about diagnostic and therapeutic interventions based on patient information and preferences, up-to-date scientific evidence, and clinical judgment.

The rapidly increasing dyspnea and oxygen requirements in this patient, given her concerning thoracic imaging studies, prompted a discussion with the surgeon about further optimizing the patient's cardiopulmonary status prior to inducing general anesthesia. Her progressing cardiac tamponade posed a grave threat and could be drained prior to the operation.

Develop and carry out patient management plans.

Prior to the operation, the patient was referred to interventional radiology for percutaneous pericardiocentesis, which produced 600 cc of straw-colored pericardial fluid.

Counsel and educate patients and their families.

The patient was counseled on the need for adequate invasive monitoring and vascular access prior to her anesthesia induction due to the potential for significant cardiopulmonary complications during the perioperative period.

Use information technology to support patient care decisions and patient education.

The patient's thoracic CT was reviewed with the thoracic surgeon, and a detailed plan for the induction of anesthesia was agreed on. Owing to the size and location of the mass, plans to perform the operation in a cardiopulmonary bypass–capable operating room (OR) were made. intraoperative surgical needs were also discussed, including the need for paralysis.

Perform competently all medical and invasive procedures considered essential for the area of practice.

Given the known right ventricular compression and superior vena cava (SVC) occlusion, the potential for cardiovascular compromise during induction was a concern. An awake radial arterial and femoral venous cannulation were planned. The patient was counseled about the need for this and was reassured throughout these procedures.

Provide health care services aimed at preventing health problems or maintaining health.

The need for appropriate antibiotics to prevent surgical site infection was discussed with the surgeon and was planned to be administered prior to skin incision.

Work with health care professionals, including those from other disciplines, to provide patient-focused care.

Plans were made to obtain an intensive care unit (ICU) bed for postop care by contacting the central intensivist and verifying bed availability. The patient's history was reported to the ICU attending who would be assuming postoperative care for the patient. The perfusionist on call was also notified to be available in the OR and prepared for cardiopulmonary bypass during the operation.

Medical knowledge

Residents must demonstrate knowledge about established and evolving biomedical, clinical, and cognate (e.g., epidemiological and social-behavioral) sciences and the application of this knowledge to patient care.

Demonstrate an investigatory and analytic thinking approach to clinical situations.

Maintaining spontaneous ventilation during induction and avoiding positive pressure ventilation if possible are two important goals for patients with large anterior mediastinal masses. The airway and shoulder girdle musculature are oftentimes maximally engaged in maintaining tracheal and vascular patency, so it is conceivable that chemical paralysis could result in sudden collapse of these two systems [1,2].

Know and apply the basic and clinically supportive sciences that are appropriate to their discipline.

Given the large size of the mass and known SVC compression, a mask induction with inhalational anesthetics was planned after an awake arterial line and femoral vein central line were placed. Since her airway exam was benign, tracheal intubation was performed via direct laryngoscopy, after the patient was adequately anesthetized with sevoflurane, while sitting at a 45° upright angle. Spontaneous ventilation was thus maintained during induction, and a stable hemodynamic response to short periods of positive pressure ventilation was ensured before administering a non-depolarizing neuromuscular blocking agent to provide paralysis for the operation [1–3].

Practice-based learning and improvement

Residents must be able to investigate and evaluate their patient care practices, appraise and assimilate scientific evidence, and improve their patient care practices.

Analyze practice experience and perform practice-based improvement activities using a systematic methodology.

Unfortunately, once the patient's upright position was removed and she was placed supine for the operation, ventilation became a significant problem. Ventilator pressures increased significantly with only 100–200 cc tidal volumes delivered. Her vital signs and oxygenation remained. However, given her large mediastinal mass, there was a great deal of concern for distal tracheal compression now that the supporting musculature had been relaxed.

Locate, appraise, and assimilate evidence from scientific studies related to their patients' health problems.

Fiber-optic bronchoscopy revealed a distal trachea that was 80% compressed, distal to the end of the endotracheal tube, and 2 cm above the carina. There are case reports documenting the use of extracorporeal membrane oxygenation (ECMO) for short periods in adults, requiring distal tracheal reconstruction due to obstruction from papillomas. ECMO is not without significant risks, and thankfully, this method of providing continuous oxygenation to the patient was not deployed [4].

Obtain and use information about their own population of patients and the larger population from which their patients are drawn.

While changing various ventilator parameters to optimize ventilation, we were able to continuously oxygenate the anesthetized patient and maintain a stable blood pressure. Ventilation improved moderately after positioning the patient in a 15° reverse Trendelenburg position. A discussion with the surgeon was initiated, and he agreed to perform the operation with the patient in a reverse Trendelenburg position.

(*First author's note*: It is worth remembering that tilting a patient head up can help with a wide variety of respiratory headaches.)

Apply knowledge of study designs and statistical methods to the appraisal of clinical studies and other information on diagnostic and therapeutic effectiveness.

In retrospect, given the patient's response to neuromuscular blockade, chemical paralysis was probably not the best course of action in this patient. Future recommendations include a closer examination of the surgeon's request for paralysis and a detailed discussion of the potential risks of this approach in patients with large anterior mediastinal masses.

Use information technology to manage information, access online medical information, and support their own education.

Previous thoracic CT scans were available in the OR, which provided the anesthesia and surgical teams ready access to information that helped in formulating a differential diagnosis, stratified according to the most likely to cause the ventilation encountered in this patient. Rapid arterial blood gas analysis also provided important information that was needed to confirm normal acid-base status and oxygenation prior to reversing the neuromuscular blockade and extubation.

Professionalism

Residents must demonstrate a commitment to carrying out professional responsibilities, adherence to ethical principles, and sensitivity to a diverse patient population.

Demonstrate respect, compassion, and integrity; a responsiveness to the needs of patients and society that supersedes self-interest; accountability to patients, society, and the profession; and a commitment to excellence and ongoing professional development.

Moments such as these help illuminate the distinct privilege it is to provide anesthesia to patients such as these, with complex medical problems. Patients are in their most vulnerable state while they are under our care, yet they place their trust in our abilities to see them safely through the operation. This trust does not come without first demonstrating respect and compassion for the patient, which is why a detailed and personable preoperative discussion is always warranted.

Demonstrate a commitment to ethical principles pertaining to provision or withholding of clinical care, confidentiality of patient information, informed consent, and business practice.

Cases such as these can easily become fodder for lunchtime discussions, but care must be taken to act as a true professional and respect the patient's right to privacy. Regardless of the educational benefit others may glean from the discussion, efforts to abide by all HIPAA regulations should be ensured.

Demonstrate sensitivity and responsiveness to patients' culture, age, gender, and disabilities.

ORs can be intimidating environments, even to those who work in health care. This patient required an awake arterial line and femoral venous line before safely inducing anesthesia and this is understandably anxiety provoking and potentially embarrassing. She

349

was draped to provide as much privacy as possible and verbally reassured throughout the procedures.

Interpersonal and communication skills

Residents must be able to demonstrate interpersonal and communication skills that result in effective information exchange and teaming with patients, their patients' families, and professional associates.

Create and sustain a therapeutic and ethically sound relationship with patients.

This relationship extends into the postoperative period, as well, and includes performing a postoperative visit the next day to ask if the patient has any lingering questions about the anesthetic and ensuring that there is no intraoperative recall and that the patient's pain has been adequately controlled.

Use effective listening skills and elicit and provide information using effective nonverbal, explanatory, questioning, and writing skills.

Demands on OR utilization oftentimes place a great deal of pressure on the anesthesiologist, but care must be taken to respect the patient and provide the patient with the time necessary to convey his or her needs and concerns. This patient, in particular, required a detailed history to plan for a safe anesthetic. Simply rushing through an anesthesia induction could have resulted in dire consequences.

Work effectively with others as a member or leader of a health care team or other professional group.

Other members of the OR team look to their physician counterparts for leadership during complex cases such as these. Keeping them informed of the sequence of events leading up to the patient's induction and including the operative course is important, especially if complications arise. For this reason, a detailed time-out that includes the entire OR team is necessary.

Systems-based practice

Residents must demonstrate an awareness of and responsiveness to the larger context and system of health care and the ability to effectively call on system resources to provide care that is of optimal value.

Understand how their patient care and other professional practices affect other health care professionals, the health care organization, and the larger society and how these elements of the system affect their own practice.

Since this patient would be transferred to the ICU after the operation, establishing and maintaining appropriate monitoring lines and delivering a problem-focused report to the ICU staff are of upmost importance to ensure a seamless transition of care. As perioperative consultants, the ICU staff also serves to benefit from our input on how best to optimize the patient's ventilation status, which, in her case, included strict upright positioning and avoidance of paralytics.

Practice cost-effective health care and resource allocation that does not compromise quality of care.

In a training institution, this point can easily be lost, but to better formulate a future practice, it is worthwhile to consider the financial cost of the anesthesiologist's decisions. Maintaining low free gas flows through the vaporizers and adequately dosing narcotics intraoperatively to limit postanesthesia care unit time spent controlling the patient's pain are two areas worth focusing on.

Advocate for quality patient care and assist patients in dealing with system complexities.

This is an area worth including in the preoperative setting and includes directing family members to waiting areas in the hospital and establishing a means of contacting them to keep them informed of their loved one's progress in the OR.

Know how to partner with health care managers and health care providers to assess, coordinate, and improve health care and know how these activities can affect system performance.

Although she was not a candidate to be downgraded to a lower status of postoperative care, it is worth reconsidering the need for ICU-level care following an operation. There is an enormous demand for ICU beds, so whenever a patient's condition is stable enough to be downgraded, it is reasonable to revisit the postoperative destination with the surgeon and keep the central intensivist appraised of the situation.

References

1. Gothard JW. Anesthetic considerations for patients with anterior mediastinal masses. Anesthesiol Clin 2008;26:304–311.

2. Prakash UB, Abel MD, Hubmayr RD. Mediastinal mass and tracheal obstruction during general anesthesia. Mayo Clin Proc 1988;63:1004–1011.

3. Cho Y, Suzuki S, Yokoi M, et al. Lateral position prevents respiratory occlusion during surgical procedure under general anesthesia in the patient of huge anterior mediastinal lymphoblastic lymphoma. Jpn J Thorac Cardiovasc Surg 2004;52:476–479.

4. Smith IJ, Sidebotham DA, McGeorge AD, et al. Use of extracorporeal membrane oxygenation during resection of tracheal papillomatosis. Anesthesiology 2009;110:427–429.

Contributions from Johns Hopkins Medical Institutions under Deborah A. Schwengel

Puff the magic dragon

Steven J. Schwartz

The case

Mr. C is an 85-year-old African American male with a history of diabetes, dementia, coronary artery disease, and multiple myocardial infarctions who is s/p coronary artery bypass graft (CABG) 5 years prior and who presented to the burn unit via ambulance. The patient presented with 15% total body surface area (TBSA) burn. Affected areas included bilateral hands, right lower extremity, and face, with an inhalation injury. The patient was intubated in the field and, when transferred to the burn unit, he was sedated and paralyzed and required blood pressure support with vasopressors. Bronchoscopy was done on admission, and his airway was full of soot and looked charred. Soot was present deep into all visual bronchi, and he required 100% FiO_2 on full mechanical support.

Patient care

Residents must be able to provide patient care that is compassionate, appropriate, and effective for the treatment of health problems and the promotion of health.

> Communicate effectively and demonstrate caring and respectful behaviors when interacting with patients and their families.

Care in the burn intensive care unit (ICU) is similar to care in the operating room. Although in most cases, families are allowed back in the rooms, each patient is isolated and draped in sterile yellow plastic. With his airway already secured, part of the battle is over, but the war is just beginning. If burns do not preclude it, conventional airway management, such as mask fit, jaw lift, and mouth opening, as well as standard induction and intubation procedures may be employed. Rapid sequence intubation is not necessary as gastric emptying is not delayed in patients with severe burns.

> Gather essential and accurate information about their patients.

Mr. C was burned in a house fire, where he was found down in the house for an unknown period of time. His wife was not burned, by report, and was transferred to the cardiac care unit for further treatment. The patient's family was not available for the first few days, and his prior history was taken from medical records at an outside institution, where he had received his medical care.

> Make informed decisions about diagnostic and therapeutic interventions based on patient information and preferences, up-to-date scientific evidence, and clinical judgment.

When burns include the face and neck, there is usually swelling and facial distortion, which makes direct laryngoscopy very difficult. The ability to mask ventilate is also difficult due to the loss of mandibular mobility. Fiber-optic intubation performed while maintaining spontaneous ventilation is safe and reliable under these circumstances. In adults, it is possible to perform fiber-optic intubation while they are awake, but pediatric patients will not be able to tolerate this because they cannot cooperate with the procedure. As most anesthetics cause collapse of the pharyngeal tissues and airway obstruction, it is very important to choose wisely from your pharmacy. Ketamine is unique among anesthetic drugs as it maintains airway patency as well as spontaneous ventilation.

> Develop and carry out patient management plans.

The ability to secure an endotracheal tube in a patient with facial burns also presents a series of problems. Taping or cross-ties over a burned area will cause irritation and dislodge grafts. One useful method involves the use of a nasal tie with one-eighth-inch umbilical tape. The umbilical tape is placed around the nasal septum using 8 or 10 French red rubber catheters that are passed through each naris and retrieved from the pharynx by direct laryngoscopy and Magill forceps. A length of umbilical tape is tied to each of the catheters, and when the catheters are pulled out of their respective naris, a loop around the nasal septum is produced. Care must be taken to ensure that the uvula is not trapped in the loop prior to tying a knot. Your knot should be snug but not tight enough to cause ischemic necrosis.

Counsel and educate patients and their families.

Prior to meeting with the family, it is important to understand that over the years, there has been a steady rise in the rate of survival from large burn injuries [1]. The vast improvement is due to early aggressive resuscitation, aggressive and early excision, and grafting as well as improved nutritional support. The development of burn centers has also been key in the survival of these patients. Modern burn care depends on the coordination of a complete multidisciplinary team, including anesthesiologists, burn surgeons, intensivists, nurse clinicians, nutritionists, and physical and occupational therapists. There is also a component of psychiatry, and pain management specialists often function on the team.

With all the efforts of the team, hard-core numbers are available. Ryan et al. identified three variables that can be used to estimate the probability of death: age greater than 60 years, burns over more than 40% of the total body surface area, and the presence of an inhalational injury [2]. Mortality increased in proportion to the number of risk factors present: 0.3%, 3%, 33%, or approximately 90% mortality, depending on whether zero, one, two, or three risk factors were present. Mortality also rose with the significant existence of coexisting disease or delay in resuscitation. Other scales include the Baux score. The Baux score is based on age plus total body surface area out of 120. This has recently been raised from out of 100. You also add points for an inhalation injury. Mr. C had a Baux score of 100 out of 120, or 83% mortality, not including his inhalational injury.

Use information technology to support patient care decisions and patient education.

Prior to going to the operating room, you are faced with multiple problems in the burn patient. Unlike your basic preoperative evaluation in stratifying risk, the burn patient will either be taken to the operating room on his initial presentation or resuscitated. During this period, you will be involved in the continued resuscitation of the patient. If your patient survives the initial burn shock and is adequately resuscitated, a state of hyperdynamic circulation develops. This systemic inflammatory response syndrome (SIRS) process is characterized by hypotension, tachycardia, and a marked decrease in systemic vascular resistance. Associated findings can include an increased cardiac output (if intravascular volume is adequate) as well as a continuum of tachycardia, tachypnea, fever, and leukocytosis. In its most severe form, you can see multisystem organ failure.

Burn patients require large-volume resuscitation in the immediate postburn period. There are standard protocols used, with the most common being the Parkland formula. The Parkland formula uses isotonic crystalloid solution and estimates the fluid requirements in the first 24 hours to be 4 mL/kg/% total body surface area (TBSA). The use of colloids within the first 24 hours has not improved outcome [3].

Nevertheless, several different formulas can be used – some use colloid and some do not. The different formulas are listed here:

- colloid formulas
- Evans – In the first 24 hours administer: normal saline 1.0 mL/kg/% burn, plus colloid 1.0 mL/kg/% burn, plus D5W 2,000 mL/24 hours
- Brooke – In the first 24 hours administer: lactated ringers (LR) 1.5 mL/kg/% burn, plus colloid 0.5 mL/kg/%burn, plus D5W 2,000 mL/24 hours
- hypertonic formulas
- Monafo – hypertonic saline – Fluid is administered at a rate sufficient to maintain the urinary output at 30 mL/hour (250 mEq Na/L)

Criteria for adequate fluid resuscitation

- normalization of blood pressure
- urine output (1–2 mL/kg/hour)
- blood lactate (<2 mmol/L)
- base deficit (less than -5)
- gastric intramucosal pH (greater than 7.32)
- central venous pressure
- Cardiac Index (CI) (4.5 L/min/m^2)
- oxygen delivery index (DO2I) (600 mL/min/m^2)

Major preoperative concerns in acutely burned patients

- age of patient
- extent of burn injuries (TBSI)
- burn depth and distribution (superficial or full thickness)
- mechanism of injury
- airway patency

- presence or absence of inhalation injury
- elapsed time from injury
- adequacy of resuscitation
- associated injuries
- coexisting diseases
- surgical plan

Perform competently all medical and invasive procedures considered essential for the area of practice.

At induction, a skilled anesthesiologist would be able to place adequate venous access and a preinduction arterial line (to monitor blood pressure on a beat-to-beat basis during induction and intubation) and would secure the airway appropriately. With all critically ill patients suffering from multiorgan involvement, the choice of monitoring in a burn patient will depend on the extent of the patient's injuries, his or her overall state, and the surgical plan. The American Society of Anesthesiologists (ASA) has documented minimum standards of monitoring, including circulation, ventilation, and oxygenation. The ability to keep a patient warm is vital in a burn patient in the operating room, and the ability to measure body temperature should be readily available at all times.

The ability to secure vascular access can be challenging even for the most skilled anesthesiologist. In the burn patient, your sites of insertion may be limited, the anatomy may be distorted, and the vasoconstriction that occurs after shock can make the establishment of peripheral lines virtually impossible. In patients with severe burns, the need to debride burned tissue is often required to establish access.

Provide health care services aimed at preventing health problems or maintaining health.

The new burn patient presents to you with no evidence of infection as the heat from the burn kills all the bacteria that can cause infection. The skin functions to protect the body from the elements. It is the natural barrier in relation to antigen presentation and entry of pathological organisms. Once the skin has been removed and grafts have been placed, the patient is at very high risk for infection. Ultimately, your patient will succumb from infection, or in an acute burn, as many as half die from lack of resuscitation [4]. There are measures recognized by the Centers for Disease Control and Prevention for reducing catheter-related bloodstream infections, including the maximum sterile barrier technique (cap, mask, sterile gown, sterile gloves, and large sterile drape with a small opening) [5].

Work with health care professionals, including those from other disciplines, to provide patient-focused care.

Modern burn care depends on coordination of a multidisciplinary team to be truly successful. Rational and effective anesthetic management of acute burn patients requires an understanding of this approach so that perioperative care is compatible with the overall treatment goals of the patient.

Medical knowledge

Residents must demonstrate knowledge about established and evolving biomedical, clinical, and cognate (e.g., epidemiological and social-behavioral) sciences and the application of this knowledge to patient care.

Demonstrate an investigatory and analytic thinking approach to clinical situations.

To manage a patient with extensive burn injuries, the resident must understand the pathophysiological changes associated with large burns. The resident must also be able to recognize the anatomical distortions that make airway management and vascular access difficult. The changes in the cardiovascular function range from initial hypovolemia and impaired perfusion to a hyperdynamic and hypermetabolic state that will develop after resuscitation. These changes will alter the response to many different anesthetic drugs.

Know and apply the basic and clinically supportive sciences that are appropriate to their discipline.

Before you cross the threshold into the burn unit, make sure that you understand all the physiology that applies to these complex cases. The supportive science for burn medicine fills entire thick textbooks. There is also a society called the American Burn Association that publishes monthly journals. For now, though, the perioperative challenges include the following:

- compromised airway
- pulmonary insufficiency
- altered mental status

- associated injuries
- limited vascular access
- rapid blood loss
- impaired tissue perfusion due to
  - hypovolemia
  - decreased myocardial contractility
  - anemia

- decreased colloid osmotic pressure
- edema
- dysrhythmia
- impaired temperature regulation
- altered drug response
- renal insufficiency
- immunosupression
- infection/sepsis

Remember to be prepared in advance. Adequate monitors, good vascular access, and availability of blood are essential. Surgical blood loss depends on the area to be excised (cm^2), time since injury, surgical plan (tangential vs. facial excision), and presence of infection [6].

Practice-based learning and improvement

Residents must be able to investigate and evaluate their patient care practices, appraise and assimilate scientific evidence, and improve their patient care practices.

> Analyze practice experience and perform practice-based improvement activities using a systematic methodology.

Many studies over the years have shown inhalation injury to be strongly associated with increased morbidity and mortality, especially in the burned patient. In one study by Shirani et al., the presence of an inhalation injury increased mortality by up to 20% and pneumonia by up to 40% [7].

Mr. C is an 85-year-old man with a questionable mental status premorbidly and with multiple medical problems, who now faces a traumatic injury with near 100% mortality.

Your team includes senior burn surgeons, senior intensivists, and attending anesthesiologists. Your decision to continue is based on multiple opinions, but the looming question has not been raised. Is this futility? Is this what the patient would want? Is this what the team would want? Is this what you would want?

> Locate, appraise, and assimilate evidence from scientific studies related to their patients' health problems.

Complications in patients with inhalational injuries alone occur secondary to the original injury and to the barotrauma that can occur from the ventilator. Every indication and every organ system in this 85-year-old man has begun to shut down. His mortality is off the charts, and his associated morbidity is even worse. If he lives, he is subject to wound infection, respiratory insufficiency, and multiple surgeries to fix scarring, in addition to retraining in relation to walking and self-care. Every scale to predict survivability says that he will not survive. Yet there is no exact science to say he will not survive. Why should you stop? When should you stop?

Mr. C was taken to the operating room for the fourth time on day 7. We performed a tracheotomy and percutaneous endoscopic gastrostomy (PEG) placement.

> Obtain and use information about their own population of patients and the larger population from which their patients are drawn.

As a resident, you draw on your own experience, and you draw on the larger world of experience, that is, the experience described in the literature. In other words, you review and keep abreast of experience with geriatric burn patients.

> Apply knowledge of study designs and statistical methods to the appraisal of clinical studies and other information on diagnostic and therapeutic effectiveness.

Much of the morbidity and mortality associated with burn injuries are related to the size of the injury. The injury is expressed as TBSA burned. The TBSA is used to guide resuscitation, which includes fluids and electrolytes and blood loss. Percentage of the skin surface that has been burned can be estimated as the rule of nines. These estimates are based on body proportion and are modified for pediatric patients. Knowledge of the burn depth is also critical to anticipate physiological changes as well as to help prepare for surgical intervention. The standard burn diagram is the Lund and Browder chart. There are many modifications to this, and the standard is in all burn textbooks. The diagram is required on presentation of all burn victims to the burn unit.

> Use information technology to manage information, access online medical information, and support their own education.

The American Burn Association has a Web site, as do the Shriners burn units. There are also multiple Web sites available to aid in your education and provide you with the tools you need to practice as an anesthesia resident functioning either in the unit or the operating room. With access to PubMed, you will be able to find any and all information available. The landmark textbook is "Total Burn Care" by Herndon. [8]

Professionalism

Residents must demonstrate a commitment to carrying out professional responsibilities, adherence to ethical principles, and sensitivity to a diverse patient population.

> Demonstrate respect, compassion, and integrity; a responsiveness to the needs of patients and society that supersedes self-interest; accountability to patients, society, and the profession; and a commitment to excellence and ongoing professional development.

Is this futility? Do we continue?

Mr. C was 14 days into his treatment. He had been debrided, he had been grafted, and he was now septic on 80% FiO_2, with a PEEP (positive end-expiratory pressure) of 10 and elevating plateau pressures. I asked for a family meeting to stop the fragmented care.

As I sat down to go over his prognosis and plan for the umpteenth time, his granddaughter looked at me and said, "I know that my granddad wants to live, because Oprah told me so." Then she started to sing loudly, and the rest of the family joined in.

So, as a clinician, what do I do? Is it futility to continue?

> Demonstrate a commitment to ethical principles pertaining to provision or withholding of clinical care, confidentiality of patient information, informed consent, and business practice.

Futility is a concept that can be hard to define. One definition says that if 99 out of the last 100 cases failed, then it is futile. When cardiopulmonary resuscitation fails, it is futile. If you are on 100% FiO_2, with a PEEP of 20 and a maximum dose of pressors, and you still have saturations in the 50s, then it can be considered futility. The patient's family says he wants to live, so for now, he will live. Remember that we have gotten very good in the year 2009 at preserving physiology, but this is not physiology – he is a man who cannot speak for himself. We are relying on next of kin and substituted judgment to proceed.

> Demonstrate sensitivity and responsiveness to patients' culture, age, gender, and disabilities.

The ability to sit and listen to a family and to a patient and empathize with them will always be what separates you from all your colleagues. Medicine is a consumer-based profession. Your patients can choose you or the guy down the street. We all have the same drugs, and it is our ability to communicate that distinguishes us.

Interpersonal and communication skills

Residents must be able to demonstrate interpersonal and communication skills that result in effective information exchange and teaming with patients, their patients' families, and professional associates.

> Create and sustain a therapeutic and ethically sound relationship with patients.

When you first meet your burn victim, your ability to establish an effective relationship will be limited to diving in and securing his airway. Patients suffering burn injuries often require surgical treatments for years after the initial injury to correct functional and cosmetic sequelae. Anesthetic management for reconstructive burn surgery presents many special problems [9], but our case focuses on the care of the acute burn and inhalational injury. The acute phase of burn injury is defined as the period from injury until the wounds have been excised, grafted, and healed.

> Use effective listening skills and elicit and provide information using effective nonverbal, explanatory, questioning, and writing skills.

Your initial evaluation of the burn injury begins by seeing the destruction of the skin. The skin is the largest organ of the body and provides an essential protective and homeostatic function. Your treatment must compensate for this loss, and your documentation will display your understanding. Your preoperative evaluation must be complete and well documented and reflect the physiological changes that you can see. In addition to loss of important functions of the skin, extensive burns result in an inflammatory response with systemic effects that alter function in virtually all organ systems. During your preoperative evaluation, special attention must be paid to the airway and pulmonary function. Remember that distortion may be present in the anatomy. The mouth and neck may be involved. Alterations in mouth opening and tongue swelling with burns to the oropharynx and larynx should all be documented. A strong clinical suspicion of an inhalational injury should be aroused by the presence of certain risk factors. The risk factors to listen for would be exposure to fire and smoke in an enclosed space or a period of unconsciousness at an accident scene, burns to the face and neck with singed facial hair, altered voice, dysphagia, oral and nasal soot deposits, or carbonaceous sputum. The most immediate threat from inhalation injury is upper airway obstruction due to edema. Early or prophylactic intubation is recommended when this complication occurs. Traditional clinical predictors of airway obstruction have been found to be relatively insensitive and inadequate for identifying early severe airway inflammation and often underestimate the severity of the injury [10]. Fiber-optic bronchoscopy is a safe and accurate method to establish a diagnosis, but what is the yield of your initial finding? Serial exams may also help in avoiding intubation. Always document your findings carefully in a clear, system-based note.

Work effectively with others as a member or leader of a health care team or other professional group.

So what happened to Mr. C and his family? Mr. C had multiple split thickness skin grafts, with over 3,000 cm^2 of graft replacement, as well as a tracheotomy and peg placement. After multiple weeks on pressor medications, antibiotics, paralytics, and ventilator support, Mr. C was liberated from the ventilator, decannulated, and finally, after 45 days, sent to rehabilitation. Mr. C beat the odds in every way. He returned to his baseline and even speaks when he feels like it.

The team did not give up, the family did not give up, and Mr. C decided that he wanted to live.

Systems-based practice

Residents must demonstrate an awareness of and responsiveness to the larger context and system of health care and the ability to effectively call on system resources to provide care that is of optimal value.

Understand how their patient care and other professional practices affect other health care professionals, the health care organization, and the larger society and how these elements of the system affect their own practice.

This burn patient has suffered what should have been a life-ending injury, but his outcome was different than the average patient. Did we practice evidence-based medicine when we saved this patient? We followed all the standards of care in relation to resuscitation. We used the most current ventilators and the strongest medications. We involved every service that our institution had to offer, and we saved one life. This patient was not ready to go, and although he gave us every indication that he wanted to go, from a bronchoscopy that showed black lungs to plateau pressures over 50, he lived. Will our practice change in relation to this patient? I doubt it, but we will continue to see that anything can be possible if there is a will to survive.

The primary resource of interest here is that the systems and protocols are in place to promote survivability. The team functions as a team and interacts in a professional and collegial manner, and the patient has every chance to do well.

Practice cost-effective health care and resource allocation that does not compromise quality of care.

To achieve the effect of adequate resuscitation, you have to have an understanding of the basics. There is no proven benefit to using invasive cardiac monitors to guide resuscitation, but you have to know when there is a time to use these devices. Be aware that measuring and trending a simple bladder pressure can help prevent and, if necessary, diagnose abdominal compartment syndrome. Understand that the incidence of acute renal failure following burn injury has been reported to range from 0.5% to 30% and is most dependent on the severity of the burn and the presence of an inhalational injury [11]. Remember that lower airway and parenchymal injuries develop more slowly than upper airway obstruction. Think about carbon monoxide and cyanide toxicity as they are major components of smoke. Treatment of cyanide toxicity begins with a high-inspired oxygen concentration. Pharmacological intervention includes methemoglobin generators, such as nitrates and dimethylaminophenol, to increase methemoglobin levels. Always maintain proper body temperature. The major components are the afferent system that senses changes in core body temperature and transmits this information to the brain; the central regulatory mechanisms, located primarily in the hypothalamus, that process afferent input and initiate responses; and the efferent limb that mediates specific biological responses to changes in core temperature. Remember your basic pharmacology and how burn injuries can change the response to medications. Clearance is the most important factor determining the maintenance dose of drugs and can influence the response to drugs given by infusion or repeated bolus during anesthesia. Drug clearance is influenced by metabolism, protein binding, renal excretion, and novel excretion pathways.

In the culture of safety, the transport of a critically ill burn patient to and from the operating room can be a formidable task. The approach should be methodical and seamless. Hemodynamic status should be optimized prior to transport, and ASA standards to evaluate, treat, monitor, and use appropriate equipment prior to attempting to move should be followed.

Advocate for quality patient care and assist patients in dealing with system complexities.

Try to do something good for each one of your patients every day. If you can't help your patient, then help the family. Provide the time and environment for these people so you can listen to them in a quiet and secure place. Most important, remember that they are not here for you; rather, you are here for them.

Know how to partner with health care managers and health care providers to assess, coordinate, and improve health care and know how these activities can affect system performance.

Use your team and a multidisciplinary approach in providing care for these people. Their ability to function in society will be a direct benefit from you and your team. Your nurse managers, caseworkers, and therapists will be your arms and legs. Treat them with the respect and professionalism they deserve.

References

1. Saffle VR. Predicting outcomes of burns. N Engl J Med 1998;338:387–388.

2. Ryan CM, Schoenfeld DA, Thorpe WP, et al. Objective estimates of the probability of death from burn injuries. N Engl J Med 1998;338:362–366.

3. Alderson P, Schierhout G, Roberts I, et al. Colloids versus crystalloids for fluid resuscitation in critically ill patients. Cochrane Database Syst Rev 2000;2: CD000567.

4. Reynolds EM, Ryan DP, Sheridan RL, et al. Left ventricular failure complicating severe pediatric burn injuries. J Pediatric Surg 1995;30:264–269.

5. http://wwwn.cdc.gov/publiccomments/comments/ guidelines-for-the-prevention-of-catheter-related-infections; accessed 11/25/09.

6. Desai MH, Herndon DN, Bromeling L, et al. Early burn wound excision significantly reduces blood loss. Ann Surg 1990;211:753–759.

7. Shirani KZ, Pruitt BA Jr, Mason AD Jr. The influence of inhalation injury and pneumonia on burn mortality. Ann Surg 1987;205:82–87.

8. Herndon DN. Total Burn Care. 3rd edition Elsevier/Saunders 2007.

9. Woodson LC, Sherwood ER, Cortiella J, et al. Anesthesia for reconstructive burn surgery. In: McCauley RL, editor. Functional and aesthetic reconstruction of burned patients. Boca Raton, FL: Taylor and Francis; 2005: 85–103.

10. Muehlberger T, Kunar D, Munster A, et al. Efficacy of fiberoptic laryngoscopy in the diagnosis of inhalational injuries. Arch Otolaryngol Head Neck Surg 1998;124:1003–1007.

11. Davies MP, Evans J, McGonigal RJ. The dialysis debate: acute renal failure in burn patients. Burns 1994;20:71–73.

Contributions from Johns Hopkins Medical Institutions under
Deborah A. Schwengel

"You mean the screw isn't supposed to be in the aorta?"

Massive bleeding during spine surgery

The case

Melissa Pant and Lauren C. Berkow

An otherwise healthy 55-year-old woman with degenerative disc disease and chronic intractable low back pain presents for a seemingly straightforward level 3 posterior spinal fusion. You and your attending come up with a reasonable plan for her anesthetic, including general endotracheal anesthesia, maintained with a combination of intravenous and inhaled anesthetic; a second intravenous line; and standard American Society of Anesthesiology monitors.

Things are going well, the line placement and flip to prone were flail-free, and the somatosensory evoked potential (SSEP) monitoring tech is happy with his signals. Hours pass uneventfully (with an expected amount of blood loss and fluid administration, given the case). Precipitously, your cuff pressure reads 70/30 (when it was 120/70), and strangely, you haven't heard any extra suctioning or the room go quiet. As you recheck it and open the fluids, you eyeball the suction canisters and peek your head over the curtain. Canisters are the same, and the surgeons don't look nervous. In fact, they are happy as they have finally finished the last screw, which was giving them problems. Your patient's pressure improves somewhat with fluid, so you turn off your remifentanil drip (they are starting to close) and chalk it up to underresuscitation.

As surgery finishes up, your patient is weaned to nitrous and is breathing (with some pressure support) on her own, but her pressure is still low, considering that you have turned off the agent. You briefly disconnect your monitors for the flip. As you are reconnecting your monitors and trying to figure out why your peak airway pressures alarm is going off, the new SSEP tech asks, "Is this patient pregnant?" As you look up in horror, you note that your patient now appears to be about 8 months pregnant!

Patient care

Residents must be able to provide patient care that is compassionate, appropriate, and effective for the treatment of health problems and the promotion of health.

> Gather essential and accurate information about their patients.

You did a thorough history and physical this morning, specifically probing for cardio and cerebrovascular disease as you know that back cases can be associated with significant blood loss and hypotension. You know that the patient's starting hemoglobin was 10 and that she has 4 units of blood available.

> Make informed decisions about diagnostic and therapeutic interventions based on patient information and preferences, up-to-date scientific evidence, and clinical judgment.

Your clinical judgment kicks in as you calmly and quickly alert the surgeon to the situation: what appears to be a belly full of blood, hypotension, and difficulty ventilating due to abdominal distension. You open your fluids, give pressor (you just got your cuff pressure back at 55/23), call for blood, and call for help. A stat chest x-ray (CXR) and bedside ultrasound are done to confirm that there is not another source for the abdominal distension. Complex fluid is seen on sonogram; compressed lungs and a large amount of abdominal fluid are seen on CXR.

> Develop and carry out patient management plans.

Anesthesia management of patient issues often needs to evolve rather quickly – you and your attending go into disaster mode and come up with a plan. Reanesthetize, place an arterial line, Cordis, and call the blood bank stat. Call additional hands to help with labs, rapid infuser, and resuscitation medications.

While doing all this, you discuss with the surgeons the plan for relieving the worsening intra-abdominal pressure while preventing further massive bleeding (currently being tamponaded by the patient's closed abdomen). A vascular cart (with aortic clamps), a vascular surgeon, and extra hands are called in to assist, given that, most likely, a great vessel has been damaged. The surgeons will wait to open until the cooler you ordered is up, a rapid infuser is primed, and you are happy with your access.

Take a half second to relish the fact that you are a senior resident now and actually know what to do.

Counsel and educate patients and their families.

You are *very* happy that you took a little extra time to explain anesthetic and surgical complications when discussing the case with your patient and her family this morning. You ask the circulating nurse to have someone update the family about the complication and the patient's current situation.

Perform competently all medical and invasive procedures considered essential for the area of practice.

As you expertly throw in an arterial line and introducer neck line, you thank the Lord for all the middle-of-the-night traumas and cardiac cases you used to complain about. You also wish you had placed an arterial line at the beginning of the case; perhaps you would have noticed the patient's hypovolemia and anemia earlier and been able to alert the surgeons.

Provide health care services aimed at preventing health problems or maintaining health.

You redose the antibiotics for blood loss, make sure the patient stays warm, and keep your central line sites clean to try to prevent later infectious complications.

Work with health care professionals, including those from other disciplines, to provide patient-focused care.

The operating room is a unique place in that all attention is on only one patient, whom all of you are desperately trying to save right now. Extra teams from nursing, surgery, and anesthesia come to help. Communication between surgery and anesthesia is paramount as a concise and calm discussion of the facts, the problem, and a differential must be done, and a plan must be decided on quickly to save your patient. An intensive care unit (ICU) bed should be obtained as her postoperative care will likely be complex – you ask the circulating nurse to page the ICU fellow.

Medical knowledge

Residents must demonstrate knowledge about established and evolving biomedical, clinical, and cognate (e.g., epidemiological and social-behavioral) sciences and the application of this knowledge to patient care.

Demonstrate an investigatory and analytic thinking approach to clinical situations.

This case is anesthesia 101: significant blood loss causing a decrease in preload, exacerbated by intra-abdominal hypertension. Hypovolemic shock: bring on the fluid, blood, and surgical control of bleeding! Monitoring of coagulation status and electrolytes is vital due to the profound coagulopathy, hypocalcemia, and sometimes hyperkalemia that can occur with massive transfusion. Monitoring of temperature is vital to prevent both the profound coagulopathy and infections associated with hypothermia.

Having just finished your neuro critical care rotation, you know that another possibility for your patient's condition is neurogenic shock (i.e., a screw accidentally placed in the spinal cord), but given her acute anemia, low central venous pressure , and other signs of hypovolemic shock, you treat the most likely cause of her instability.

Know and apply the basic and clinically supportive sciences that are appropriate to their discipline.

As the cooler arrives, you plan when you will dose calcium (knowing that the citrate from all the blood products you are about to give will bind it) and your escalation of pressors based on mechanism of action. You set a reasonable mean arterial pressure and hemoglobin goal to balance the surgeon's need for less blood in the field against the patient's need to perfuse her vital organs.

Practice-based learning and improvement

Residents must be able to investigate and evaluate their patient care practices, appraise and assimilate scientific evidence, and improve their patient care practices.

Analyze practice experience and perform practice-based improvement activities using a systematic methodology.

It's not the time right now, but later, as a team, the case should be discussed. Anesthetic as well as surgical issues should be included in the discussion, including whether preparation and access were appropriate given the risk of the case (i.e., are we underpreparing as large blood loss is often associated with this case, or was this an outlier)? Was there a way to identify that the screw was malpositioned? Should you have mentioned something earlier when the blood pressure dropped as they were having difficulty with the screw?

> Locate, appraise, and assimilate evidence from scientific studies related to their patients' health problems.

You do recall something about last week's journal club about large back surgery and coagulopathy. You have your tech send off coags with the next draw, and you also start giving blood: fresh frozen plasma in a 1:2 ratio. You also recall an article on factor VII and massive bleeding, indicating that it did improve massive bleeding, however, it did not improve mortality, and in some cases, it even caused higher mortality due to acute thromboembolic events[1–4].

> Use information technology to manage information, access online medical information, and support their own education.

You use Micromedex to quickly look up the standard concentration and starting dose for a vasopressin infusion.

Professionalism

Residents must demonstrate a commitment to carrying out professional responsibilities, adherence to ethical principles, and sensitivity to a diverse patient population.

> Demonstrate respect, compassion, and integrity; a responsiveness to the needs of patients and society that supersedes self-interest; accountability to patients, society, and the profession; and a commitment to excellence and ongoing professional development.

When the case is done and the patient is safely in the ICU, go talk to the patient's family with the surgeon. Tell them what happened, what you did, and what will be done for their loved one. Make it clear that you are available to talk later if they have questions.

> Demonstrate a commitment to ethical principles pertaining to provision or withholding of clinical care, confidentiality of patient information, informed consent, and business practice.

Don't talk about this case in the elevator on the way home. Do talk about this case in a morbidity and mortality conference so that you and your colleagues can learn from it.

Interpersonal and communication skills

Residents must be able to demonstrate interpersonal and communication skills that result in effective information exchange and teaming with patients, their patients' families, and professional associates.

> Create and sustain a therapeutic and ethically sound relationship with patients.

This can sometimes be tricky in anesthesia, but it can be done (there are request cases, after all). Your patient should know your name, what you do, and trust you to take care of him or her while unconscious and completely defenseless.

> Use effective listening skills and elicit and provide information using effective nonverbal, explanatory, questioning, and writing skills.

Your effectiveness in calmly but quickly alerting the entire team to the need for surgical reintervention sets the tone for the rest of the case. If the anesthesiology team is freakin' out, then you had better believe that the rest of the team is 100 times worse.

> Work effectively with others as a member or leader of a health care team or other professional group.

Be respectful and polite to your surgical team members. Actively participate in the time-out, making sure that you are in fact doing the right surgery for the right patient, that appropriate antibiotics have been given, and that potential problems (including blood loss) have been discussed before surgery begins. Know the names of the rest of the providers in the operating room.

And yes, be polite and respectful to the blood bank (who, despite their molasses pace, are making sure that the patient is not exposed to another complication related to a transfusion reaction).

Systems-based practice

Residents must demonstrate an awareness of and responsiveness to the larger context and system of health care and the ability to effectively call on system resources to provide care that is of optimal value.

> Practice cost-effective health care and resource allocation that does not compromise quality of care.

At this point, you realize that your patient's hospital bill just got *a lot* bigger, and you consider all the products you are using for only one patient. You know,

however, that if surgical control of bleeding can be attained, along with adequate upkeep with blood loss, your patient will likely be fine. So bring on the blood products, calcium, neo, epi, and vasopressin!

Your hard work pays off – the vascular surgeon finds and repairs the aortic tear, and the orthopedic surgeon fixes the aberrant screw.

> Advocate for quality patient care and assist patients in dealing with system complexities.

Quality care in anesthesia is all about the details. During the case, you still managed to clean off and cap line ports; check your patient's head, arms, and eyes; and detangle your lines prior to arrival in the ICU. In the ICU, you give a thorough report of the case and give the accepting team time to ask questions, even though you just want to go home and sleep now!

References

1. Berkhof FF, Eikenboom JC. Efficacy of recombinant activated factor VII in patients with massive uncontrolled bleeding: a retrospective observational analysis. Transfusion 2009;49:570–577.

2. Stanworth SJ, Birchall J, Doree CJ, Hyde C. Recombinant factor VIIa for the prevention and treatment of bleeding in patients without haemophilia. Cochrane Database Syst Rev 2007;2:CD005011.

3. Rizoli SB, Nascimento B Jr, Netto FS, et al. Recombinant activated coagulation factor VII and bleeding trauma patients. J Trauma 2006;61:1419–1425.

4. Horlocker TT, Nutall GA, Dekutoski MB, Bryant SC. The accuracy of coagulation tests during spinal fusion and instrumentation. Anesth Analg 2001;93:33–38.

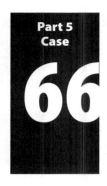

66

Contributions from Johns Hopkins Medical Institutions under Deborah A. Schwengel

Oh *no*, someone get the NO!

Rabi Panigrahi, Brijen L. Joshi, and Nanhi Mitter

The case

Twenty-nine-year-old Anita Heart (5 feet 2 inches, 65 kg) comes to the operating room (OR) for a heart transplant. After giving birth to her baby, she develops peripartum cardiomyopathy and is ready to sign the adoption papers for her child, when she finds out that a transplant has just become available. You take her to the OR and insert an awake arterial line and induce and intubate her. You decide to line her up and perform a transesophageal echo. Her baseline data are stable: heart rate in the 50s, blood pressure in the 100s (50s PASP [PADP 48/20s]), and CVP 10–15. The case proceeds, and after you come off pump and give the protamine, the cardiac surgery fellow asks her attending if the right ventricle (RV) is supposed to look so large and bulky. The cardiac surgeon looks across the drapes at you and screams at you to do something fast! Save the RV, she says!

Patient care

Residents must be able to provide patient care that is compassionate, appropriate, and effective for the treatment of health problems and the promotion of health.

> Make informed decisions about diagnostic and therapeutic interventions based on patient information and preferences, up-to-date scientific evidence, and clinical judgment.

Treatment of right ventricular failure is aimed at increasing forward flow as well as avoiding additional insults to the right ventricle. This can be managed by decreasing any outflow obstruction, that is, pulmonary hypertension that may be present. Physiologically, hyperventilating, minimizing airway pressures, and correcting any hemodynamic or metabolic derangements will help to attain this goal; this is easier than it sounds, though. Drugs that have been used as selective pulmonary vasodilators include nitric oxide and prostacyclin analogues. Epoprostenol is a prosta-

cyclin analogue, and it is only approved for primary pulmonary hypertension. Cost is one deterrent to the use of the prostacyclin analogues. Nitric oxide (NO) has also been used, but it is not approved by the U.S. Food and Drug Administration (FDA) for this use. That doesn't seem to stop us, though. In the setting of RV failure after orthotopic heart transplant, one must weigh the evidence. On one hand, you have the use of a drug (off-label) that may or may not help. On the other hand, you are using a drug that may help save Anita's heart! It is a tough call. Although both drugs have been used extensively, prophylactic use still remains controversial.

The current FDA approval for nitric oxide is for neonatal respiratory failure, perinatal hypoxia, and neonatal pulmonary hypertension. Off-label use in adults has been described and includes use in cardiovascular surgery, acute respiratory distress syndrome, pulmonary hypertension, congestive heart failure, high-altitude pulmonary edema, primary pulmonary hypertension, and right-sided heart failure after implantation of a left-ventricular assist device in patients with reversible pulmonary hypertension.

Nitric oxide relaxes vascular smooth muscle. It binds to intracellular heme moieties and activates guanylate synthase. This results in the increase of cyclic guanosine 3′,5′-monophosphate (cGMP), and ultimately, smooth muscle relaxation. When it crosses the alveoli to enter into the bloodstream, it immediately interacts with hemoglobin to form methemoglobin and nitrates and therefore is inactivated. Its half-life is about 6 seconds, and that is why it needs to be administered continuously via a special ventilator. Owing to this inactivation, inhaled nitric oxide can selectively vasodilate the pulmonary vasculature and doesn't seem to cause massive systemic hypotension.

Inhaled nitric oxide (iNO) is very popular. Did you know that it was termed "Molecule of the Year" in 1992? Yes, it has been used extensively off-label so much so that sometimes we hear from the cardiac surgeons, "Can we come off pump with some epi and some iNO?"

Most important, when you use it, know why you are using it!

Perform competently all medical and invasive procedures considered essential for the area of practice.

Hopefully the patient has already been "lined-up" but if not, a pulmonary artery catheter would be helpful in order to ascertain pulmonary pressures and the effectiveness of treatment modalities. Transesophageal echocardiography is also useful in that you can directly visualize the right ventricle as well as ascertain left ventricular function and rule out any other causes of right heart failure.

Work with health care professionals, including those from other disciplines, to provide patient-focused care.

In some hospitals, one cannot even speak of nitric oxide much less use it without explicit permission by the powers that be. To use it, different disciplines need to communicate – pharmacy, respiratory, surgery, ICU, and anesthesia. Special ventilators are required for the administration of nitric oxide and special circuits are needed to attach to the anesthesia circuits. These need to be attached appropriately prior to the accurate administration of nitric oxide. These special attachments are the way to actually give the nitric oxide as well as measure how much nitric oxide is being given. You may want to check with your hospital respiratory staff and pharmacy to determine who needs to be alerted ahead of time so that you are not making the arrangements in the heat of the moment.

Medical knowledge

Residents must demonstrate knowledge about established and evolving biomedical, clinical, and cognate (e.g., epidemiological and social-behavioral) sciences and the application of this knowledge to patient care.

Demonstrate an investigatory and analytic thinking approach to clinical situations.

So here is when you start wishing that you did internal medicine and all of you could sit around the conference room at the drug rep lunch and fill up the dry-erase board with the longest differential diag-

nosis possible for RV failure, but right now is the time to focus – so esoteric causes like fibrosis of the myocardium are going to be placed on the back burner, and things like pulmonary hypertension and myocardial stunning are on the front burner. Contributors for hemodynamic instability after orthotopic heart transplantation include myocardial stunning, hyperacute rejection, primary allograft failure, arrhythmias, and right ventricular failure. One of the most dreaded complications is right ventricular failure. When the right ventricle goes, so does the rest of the case. There is a high mortality rate associated with RV failure post–cardiac transplant.

RV failure can present with hemodynamic instability and can be due to preexisting pulmonary hypertension, transient pulmonary vasospasm, air in the right coronary artery, tricuspid (pulmonary valve insufficiency), donor-recipient heart size mismatch, prolonged ischemia time, edema from surgical manipulation, and acquired obstructive causes.

The goal of treatment is getting the RV back to its normal self as soon as possible. Treatment modalities include, but are not limited to (do I sound like the fine print?), correcting hemodynamic and metabolic derangements, decreasing pulmonary resistance, and using selective pulmonary vasodilators.

Professionalism

Residents must demonstrate a commitment to carrying out professional responsibilities, adherence to ethical principles, and sensitivity to a diverse patient population.

Demonstrate respect, compassion, and integrity; a responsiveness to the needs of patients and society that supersedes self-interest; accountability to patients, society, and the profession; and a commitment to excellence and ongoing professional development.

So when the surgeon starts screaming at you, do you scream back? No, certainly not. Most of the time in the operating room, screaming and stress go hand in hand, and it is usually hard to tell which came first. One thing for sure is that communication diminishes exponentially once someone starts screaming at another person. Handling patients with RV failure intraoperatively can be stressful in and of itself, and having someone scream at you just adds to the stress. Screaming back at the person just adds fuel to the fire.

The important thing to understand is that the patient comes first, and keeping things like that in perspective can help maintain calm in the operating room. Another lesson to be learned is that this is not the time to win the arguing battle – again, focusing on the patient helps to keep you from getting into that screaming match.

Generally, reverting to crisis mode is what gets you in gear. As an anesthesiologist, you will be team leader when it comes to codes and other critical situations. Things to keep in mind are closed-loop communication; clear communication; being open to ideas; asking for information about the patient, implementing intervention strategies; and finally, maintaining a calm, professional, and – possibly most important – mutually respectful environment in the operating room.

Interpersonal and communication skills

Residents must be able to demonstrate interpersonal and communication skills that result in effective information exchange and teaming with patients, their patients' families, and professional associates.

> Work effectively with others as a member or leader of a health care team or other professional group.

Like we mentioned earlier, just getting on the hospital intercom and screaming for some nitric oxide stat to OR A is probably not the best way to go. Communicating with all members of the team is necessary. As important as this is in terms of arranging to have it used intraoperatively, one must also keep in mind that educating other staff about it is useful. For example, if you shut it off all at once (rather than weaning it), then the patient can experience some pretty scary rebound pulmonary hypertension, and you could end up with the same problem you were looking to avoid in the first place. Furthermore, it can result in methemoglobinemia, so it is important to communicate this to the entire team.

Systems-based practice

Residents must demonstrate an awareness of and responsiveness to the larger context and system of health care and the ability to effectively call on system resources to provide care that is of optimal value.

> Know how to partner with health care managers and health care providers to assess, coordinate, and improve health care and know how these activities can affect system performance.

The most important lesson in using these drugs is in understanding how to coordinate with others to improve patients' outcomes. Because inhaled nitric oxide is a selective vasodilator and has been proven to decrease pulmonary vascular resistance, coordinating its efficient use is paramount in its administration. Sometimes system hurdles that need to be overcome can be done so by communicating early with respiratory therapy or pharmacy (whoever is in charge of the drug at your hospital) and by demonstrating the "appropriate" use of the drug. Although prophylactic use remains controversial, one of the off-label indications is intraoperatively during cardiac surgery. Again, it is important to weigh the risks versus benefits versus costs. At our hospital, the cost of iNO is around $150 per hour. Yikes! Using this drug appropriately can help manage hospital costs. Hospital costs? you ask. Well, as a resident, this is not a priority, but to an attending, this may be the difference between a covered, heated, reserved parking spot near the coffee shop entrance to the hospital versus taking a bus to work due to expensive parking costs!

Additionally, any time this patient is transported while on inhaled NO – whether it is from the OR to the ICU (or, unfortunately, vice versa!) or from the ICU to any imaging locations – she will need a special transport ventilator to go with her so that the iNO is not prematurely and abruptly discontinued. As we stated earlier, premature and abrupt discontinuation can lead to some pretty ugly consequences, that is, rebound pulmonary hypertension. Therefore partnering with nursing, respiratory, and ICU staff is key.

Additional reading

1. Belikov S, Hoftman N, Mahajan A. Anesthesia for heart transplant patients. Sem Anesth Periop Med Pain 2004;1:23–33.

2. Frogel J, Vodur S, Applefield A, et al. An unusual case of right ventricular failure after orthotopic heart transplantation. J Cardiothorac Vasc Anesth 2008;22:913–919.

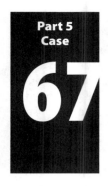

Contributions from Johns Hopkins Medical Institutions under
Deborah A. Schwengel

What to do when HITT hits the fan

Ira Lehrer and Nanhi Mitter

The case

A 58-year-old male presented to the emergency department (ED) on a Saturday after he developed crushing substernal chest pain while attending a football game and yelling at his favorite football team, the Baltimore Ravens. On his electrocardiogram, he had sinus tachycardia (ST) elevation in his anterior-lateral leads. After being stabilized in the ED and getting relief from his chest pain, he was brought to the cardiac catherization lab and was found to have severe three-vessel disease. He was bolused with heparin and scheduled for an elective coronary artery bypass graft (CABG). He was admitted for 3 days and discharged home with metoprolol, aspirin, Plavix, Lipitor, and hydrocholorthiazide.

In the anesthesia preoperative clinic, the anesthesiologist noted that the patient had been diagnosed with heparin-induced thrombocytopenia and thrombosis (HITT) by hematology and was scheduled to consult with you regarding management plans on intraoperative anticoagulation during surgery. You contact the surgeon's office to discuss the diagnosis, and she says, "I haven't had a HITT patient in the last 10 years of my practice. What should we do?"

(*First author's note*: Once again, we see "same problem, different institution." See how the Hopkins' approach is similar to yet distinct from Stony Brook's.)

Patient care

Residents must be able to provide patient care that is compassionate, appropriate, and effective for the treatment of health problems and the promotion of health.

Communicate effectively and demonstrate caring and respectful behaviors when interacting with patients and their families.

Your patient has just been discharged from the hospital after having a heart attack and is scheduled for open-heart surgery. If that is not anxiety provoking enough, now you must communicate that he has developed a complication from a medication that can become an additional life-threatening problem during an already high-risk surgery. It is important to keep your patient involved in the decision-making process of his medical care.

HITT can be a devastating complication in the cardiac surgical patient population. It should be explained to the patient that if he proceeds with surgery, he has a higher risk of perioperative complications. These possible complications include bleeding and thromboses. Owing to their already established accelerated arteriosclerosis, these patients are at an especially higher risk of life- and limb-threatening thrombosis.

HITT antibodies are usually transient and decline to undetectable levels in 100 days. If the surgery can be delayed, then the recommendation according to the American College of Chest Physicians is doing just that. However, this is after all cardiac surgery, and sometimes it cannot be delayed.

If your patient decides to proceed with surgery, it would be prudent for the surgeon to discuss the option of on- versus off-pump CABG. Off-pump CABG requires smaller dosing regimens of unfractionated heparin (UFH). Other options, such as percutaneous intervention, should also be entertained.

Gather essential and accurate information about their patients.

When entertaining the diagnosis of HITT, it is essential to obtain a detailed history and physical from your patient. Besides eliciting a history of heparin exposure, it is important to obtain the exact date when the patient was first exposed to heparin. When HITT occurs, it results in a drop in platelet count greater than 50% 5–10 days after exposure to heparin. Additionally, patients given heparin can develop an abrupt drop in their platelet count (median time 10.5 hours after the start of heparin) if they were exposed to heparin in the past 100 days. This is due to the persistence of circulating HITT antibodies.

On physical exam, some of these patients can develop skin lesions at injection sites ranging from painful erythematous plaques to skin necrosis. This diagnostic finding can help confirm the diagnosis of HITT when further confirmatory tests are not available.

A full set of labs should be drawn, including a complete metabolic profile to assess the patient's renal and hepatic function. In addition to using this pertinent information for all high-risk surgeries, these data will be used to help determine what type of anticoagulation is optimal for this patient.

Additionally, the patient's cardiac cath report, echocardiogram, carotid Dopplers, electrocardiogram, and chest X-ray should be obtained, which will provide the anesthesiologist with important information to direct the intraoperative anesthetic management.

Make informed decisions about diagnostic and therapeutic interventions based on patient information and preferences, up-to-date scientific evidence, and clinical judgment.

Now that we have three pieces of information – heparin exposure, a relative thrombocytopenia (50% in platelet count), and a positive HITT antibody – you have to decide what additional information is needed that will help make your clinical diagnosis and direct further medical management and surgical intervention.

The HITT antibody can be detected using a solid phase enzyme-linked immunosorbent assay (ELISA) immunoassay, which is a very sensitive test (up to 97%). This assay has a high false-positive rate; that is, several people that have HITT antibodies may not actually have the clinical entity. Ordering more specific diagnostic tests, such as the platelet serotonin release assay or heparin-induced platelet aggregation assay, can help to confirm the diagnosis. The only catch is that it may take some time to receive these results, and results may not be ready prior to the scheduled surgery date.

Develop and carry out patient management plans.

Without a definitive diagnosis of HITT, several decisions need to take place before further medical or surgical management of your patient can proceed. First, it needs to be decided how urgently your patient needs surgery. Can it be delayed long enough for a more confirmatory diagnostic test? If a diagnosis of

HITT is positive, can surgery be delayed long enough for the antibody to clear? Second, if it is decided to proceed with surgery, what are the plans for anticoagulation while on CPB? Can his surgery be performed as an off-pump CABG? Third, what are plans for postoperative deep venous thrombosis(DVT) prophylaxis?

To help make these decisions, a multidisciplinary approach should be taken. The other players involved should be the cardiothoracic surgical team, cardiology, hematology, perfusion, laboratory medicine, transfusion, and the pharmacy.

You should determine what laboratory capabilities your hospital has to monitor the level of anticoagulation of nonheparin anticoagulants. Also, you should discuss with the surgeon what experience he or she has with using other types of anticoagulation.

Once the diagnosis of HITT is made, the first intervention is to stop all exposure to heparin. Low-molecular-weight heparin (LMWH) should also be avoided because it can cross-react with heparin antibodies. Warfarin should also be avoided in patients diagnosed with acute HITT because they can develop limb necrosis from protein C depletion. After thrombocytopenia resolves, if long-term anticoagulation is needed, oral anticoagulation can be initiated after 5 days of anticoagulation with a nonheparin anticoagulant.

Counsel and educate patients and their families.

The patient should understand the importance of letting all future medical providers know that he has a history of HITT. Although this may or may not change the management 10 years down the line, it is important information for his health care providers. Patients in whom the antibodies have cleared can receive heparin safely.

Provide health care services aimed at preventing health problems or maintaining health.

When patients have HITT, it is a setup for a perfect storm. You certainly want to make sure that this patient doesn't get heparin. It is important to educate your patient that it is still possible to receive UFH in the future, especially for procedures for which it is the drug of choice. HITT antibodies are transient and usually drop to undetectable levels by 100 days. In this circumstance, it is important for these patients not to receive UFH perioperatively, and an alternate form of anticoagulation should be used postoperatively. Not educating these patients presents the opportunity for future harm. For future procedures that require heparin anticoagulation, as long as the appropriate time has elapsed since last exposure and appropriate preoperative screening is done, they should still be able to receive heparin.

Once the diagnosis of HITT is made, to prevent any further complications, the patient's chart should be marked as having a heparin allergy, and signs should be posted at the bedside to avoid heparin flush administration.

Work with health care professionals, including those from other disciplines, to provide patient-focused care.

Having a multidisciplinary approach that includes cardiothoracic surgery, anesthesiology, hematology, perfusion, pharmacy, laboratory, and transfusion medicine as well as the ICU intensivist is essential in this group of patients. A hematologist can help rule out other causes of thrombocytopenia. If a diagnosis of HITT is confirmed, a hematologist can help determine the best form of anticoagulation based on your hospital's monitoring capabilities. Additionally, it is important that the intensivist be involved early to make sure appropriate anticoagulation is implemented postoperatively to decrease the risk of DVT/pulmonary embolism and catheter thrombosis. Finally, the nurses should understand that heparin flushes and other heparin-impregnated devices are to be avoided.

Medical knowledge

Residents must demonstrate knowledge about established and evolving biomedical, clinical, and cognate (e.g., epidemiological and social-behavioral) sciences and the application of this knowledge to patient care.

Demonstrate an investigatory and analytic thinking approach to clinical situations.

When presented with a patient with thrombocytopenia and recent heparin exposure, it is important to develop a differential diagnosis of the cause of thrombocytopenia. As you know, not everyone exposed to heparin develops a drop in his or her platelets. Breaking your differential down to a defect in platelet production versus increased consumption and destruction is a good way to remember the causes of thrombocytopenia.

Be sure to review your patient's medicine list, especially newly prescribed ones, as drugs are a common cause of reversible thrombocytopenia. Look at the rest of the complete blood count. If other cell lines were depleted, one would lean toward a diagnosis of a production problem. Looking at a coagulation profile can also be helpful in the differential diagnosis of thrombocytopenia. If the aPTT and PT are elevated, a consumptive process, such as disseminated intravascular coagulation, would be more likely. Ordering a blood smear and hemolysis labs can help diagnosis disorders like idiopathic thrombocytopenic purpura and thrombotic thrombocytopenic purpura. Last, but not least, it can't hurt to repeat a platelet level to make sure that it is accurate. EDTA tubes used for blood collection can cause pseudothrombocytopenia secondary to platelet clumping

---

Know and apply the basic and clinically supportive sciences that are appropriate to their discipline.

Heparin-induced thrombocytopenia is an adverse reaction to heparin consisting of thrombocytopenia with or without thrombosis. Historically and in the literature, it is very confusing, because there are loads of names that we use to define this entity such as HIT I, HIT II, and HITT. What it basically boils down to is that there are really two types of HITT: immunologically mediated HIT and nonimmunologically mediated HIT. Nonimmunologically mediated HIT is a transient drop by less than 50% of platelets 1–2 days after exposure to heparin. No treatment is required.

Immunologically mediated HITT develops after heparin binds to circulating platelet factor 4 and you develop antibodies to this heparin-PF4 complex. The tail end of the antibody binds to Fc receptors on platelets, causing them to be activated and then aggregate. This results in the thrombocytopenia and the paradoxical thrombosis. Additionally, if your patient does develop thrombocytopenia secondary to heparin, it doesn't mean that he or she will definitely develop clinical thrombosis. That is what is most mind-boggling about this entity.

HIT II is an immunologically mediated response that occurs after approximately 5–10 days of heparin exposure, resulting in a drop in platelet count (usually more than 50%) and (sometimes) limb- or life-threatening thrombosis (HIT II with thrombosis).

The thrombocytopenia that develops from HITT usually does not lead to clinical bleeding; rather, these patients are at high risk of thrombosis. Most patients have platelet count nadirs between 20 and 150 × 109/L (median 60 × 109). A few will have platelet levels below 20 but still will not develop thrombocytopenic bleeding. Another small population will have platelet levels that stay above 150 but which have dropped more than 50% from their prior levels.

Practice-based learning and improvement

Residents must be able to investigate and evaluate their patient care practices, appraise and assimilate scientific evidence, and improve their patient care practices.

Locate, appraise, and assimilate evidence from scientific studies related to their patients' health problems.

Given the limited experience most anesthesiologists and surgeons have at providing an alternate form of anticoagulation, physicians should seek the expertise of those more experienced. Using PubMed to search for case reports and, ultimately, multicentered, large, population-based, randomized, controlled trials is a rational approach to find the safest and most efficacious method of providing anticoagulation for cardiopulmonary bypass for patients with HITT. It is also prudent to use current guidelines put together by experts in the field.

For those patients who have HITT or are strongly suspected to have HITT, the American College of Chest Physicians has recommended alternative non-heparin anticoagulant over the continuation of UFH or LMWH or the initiation or continuation of a vitamin K antagonist [1]:

1. danaparoid (grade 1B)
2. lepirudin (grade 1C)
3. argatroban (grade 1C)
4. fondaparinux (grade 2C)
5. bivalirudin (grade 2C)

In those patients with strongly suspected HITT or with acute confirmed HITT, the following (in descending order of preference) are recommended over the use of UFH for cardiac surgery:

1. Wait, if possible, until HITT is resolved and a HIT antibody test is negative or weakly positive (Grade 1B).

2. Use bivalirudin if techniques of cardiac surgery and anesthesiology have been adapted to the unique features of bivalirudin pharmacology (Grade 1B).
3. Perform off-pump coronary artery bypass grafting (Grade 1B).
4. Use lepirudin only if ecarin clotting time (ECT) is available and renal function is normal and the patient is at low risk for postoperative renal dysfunction (Grade 2C).
5. Use UFH and epoprostenol if no ECT is available for intraoperative use or the patient has renal dysfunction (Grade 2C).
6. Use UFH and tirofiban (Grade 2C).
7. Use danaparoid for intraoperative coagulation for off-pump coronary artery bypass grafting (Grade 2C).

Apply knowledge of study designs and statistical methods to the appraisal of clinical studies and other information on diagnostic and therapeutic effectiveness.

An important question one might ask follows: "My patient has thrombocytopenia with a platelet level of 60 undergoing surgery where bleeding can be a detrimental complication. Should I give a platelet transfusion?" Given that HITT is a pathologic condition causing hypercoaguablity, rather than bleeding, one might be concerned that giving platelets could trigger or increase the patient's risk of developing a thrombotic event.

Hopkins and Goldfinger [2] report a somewhat unsubstantiated risk of thrombotic events associated with platelet transfusions in patients diagnosed with HITT and did not find an increased risk of this dreadful complication in their study – although this may be attributable to the small study size and it being retrospective in nature. Further studies need to be done to identify the true risk of adding insult to injury, as Hopkins and Goldfinger point out. According to the American College of Chest Physicians (ACCP), in patients who are actively bleeding or at risk thereof, where the clinical diagnosis of HITT is not apparent, platelet transfusions in the setting of HITT or probable HITT may be appropriate. According to the ACCP recommendations, prophylactic platelet transfusions should not be given in patients without active bleeding with strongly suspected or confirmed HITT.

Interpersonal and communication skills

Residents must be able to demonstrate interpersonal and communication skills that result in effective information exchange and teaming with patients, their patients' families, and professional associates.

> Work effectively with others as a member or leader of a health care team or other professional group.

If you have any people skills, this is the time to put them into action. Coordinating the different teams and making sure you know your plan as well as alternatives are very important prior even to getting to the OR with this patient. One of the most important things during the case will be to recognize problems with the drug that you are using for anticoagulation and having a plan in place for combating these problems and/or complications. During every case, but especially this case, keeping open communication with the surgeon, perfusionist, laboratory personnel, blood bank, and nursing staff is very important.

Systems-based practice

Residents must demonstrate an awareness of and responsiveness to the larger context and system of health care and the ability to effectively call on system resources to provide care that is of optimal value.

> Know how to partner with health care managers and health care providers to assess, coordinate, and improve health care and know how these activities can affect system performance.

Again, partnering, communicating, and making up plans A, B, and C prior even to coming to the OR is going to be what helps ensure this patient's safety and outcome. The pharmacy will play a role by providing the nonheparin anticoagulant that you have available in your hospital. The hematologist will help guide the diagnosis and aid in drug usage. The surgeon will lose his or her temper but, more important, will determine what type of surgery (on- or off-pump bypass) he or she will do. The perfusionist will be aware of the specific drug properties during bypass. The laboratory and blood medicine departments will help with monitoring, if needed, for the drug of choice and blood product administration and availability. You will be the captain of this ship, guiding it through this storm of a case (as these cases can sometimes be!). Finally, the intensivist will be on the receiving end and will determine the type of nonheparin anticoagulant in the ICU postoperatively. So it can be sort of like trying to gather little children in a candy store, but it certainly can be done, and oftentimes very safely. The work for these cases starts well before in-room time.

References

1. Warkentin TE, Greinacher A, Koster A, et al. Treatment and prevention of heparin-induced thrombocytopenia: American College of Chest Physicians evidence based clinical practice guidelines (8th edition). Chest 2008;133:340–380.

2. Hopkins CK, Goldfinger D. Platelet transfusions in heparin-induced thrombocytopenia: a report of four cases and review of the literature. Transfusion 2008;48:2128–2132.

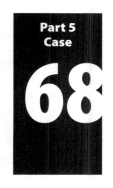

Contributions from Johns Hopkins Medical Institutions under Deborah A. Schwengel

"Just don't stop my achy, breaky heart ..."

Sapna Kudchadkar and R. Blaine Easley

The case

A 13-year-old girl with a history of congestive heart failure underwent device closure of her atrial septal defect (ASD) about 3 months ago. Now she presents with worsening cardiac function, and the cardiologist thinks she might have myocarditis. She presents today for a diagnostic cardiac catheterization. "She's very nervous, doctor. She can't lay still for 10 minutes, there's no way she's going to be able to lay still for 1 hour," her mother explains. "She definitely needs general anesthesia – and that's what she wants." The patient is sitting quietly next to her mother with her head down and won't look at you when you address her. As you go through the preop questionnaire, you learn that she can only go up one flight of stairs before she "looks like she's gonna faint!" Yesterday's echocardiogram showed a whopping ejection fraction (EF) of 20%. "The cardiologist assured us that she would be totally asleep for this."

Patient care

Residents must be able to provide patient care that is compassionate, appropriate, and effective for the treatment of health problems and the promotion of health.

Communicate effectively and demonstrate caring and respectful behaviors when interacting with patients and their families.

Here we have a very nervous teenager and her equally, if not more, nervous mother – who has been told by another physician (a nonanesthesiologist) how *you* are going to perform this anesthetic. Nice. This is the point at which a caring and respectful attitude will get you very far with a patient and her family. It's obvious why this teenager is nervous – she's smart enough to know that she has a ticker that just doesn't tick well and that she's at higher risk for any procedure, particularly one that involves her heart.

You know that a general anesthetic in a patient with horrible cardiac function carries a very high risk of complication – but how does one couch this with an *extremely* nervous teenager? She's established that she's letting her mom do the talking – and boy, is mom talking. This is the point at which acknowledging the patient and her mother's concerns is priceless.

"I know that you are extremely nervous about this procedure, and I *completely* understand. You've been through a lot over the last few months, and I don't blame you for wanting to be asleep for the whole thing. What are your major concerns, and what questions can I answer before I explain what I feel is the safest plan for today's procedure?" If you look directly at the teenager, she may be more willing to respond and ask her questions – or she may continue to be quiet. Either way, you are acknowledging that she is a young adult who is able to voice her opinions, help make decisions, and play an important role in her own medical care.

Gather essential and accurate information about their patients.

For this case, it's pretty obvious what you need to know – you already know that her exercise tolerance is virtually nil. The routine preop questionnaire should suffice here. You find out that she's otherwise had an unremarkable medical history until she went to camp and got this "viral syndrome" that ended in myocarditis. Of course, her medications are important. You find out that she is on captopril, furosemide, hydrochlorothiazide, and spironolactone but that she did not take any of her meds this morning.

Make informed decisions about diagnostic and therapeutic interventions based on patient information and preferences, up-to-date scientific evidence, and clinical judgment.

At this point, it's important to make sure that the patient and her mother understand what general anesthesia means as many people just think it means being asleep and not remembering anything. If you take the position mentioned in the chapter on cardiomyopathies in *Pediatric Cardiac Anesthesia,* "the only procedure for which [patients with severe dilated cardiomyopathy] should have an anesthetic is cardiectomy for heart transplantation" [1, p. 530]. You know that she would probably benefit from a moderate sedation technique with green mask – keeping her cardiac function in mind, a full-on vapor anesthetic and the medications needed for intubation and maintenance put her at higher risk for significant hypotension and potential arrhythmias during the procedure. Of course, moderate sedation can include a number of options for drugs. A benzodiazepine-opioid combination is feasible but still carries a risk of hypotension in the doses this young woman might require to be still for the procedure. As long as she is not catecholamine depleted, ketamine is an excellent choice as it enables you to have a spontaneously breathing patient with some analgesia and likely no major cardiac effects. You explain the risks and benefits of both options to the mom and patient and answer all their questions. Either way, you want an intravenous catheter in place to titrate the medications.

Develop and carry out patient management plans.

The patient and her mother agree to the sedation plan – she's going to need a benzo either way, so you give her some PO Versed before bringing her into the room, and you are mindful of the dose because of her hemodynamics. The caveat is how she will do with obtaining intravenous (IV) access. If she will tolerate it, a little subcutaneous lidocaine might be sufficient. Otherwise, she might benefit from a little nitrous oxide by mask. After IV access has been established, green mask oxygen, and don't forget to give some glycopyrrolate so you don't have a drool fest on your hands! Ketamine in, nystagmus hello! You see a nice minor bump in her blood pressure – you'll take it!

If general anesthesia is the agreed on choice (or sedation fails secondary to movement), you have the option of using ketamine or etomidate to maintain stable hemodynamics during the induction. Propofol or thiopental can be done but should be administered with extreme caution as they can quickly put you in a lowly place when it comes to blood pressure. For maintenance anesthesia, a low-dose isoflurane or sevoflurane (0.5% to 1% MAC) will probably be sufficient for

a minimally invasive and (it is hoped) short procedure. A laryngeal mask airway or endotracheal tube? your choice.

There are many ways to do this anesthetic, and almost any of them can lead to trouble. Definitely prepare the patient and family for the possibility of needing a breathing tube and monitoring after the procedure, even if all goes well. Though the plan is to go to the inpatient floor, you should prepare the child and her parents for the possible hemodynamic problems and have an intensive care unit (ICU) bed available.

Counsel and educate patients and their families.

You did an excellent job with this prior to the procedure, and the case is going swimmingly, so you ask the operating room (OR) nurse to update the family.

Use information technology to support patient care decisions and patient education.

This is something you took care of in your preop – you personally read the echo report, examined her chest X-ray, and looked up her computerized patient record, which included her course in the pediatric intensive care unit (PICU) when she was admitted for worsening heart failure and they noted her decrease in cardiac function and suspected a myocarditis. Her last set of labs is also important given her medication list – you're not surprised about a potassium of 5.5 mg/dL or a hemoglobin of 11 g/dL going into the cath lab with her diuretic usage. She *is* on spironolactone, a K^+ sparing diuretic, so you need a plan for treating hyperkalemia were it to become an issue – have calcium available as a myocardial stabilizer and insulin and glucose at the ready in case you do observe the classical peaked *T*-waves or widened QRS associated with hyperkalemia.

Perform competently all medical and invasive procedures considered essential for the area of practice.

You've obtained venous access – for a simple diagnostic cath, a preinduction arterial line is probably not necessary as long as you have good cuff pressures. However, with her degree of cardiac dysfunction, a radial arterial line would be a reasonable consideration. You are correct in anticipating cardiac issues such as hypotension and arrhythmia. Getting yourself familiar with the emergency equipment (i.e., a defibrillator – how to turn it on and charge), drugs (i.e., epinephrine), and personnel (like the circulating nurses and radiation technicians) that are immediately available is a good proactive plan. You must make sure you have an appropriate backup plan to secure the airway, if needed, and may consider discussing with your attending whether having the cardiologist in the room would be a good idea before inducing anesthesia.

Provide health care services aimed at preventing health problems or maintaining health.

The parent hands you a 1998 American Heart Association card and says, "I don't know if she still needs antibiotics now that her ASD is closed." In this case, the most important preventative care measure you can provide is subacute bacterial endocarditis (SBE) prophylaxis. Multiple recommendations have changed regarding SBE treatment. Though her ASD closure will ultimately exclude her from needing prophylaxis, she is still in the 6-month period following treatment, in which current recommendations advise coverage. The reason for the change in guidelines is based on current risk-benefit studies that demonstrate that the risk of anaphylaxis from an antibiotic is greater in most at-risk cardiac patients than developing SBE after a nondental procedure. If this were for a simple diagnostic cath, SBE would not be indicated, even if the ASD were open. Point being, double-check the guidelines [2] (available at http://www.americanheart.org/presenter.jhtml?identifier=3047051).

Another issue regarding health maintenance and this particular patient's future – is she a potential transplant recipient? It sure sounds that way, with her worsening function. If this is the case, you need to think about how to optimize her care to provide the easiest possible conditions for a transplant. The main thing here is to avoid blood products, if at all possible, to minimize her antibody load. All decisions are a balance of risks and benefits for this patient, even a blood transfusion. Involve the other physicians, like the referring cardiologist and procedural physician, when deciding about the blood transfusion. In addition, this procedure, with the increased vascular access, may facilitate certain testing that would be important to her evaluation (just as much as the cath) and that may not have been considered.

Work with health care professionals, including those from other disciplines, to provide patient-focused care.

As mentioned earlier, you are in a remote location, and this is a very important aspect of providing safe patient care. You *must* make sure you have all the resources you need in case things get hairy. Communicating with the cardiologist performing the cath about his or her availability during induction and discussion with the cath lab nurses and techs regarding your expectations for this patient and worst-case scenarios are imperative. That way, there are no surprises if things start to go downhill. Make sure everyone knows his or her role *prior to* beginning – it will make everything much easier down the line.

This is also where you make sure that you know exactly what the cardiologist has planned for the patient – is this simply a diagnostic cath, or are they doing a biopsy, as well? Where do they plan on getting access? Jugular? Femoral? If they are planning access in the neck, it will be a little more challenging because the patient will not have a secure airway and would need to be completely covered with drapes up top; it is important to discuss these things *before* you get started.

Medical knowledge

Residents must demonstrate knowledge about established and evolving biomedical, clinical, and cognate (e.g., epidemiological and social-behavioral) sciences and the application of this knowledge to patient care.

Demonstrate an investigatory and analytic thinking approach to clinical situations.

Having an algorithm in your head (much like the difficult airway algorithm) for case-specific complications is imperative. You start with a "healthy" patient and move down the algorithm with management options for various situations. If she becomes hypotensive on induction, what are your choices? Drugs (epi, ephedrine, phenylephrine)? Fluid (bolus)? Remember, her heart may not handle a large fluid bolus without some accompanying pulmonary edema – and you are not planning on having a secure airway initially. What about arrhythmias? Which drugs should you have available for this highly possible event? Lidocaine, amiodarone, adenosine? Also, consider electrolyte repletion in the event of arrhythmia. Having calcium (to stabilize the myocardium), magnesium, and potassium available is important, keeping in mind you probably won't have access to a fully stocked pharmacy in your remote location. Also, consider afterload reduction – a readily available milrinone drip might be a life-saver – and keep in mind that the patient was on captopril prior to the procedure!

> Know and apply the basic and clinically supportive sciences that are appropriate to their discipline.

You have already read the requisite textbook chapters on anesthesia for the cardiac patient- specifically dilated cardiomyopathy. The basic physiology here is pretty simple, not like a complicated congenital cardiac anomaly where the blood goes in all different directions. Simply put, the pump ain't workin' well. So you need to know how to do the appropriate thing to prevent and treat:

1. hypotension: gotta keep the brain and heart perfused!
2. arrhythmias: the brain doesn't like these either, and throwing clots is no fun
3. pulmonary edema: unsecured airway, worsening tachypnea, and hypoxia in a sedated patient – yuck

Practice-based learning and improvement

Residents must be able to investigate and evaluate their patient care practices, appraise and assimilate scientific evidence, and improve their patient care practices.

> Analyze practice experience and perform practice-based improvement activities using a systematic methodology.

Every hospital is different, but in general, anesthesia and procedures *not* performed in an operating room suite have a higher rate of complications that are attributed to *inappropriate resources*. You will not usually have 10 anesthesiologists barrel into your room if you page "anesthesia stat" when things hit the fan. Your full pharmacologic arsenal will likely not be at your immediate disposal, unless you already planned ahead and brought every possible drug you might ever need. If she goes into pulseless V tach and advanced cardiac life support does not bring her back, an extracorporeal membrane oxygenation (ECMO) circuit isn't standing outside the room ready to roll. This is why the preoperative briefing among all staff involved in the case is so crucial. "Expect the unexpected." Cliché, but if you plan for it, and it doesn't happen – awesome. But if you don't plan and it does – *crap!* Now, we're not saying that you should have an ECMO circuit primed and

outside the room; you should simply know your case, know the potential for complications, and have a plan of action for every possible scenario. Your attending, having probably done many more of these remote procedures than you have, will probably have many useful tidbits in this regard – after all, "ya learn by being burned."

> Locate, appraise, and assimilate evidence from scientific studies related to their patients' health problems.

There are many reviews on anesthetic management of cardiomyopathy, specifically diastolic dysfunction, out there on PubMed. Reading case reports is also very useful in these circumstances to draw your attention and educate you on some unusual complications that may arise in this patient population [3].

> Obtain and use information about their own population of patients and the larger population from which their patients are drawn.

Your attending probably spends a good deal of his or her clinical time doing cardiac cases and patients with cardiac pathology. Drawing on your attending's breadth of experience as well as your own, and reading the literature, as described earlier, will enable you to provide the best patient care possible.

> Apply knowledge of study designs and statistical methods to the appraisal of clinical studies and other information on diagnostic and therapeutic effectiveness.

You know this is important – but for this case, you're likely concentrating on reviews and case reports to manage this specific patient.

> Use information technology to manage information, access online medical information, and support their own education.

Computers are awesome, as is that fine thing called the Internet. When you have time between cases, when a case is canceled, and you're trolling for something to do, you have a portable source of endless information at your fingertips. The challenge is using the right sources – the Internet is full of pages from people who claim to know what they're talking about. PubMed, of course, is your main source for up-to-date literature searches on any medical topic, but don't leave out so many other important databases, for example, the Cochrane Database. Virtually every anesthesia textbook is probably available to you online through your institution's library subscription, so you can read *Faust*'s chapter on automated implanted cardioverter-defibrillator [4] for a quick review – by the way, does this patient have one?

Professionalism

Residents must demonstrate a commitment to carrying out professional responsibilities, adherence to ethical principles, and sensitivity to a diverse patient population.

> Demonstrate respect, compassion, and integrity; a responsiveness to the needs of patients and society that supersedes self-interest; accountability to patients, society, and the profession; and a commitment to excellence and ongoing professional development.

Your responsiveness and bedside manner when dealing with the patient and her mother during the preop are a prime example of respect, compassion, and integrity. You made a recommendation based on your patient's best interests and safety.

> Demonstrate a commitment to ethical principles pertaining to provision or withholding of clinical care, confidentiality of patient information, informed consent, and business practice.

Before the case, make sure informed consent, site of surgery, and all the paper work are in order. Observe all HIPAA regulations (don't talk about the case where others can overhear and don't reveal any confidential patient information). When filling out your billing slips, be ethical. Bill for what you did and nothing more.

As noted earlier, this is background behavior that applies to all cases.

> Demonstrate sensitivity and responsiveness to patients' culture, age, gender, and disabilities.

As a teenager, you understand that your patient is in a place of delicate balance – she is expected to be mature and understand what is going on, but she is still a child trying to make sense of a very heavy diagnosis. Approaching her as such and giving her a sense of independence and respect in medical decision making, while at the same time keeping her mother equally involved, takes a heavy feeling of responsibility off the patient without making her feel like a kid.

Interpersonal and communication skills

Residents must be able to demonstrate interpersonal and communication skills that result in effective information exchange and teaming with patients, their patients' families, and professional associates.

> Create and sustain a therapeutic and ethically sound relationship with patients.

Comforting the patient from the get-go and making her feel like an adult is the most therapeutic, ethically sound relationship you can formulate with this teenager.

> Use effective listening skills and elicit and provide information using effective nonverbal, explanatory, questioning, and writing skills.

If she does have questions, *really* listen – if she has a concern that may seem silly to you, make it seem like the most valid concern in the world, which will make her even more comforted. In the cath lab, *listen!* The interventionalists are in their own little world and may not scream out if they have an issue or, "oops," their wire pokes a hole in the myocardium. It's your job to be keyed in to every aspect of the procedure – watching the cath to see where they are in the vasculature and what issues you might have to anticipate.

> Work effectively with others as a member or leader of a health care team or other professional group.

If you are having issues with hypotension or desaturation, let the interventionalists know! This is no time for quiet management because *they* might be the reason you're having issues. They have access to the femoral sheath if you need immediate central access – plan, plan, plan for emergency readiness. It is vital to talk through any problems that are occurring.

Systems-based practice

Residents must demonstrate an awareness of and responsiveness to the larger context and system of

379

health care and the ability to effectively call on system resources to provide care that is of optimal value.

> Understand how their patient care and other professional practices affect other health care professionals, the health care organization, and the larger society and how these elements of the system affect their own practice.

Safely taking care of this patient by providing an anesthetic with minimal risk and communicating with the entire team involved in taking care of her are of the essence. The complexity of this case should suggest it be carried out at a facility that can provide an ICU level of care to the patient. Recognition of this need is paramount to providing optimal and safe care to this patient and advocating for her to have this procedure elsewhere. You and the other physicians may be capable, but the resources (a *pediatric* ICU bed; extracorporeal support measures like an aortic balloon pump or ventricular assist device) may be lacking.

> Know how types of medical practice and delivery systems differ from one another, including methods of controlling health care costs and allocating resources.

Keep in mind that things are done differently everywhere – there is the (insert your hospital's name) way – and we frequently forget that practice is very different in the real world. Be open to many possibilities and weigh the pros and cons of each – it *is* easier to practice medicine the way you're used to, but in the appropriate situations, it's important to broaden your experience, without *experimenting*. This patient clearly needs to be at a center that can provide tertiary, pediatric-focused cardiac care that may include esca-

lating levels of support, including cardiac transplantation. These centers are willing to be dedicated.

> Practice cost-effective health care and resource allocation that does not compromise quality of care.

Minimize costs in this case as much as possible. If you don't need a remifentanil drip, don't use one – low-dose vapor (isoflurane is most cost-effective, if she tolerates it) will be just fine. However, if problems develop, "cost-effective" may be a fairly remote issue.

> Advocate for quality patient care and assist patients in dealing with system complexities.

By making the patient and her mother feel comfortable with your plan and helping them navigate through the risks of the various anesthetic options, you have made a potentially scary time an easier experience.

> Know how to partner with health care managers and health care providers to assess, coordinate, and improve health care and know how these activities can affect system performance.

If there are any concerns with this patient's management and/or things that you feel should have been done differently, it is important to cover this in debriefing at the end of the procedure and to speak with the appropriate channels about correcting the problem – do you need a Pyxis machine in the cath lab to access a comprehensive pharmacy of drugs immediately? Patient care should not be compromised simply because you're in a remote location. If you feel that there are improvements that can streamline patient care in this setting, let the powers that be know!

References

1. McKenzie I, Weintraub R. Cardiomyopathies. In: Lake C, Booker P, editors. Pediatric cardiac anesthesia. Philadelphia: Lippincott, Williams, and Wilkins; 2005: 530–535.

2. Wilson W, Taubert KA, Gewitz M, et al. Prevention of infective endocarditis: guidelines from the American Heart Association. Circulation 2007;116:1736–1754.

3. Kipps AK, Ramamoorthy C, Rosenthal DN, Williams GD. Children with cardiomyopathy: complications after noncardiac procedures with general anesthesia. Paediatr Anaesth 2007;17:775–781.

4. Trankina MF. Automatic implantable cardioverter-defibrillator. In: Anesthesiology Review. 3rd ed. Faust RJ, editor. Philadelphia: Churchill Livingstone; 2002; 343–345.

Contributions from Johns Hopkins Medical Institutions under Deborah A. Schwengel

Too bad, so sad … it's Friday afternoon with a VAD

Jeremy M. Huff and Theresa L. Hartsell

The case

It's a Friday afternoon; you are tired and ready for a much deserved weekend retreat. You have been working the GI suites all day and have been as efficient as you could be to get done early and have a head start on your weekend.

Just as you finish your last case, you start creeping toward the door, when you notice another patient in the preoperative area. You question the administrative assistant, and she says that it is a last-minute add-on and that she knows nothing about the patient, except that he is scheduled for a percutaneous endoscopic gastrostomy/jejunostomy(PEG/J) tube placement.

You curse, put down your bag, and proceed to rummage through the various stacks of paper work, looking for the patient's chart. There are a couple of papers bound with a paper clip that represent the "extensive" chart available on this patient.

As you approach the patient, you notice a peculiar-looking device at the side of the bed with various digital readings. On further evaluation, you notice the word *THORATEC* etched across the machine, and your worst fears are realized – this patient has a ventricular assist device (VAD).

The patient is a 55-year-old who appears awake but drowsy. He has a tracheostomy in place without supplemental oxygen. He is afebrile and has vital signs as follows: heart rate 65, blood pressure 95/60, RR 10–20, SpO_2 96%. You notice a single 20-gauge peripheralIV in his hand and a weak smile on his face.

Patient care

Residents must be able to provide patient care that is compassionate, appropriate, and effective for the treatment of health problems and the promotion of health.

> Communicate effectively and demonstrate caring and respectful behaviors when interacting with patients and their families.

OK. Don't react. Remember that first and foremost, it is not your patient's fault that he was scheduled at the last minute for this procedure. He is not to blame for the scheduling fiasco, or his inappropriate transport and desertion, or the ruining of your early vacation plans. It is imperative that you first evaluate and then react to the situation, remembering to always act professionally and be caring, despite your inconvenience.

The patient is drowsy and, due to the lack of available medical information, it is best to approach the patient and determine his mental status. If you assess that it is altered, it will be necessary for you to contact a legal guardian or next of kin prior to proceeding. You will need him or her for consent purposes.

> Gather essential and accurate information about their patients.

From the time you became aware of the patient, you have begun to gather information that is essential. You secured the available paper records, the proposed intervention, and, from your brief visual survey, some vital information about the patient's medical history. In that brief interval of patient contact, you determined, based on vital signs and interviewing, that the patient is, at least for the moment, stable.

Other information that you likely need includes family contact information, the name of the surgeon or gastroenterologist performing the procedure, an extensive medical history and indications for the proposed procedure, medications (specifically anticoagulation status), availability of blood products, results of any recent testing, and specific information regarding the settings of the patient's VAD. In other words, you aren't rushing this one through the door without gathering more complete information about the whole situation.

It is important to gather and utilize all available resources. An important resource includes the VAD care team, which consists of multiple people who are involved in various aspects of care. Your VAD coordinator can help you efficiently locate information about the patient and the VAD as well as assist in mobilizing other resources.

Make informed decisions about diagnostic and therapeutic interventions based on patient information and preferences, up-to-date scientific evidence, and clinical judgment.

Remember in medical school when they said that you can make the majority of diagnoses from history alone? Well, they were right. But this guy has a VAD and a lot of stuff you can't get from history alone, especially if he is too sleepy to talk. You are going to need accurate information from multiple sources to determine the patient's current status, his ability to tolerate the rigors of the proposed procedure, and what you can do to facilitate the proposed plan.

Develop and carry out patient management plans.

Development of the patient management plan occurs after you have gathered all applicable information. If you would choose to proceed without this information, please contact your insurance carrier and lawyer prior to starting the case. You may need a moment to review VAD physiology, which can be done by pursuing a review article [1–4], opening a textbook (scary, I know), or contacting an appropriately knowledgeable colleague.

Once all the available information is on the table, you make an *informed* decision as to the patient's status and the risks and benefits of proceeding with the planned procedure. Review probable complications for this patient and the means by which you will address them.

Counsel and educate patients and their families.

The preoperative discussion is an ideal venue to instill confidence and treat the anxieties of both the patient and his or her family members. This discussion should include a complete disclosure of your anesthetic plan with associated risks and benefits as well as discussion and responses to patient and family member questions. You must decide if the patient has a clear understanding of the risks, their implications, and any future consequences; if you detect faulty understanding or impaired capacity for judgment – whether from decreased mental status, psychiatric disease, baseline cognitive function, medication use, or any other reason – you should not consider the patient as able to give informed consent. If the patient is not competent to give consent and there are no legally appropriate representatives available, then you should approach the primary team regarding your inability to secure informed consent.

Use information technology to support patient care decisions and patient education.

Part of your preoperative evaluation consists of locating any applicable test results, radiologic findings, surgical notes, visit summaries, and so on that can help you formulate a complete assessment of the patient. This may involve a paper chart; however, this day and age, typically, you are going to get on a computer and look some stuff up. Obviously, you want any information regarding the cardiovascular status of this particular patient – keep an eye out for anything pertaining to the VAD.

Many of your medical reference resources regarding physiology and treatment methods are now readily available via information technology means. You may not have to lift that hefty textbook after all. Remember that the mark of a good physician isn't necessarily always knowing, but knowing what you don't know and where to find it.

Perform competently all medical and invasive procedures considered essential for the area of practice.

So, you have now decided that it is appropriate to proceed. Now you must decide what kind of monitoring is necessary to ensure patient stability. Obviously, the standard American Society of Anesthesiology (ASA) monitors are appropriate (temperature, $ETCO_2$, three-lead EKG, pulse oximeter, and noninvasive blood pressure monitor). You must decide if there will be significant fluid shifts during the procedure to warrant more invasive monitoring. With this particular case, it is unlikely that you would need to add an arterial line or CVP/PA catheter as fluid shifts will be likely minimal and you will have some idea of the patient's overall forward flow measured from the VAD itself.

Seems like a 20-gauge peripheral IV may be a bit weak for someone who will need fluid in the event of decreased cardiac output (see the medical knowledge section). You probably aren't going to need a cordis, but an 18-gauge wouldn't hurt. Remember that the patient is likely anticoagulated (he has a Thoratec), so if the surgeons encounter bleeding, it is likely to be more profound than your bread-and-butter PEG/J.

Provide health care services aimed at preventing health problems or maintaining health.

Do no harm! This includes proceeding with the procedure only when the benefits are greater than the risks. Minimize the number of invasive monitors; however, do what is necessary to keep the patient safe. Remember to give your preoperative antibiotics; after all, this patient has endovascular hardware! Be *vigilant* and identify trends that may be intervened on prior to the patient coding.

Work with health care professionals, including those from other disciplines, to provide patient-focused care.

This patient is likely going to need some additional TLC from the whole team. Identify and utilize resources that will allow you to focus better on patient care. You may need an additional coordinator in the room to manage the other team members so that you can focus on the patient's stability. Get the cardiac team on board (they know the VAD) and get the GI team in the room and intimately aware of your concerns about patient status, positioning, and so on. There should be *active* communication on your and their part – you are the one who should facilitate that. Remember that nursing is your best friend or worst enemy, and you need all the friends you can get.

Medical knowledge

Residents must demonstrate knowledge about established and evolving biomedical, clinical, and cognate (e.g., epidemiological and social-behavioral) sciences and the application of this knowledge to patient care.

Demonstrate an investigatory and analytic thinking approach to clinical situations.

Admit it – your first impulse when you saw the VAD was to run. Don't worry; you wouldn't be the only one. VADs are foreign objects for both the patient and most medical providers. When you truly break down the mechanics of ventricular support, however, you may find their management surprisingly simple.

What is a VAD? If you don't know the answer to this question, you should be on the phone with one of your superiors and getting someone knowledgeable to

assist you. VADs are implanted devices that replace or assist the body's normal ventricular output. The device flow aims to ensure optimal organ perfusion and ventricular decompression. They are implanted with an "inflow" tract in a ventricle that collects blood into the VAD; the blood passes into a pneumatically powered chamber or through a rotary flow device. In the case of the Thoratec, which your patient has, the blood fills in the chamber, and at a set volume, the device forces blood through an outflow tract into the pulmonary artery (as in the case of an RVAD) or the aorta (as in the case of an LVAD). BiVAD is a term for a situation in which a patient has both an LVAD and an RVAD, meaning that both the right and left ventricles are assisted. Newer devices, which may be fully implantable, use rotary propulsion mechanisms and are notable for continuous flow; these devices support a mean arterial pressure without significant pulse pressure.

VADs generally collect blood passively by siphoning from available preload and are therefore dependent on preload. Your patient's Thoratec is likely set on "fill to empty" mode, in which case, the VAD ejects its contents only after filling to the set level. It does this independent of the heart function (i.e., unsynchronized). The rate of ejection is capped at a set maximum; however, the true rate is determined by speed of passive filling of the device. Higher preload means quicker filling, which equals a quicker rate of ejection up to the device maximum. For rotary flow devices, the cardiac output is dependent both on preload as well as rotary flow speed [3].

That's the preload part of the physiology. VADs also respond to changes in afterload; most specifically, increases in vascular resistance can decrease forward flow and may result in excess wear and tear on the VAD mechanism. Most patients are maintained at the minimum blood pressure required to sustain end organ perfusion; however, it is certainly appropriate to support blood pressure with titration of pressor agents in the setting of hypotension. From a contractility standpoint (and rate/rhythm), the patient with a BiVAD will be perfectly fine, unless there is a mechanical issue. However, patients with only one ventricle supported may need inotropic agents or arrhythmia management to support the nonmechanically assisted side of the heart.

The first thing in medical management is to know when to get help. You need to discover who in your hospital is the VAD team. Odds are pretty good that if you contact any of the cardiothoracic surgeons, they will know the VAD coordinator's contact information. You need the contact information to tease (no harassment, please) vital medical history and device characteristics from that person. The VAD coordinator will surely know the patient. He or she will also be able to tell you key pieces of information to help in the case of device failure such as how to manually sustain the cardiac output while someone is running for a replacement console!

Preoperatively, things important to know include the following:

- type and location of VAD: there are various types with some subtle differences that are important to understand. You should know where the VAD is located (i.e., LVAD, RVAD, and BiVAD). You should also know whether the VAD is a pulsatile system, like this patient has, or a rotary device, in which case the patient will have nonpulsatile flow. This can be a bit disconcerting if you feel for a pulse or if you only get a "mean" as you measure blood pressure. You should also know the location of a replacement console (if appropriate, as it would be for your patient with a Thoratec) and/or replacement batteries. A quick lesson in how to hand pump the Thoratec may be appropriate, as well – hope for the best, but always prepare for the worst!

- anticoagulation status: if the patient has a VAD that requires anticoagulation, you should know about it. Check coagulation studies. Is the patient on heparin, coumadin, or aspirin? If he is on coumadin, then you can pretty much assure yourself that you may just make that vacation early after all as it is generally inappropriate to proceed with an elective surgery.

- overall stability: VAD patients are generally some of the most stable patients when optimized. This gentleman was left in the GI preop area alone with a VAD, which is unacceptable, by most standards. Who would have dared to do such a thing? Contacting the VAD team will verify this, in addition to your own thorough evaluation of the patient. Those who know the patient well can also give you key information such as his underlying heart function (less important for BiVADs but very important in a patient with only one ventricle supported) and particular issues or situations that tend to cause decompensation.

- proposed case: when tailoring your anesthetic plan to the needs of the patient and the demands of the procedure, it is important to understand the risks and benefits. A long case that will involve significant fluid shifts is likely to be much more complex than the simple proposed PEG tube with our patient.

Intraoperative concerns are preload, preload, and preload:

- anesthetic technique: anesthetic plans should emphasize balance as there is little research to support one particular technique over another. As preload is vital to proper VAD functioning, a plan that would minimize changes in preload (or venous capacitance) is recommended. Neuraxial anesthesia can be performed; however, the anticoagulation status and the ability to maintain stable hemodynamics with vasodilatation make this choice less popular. Invasive monitoring may be needed if large fluid shifts are of concern or if the nonsupported ventricle is functioning poorly. You lucked out in our case: the patient would not likely need a pulmonary artery catheter placed for a PEG. (Can you imagine trying to explain yourself if you did? Not pretty!)

- positioning: because the device is preload-dependent, changes in position that affect preload will also alter hemodynamics. In addition, although the cannulae for VADs are structured to prevent kinking, attention to these and to drivelines can be important.

- hypovolemia: if asked how you would treat the majority of issues with VAD patients, the answer will invariably be give blood, give fluid, or give blood and fluid. Stability of VAD patients hemodynamically is directly related to – you guessed it – *preload*.

- arrhythmias: patients with arrhythmias can be monitored – that's right, monitored – so long as the arrhythmia does not compromise VAD flows. Follow normal ACLS protocols when defibrillating or performing cardioversion. NO CHEST COMPRESSIONS! You don't want to displace an inflow or outflow cannula, unless you want to spend the rest of your evening on cardiopulmonary bypass repairing the damage. There is a particular protocol regarding each type of VAD device when it comes to cardioversion and defibrillation. You will need to get this information from the VAD coordinator or particular VAD representative.

Know and apply the basic and clinically supportive sciences that are appropriate to their discipline.

It is critical to understand VAD physiology to manipulate that function to your, and the patient's, advantage.

Practice-based learning and improvement

Residents must be able to investigate and evaluate their patient care practices, appraise and assimilate scientific evidence, and improve their patient care practices.

Analyze practice experience and perform practice-based improvement activities using a systematic methodology.

You don't have "the night before" to bolster your patient- or case-specific knowledge, but rather than shooting from the hip, take a moment to think about what you've learned before about VADs and their management. Perhaps during cardiac anesthesia or a cardiac SICU (surgical intensive care unit) rotation?

It may be well worth your time to do a little targeted learning before stepping into the case itself. Here it may be higher yield to find an expert (the VAD coordinator or a cardiac anesthesia attending) to give you some quick pointers, rather than looking up a review article, but even the latter may be worthwhile.

Once the case is done, presuming it goes well, you can pat yourself on the back for taking care of the patient. However, this was clearly a suboptimal situation, and ideally, it shouldn't happen again. So even if there were no medical errors, it's worth making sure that the anesthesia, GI, and cardiac surgery departments review this case to decide if guidelines or protocols should be developed. These protocols should include guidelines for posting VAD patients, mandatory preoperative evaluation, consideration of surgical venue, a checklist of required and readily available resources, and a VAD team representative present during interventions. Don't assume that this will happen automatically – there's actually a lot of learning to be had from being proactive and being the multidisciplinary liaison to these review sessions. This is also a

systems-based practice issue (see how those competencies overlap!).

It occurs to you that many of your fellow residents (and some attending anesthesiologists) would not have known even how to approach this case, so perhaps it's worth putting in some effort to create a short fact sheet or educational review about taking care of a VAD patient having noncardiac surgery. It'll make you the local expert and give you the opportunity to do some teaching.

Obtain and use information about their own population of patients and the larger population from which their patients are drawn.

With the lack of available hearts for transplant and an ever increasing need for viable tissue, VADs have become ever more prevalent. There is a serious likelihood that you will encounter a VAD at some point during your career.

However, in this case, a quick review of the literature will reveal that there's not much information about "anesthesia for the VAD patient having noncardiac surgery," and certainly nothing evidence based. So perhaps that's a niche you'd like to fill? This is how scholarly ideas (and trips to ASA meetings) are born!

Use information technology to manage information, access online medical information, and support their own education.

This will be key as the major textbooks don't have great material in this area yet, and even if they did, you wouldn't be hauling them around in your backpack, would you? So here, either before or certainly after the case, you need to do a quick search for resources. In this case, PubMed is a place to start, but specialty societies or other academic institutional Web sites may be useful, as well. Or perhaps that departmental Web site library section where last year's PowerPoint lectures on various topics are housed. If all this fails, consider a number of forums designed to discuss difficult clinical cases (just remember HIPAA at all costs). Last, just Google it and be amazed.

Professionalism

Residents must demonstrate a commitment to carrying out professional responsibilities, adherence to ethical principles, and sensitivity to a diverse patient population.

Demonstrate respect, compassion, and integrity; a responsiveness to the needs of patients and society that supersedes self-interest; accountability to patients, society, and the profession; and a commitment to excellence and ongoing professional development.

Ancient Chinese proverb say, "It ain't all about you." The truth is, however, that it is the little things that you do that affect your patient, your profession, and society as a whole. A true professional recognizes this responsibility and opportunity to leave a positive mark on the lives of many.

In this case, you step up and adhere to practice guidelines, hospital policies, patient wishes, and ethical standards. Ultimately, you honorably perform your responsibility to all entities by providing the best possible care. If you have complaints with the manner in which the case is proceeding, maintain perspective and attempt to change the system at a later date, focusing your immediate attention on patient care. Believe me, there will always be an opportunity to deal with the system.

Demonstrate a commitment to ethical principles pertaining to provision or withholding of clinical care, confidentiality of patient information, informed consent, and business practice.

In a few short lines, I have to give you an ethics lesson that some spend years as undergrads studying. Ethics in medicine is about doing the right thing, which would be easy if the world were black and white. Medical ethics are never black and white. You must, in the course of your clinical experience, develop some moral integrity and common sense. With that compass, you navigate the endless decisions regarding clinical care, conduct ethical business, defend patient confidentiality, and truly inform patients of that which can happen and that which did happen.

Remember that this is an elective case. Just because the patient is sitting in the preoperative area does not mean that corners should be cut. Be sure of your patient's preoperative status and preparation and ensure that informed consent has been obtained.

Demonstrate sensitivity and responsiveness to patients' culture, age, gender, and disabilities.

In other words, *don't be a jerk*! This patient, as any other patient you work with, deserves to be treated with the dignity and respect of a fellow human being. In this age, we need to identify differences and be mindful of the effect of those differences to the care plan. We can't control many things about patient care, but we can control how we act. We need to learn to be sensitive, have a little tact, and show some respect.

Interpersonal and communication skills

Residents must be able to demonstrate interpersonal and communication skills that result in effective information exchange and teaming with patients, their patients' families, and professional associates.

Create and sustain a therapeutic and ethically sound relationship with patients.

For some, this is second nature; for others, this is easy. Basically, we must learn to enter a room, put patients at ease in limited time, and build a relationship of trust. The patient may have already sensed an atmosphere of fear, and even been depersonalized. It is important that your communication be patient centered and confidence inspiring.

Use effective listening skills and elicit and provide information using effective nonverbal, explanatory, questioning, and writing skills.

This case is a fine example of learning to utilize listening skills. You have no chart, and hence no information, so who better to ask than the patient himself? You can learn a lot by listening to patients. Weren't we always told that the majority of medical diagnoses could be made on information gathered from a thorough medical history alone? Learn to ask the right questions so you get to the meat (sorry, vegans) of the information and direct the conversation with patients to discourage rambling. We listen to various team members to determine needs and better patient care.

Nonverbal skills equal body language. Whether with your patient or with your team, what your body tells them can strengthen or weaken your credibility as a provider.

Work effectively with others as a member or leader of a health care team or other professional group.

Once upon a time, rants and tirades were tolerated in medicine. Now even Joint Commission on the Accreditation of Healthcare Organizations (JCAHO) has policies regarding the "disruptive physician." You can conform on your own or be compelled to change – remember, Big Brother is always watching.

Seriously, is it all that difficult to work cooperatively as a group? When egos are checked at the door, it seems that everything is more efficient. When communication is good, attitudes are optimal, and cooperation/collegiality is present, patient care is improved. (No need to do a study on that one – just use your noggin.)

Be sure to listen to the concerns of all team members and even facilitate this interaction. Hold a preoperative meeting/discussion that outlines concerns, expected courses of action, individual roles and responsibilities, and even worst case scenarios. A postoperative discussion can provide meaningful feedback to team members and instill a culture of cooperation that will serve to facilitate optimal health care delivery on future patients. Structure tends to decrease anxiety. A sensitive, open-minded, confident leader can inspire the masses to greatness.

A Boy Scout leader said, or maybe he yelled, that we are "only as fast as our slowest man." Recognize that you are a team leader and that like any elite team, you must encourage, reward, and motivate.

Systems-based practice

Residents must demonstrate an awareness of and responsiveness to the larger context and system of health care and the ability to effectively call on system resources to provide care that is of optimal value.

> Understand how their patient care and other professional practices affect other health care professionals, the health care organization, and the larger society and how these elements of the system affect their own practice.

This one is easy. The very decision to use VADs is known as a "bridge to transplant therapy." The continued use of VADS buys a patient time and allows him the possibility of a longer time on the transplant list and, subsequently, a higher probability of finding a tissue donor who matches. Some studies have shown that VADs actually unload the heart to a degree such that remodeling is able to occur, leaving the heart in better condition than it was found. This length of life

increase is what medicine is all about, right? (Surgeons, pat yourselves on the back now.)

What I am about to say is going to make me some enemies for sure. What does the increased length of life cost society? (GASP!) This cost can be monetary: the cost for periodic ICU level of care, endless office visits, medications. The cost can be nonmonetary: increased time on the transplant list means that someone who would have been higher on the list must wait potentially longer. Larger transplant demands ultimately mean that less quality organs are transplanted to supply the demand and lead to repeated use of limited resources such as ICU beds.

> Practice cost-effective health care and resource allocation that does not compromise quality of care.

Let's face it: we have limited resources in our society. These resources must be allocated and partitioned appropriately to ensure that the best needs of the whole of society are being met. Physicians and other health care providers decide to allocate a portion of these resources every day; be mindful of your decisions.

> Advocate for quality patient care and assist patients in dealing with system complexities.

Our patient has undoubtedly seen the inefficiencies and complications that exist in the medical system. Quality patient care involves not only providing quality medical care, but also the way in which it is provided. We know the system better and therefore have the responsibility to help our patients navigate it as easily as possible. Honestly, how can we say we improve a patient's quality of life if we leave him or her to navigate our infuriatingly complex and unintuitive medical system?

> Know how to partner with health care managers and health care providers to assess, coordinate, and improve health care and know how these activities can affect system performance.

Probably the most obvious defect in this patient's course is the lack of a coordinated transfer of care. Handoffs between health care providers are increasingly seen to be the weak link in the chain of quality patient care. When poorly done, they can and do often lead to serious patient safety issues. In this circumstance, it's likely that the team caring for the patient on the floor didn't consider a quick trip to the endoscopy suite as a transfer of care – yet another reason that education and a protocol for such situations would be important! In anesthesiology, some form of handoff is inherent at the beginning and end of almost all our cases. Be involved! This whole section on systems-based practice deals with the need for us to work with others on committees, societies, groups, and so on to identify and improve the medical system as a whole, even if it's one patient handoff at a time.

References

1. Lawrence JP. Preanesthetic assessment of the patient with an artificial circulation device. Anesthesiol News 2002;28:123–128.

2. Nicolosi AC, Pagel PS. Perioperative considerations in the patient with a left ventricular assist device. Anesthesiology 2003;98:565–570.

3. Stone ME. Current status of mechanical circulatory assistance. Sem Cardiothorac Vasc Anesthesiol 2007;11:185–204.

4. Stone ME, Soong W, Krol M, Reich DL. The anesthetic considerations in patients with ventricular assist devices presenting for noncardiac surgery: a review of eight cases. Anesth Analg 2002;95:42–49.

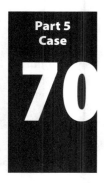
The disappearing left ventricle

A double lung transplant in a patient with severe pulmonary hypertension

The case
Kerry K. Blaha and Dan Berkowitz

The patient is a 43-year-old female who has had a history of idiopathic pulmonary hypertension for many years. Her home treatment regimen consisted of numerous medications, including a continuous IV infusion of Flolan delivered by a patient-controlled pump. A recent echocardiogram revealed a RVSP (right ventricular systolic pressure) of 127 mmHg, and right heart catheterization was significant for pulmonary artery pressures greater than her systemic blood pressures. A decline in her functional status over the past 2 weeks landed her a top spot on the lung transplant list and a "luxurious" room on Osler 4.

She is the youngest of many children and is surrounded by her entire family awaiting the news: will these lungs be good enough? She has been in this position before, anxiously anticipating her new set of lungs. She has been disappointed once before and remembers the words "I'm sorry, but it's a no-go" all too clearly.

You thoroughly discuss the anesthetic plan with the patient and her family. They are quite intelligent and ask some pretty in-depth questions. You breathe a sigh of relief as you answer the final question. You explain that you will take excellent care of the patient as you try to put them at ease. They smile, and you feel as if you gained their trust. However, now that *their* fears have been allayed, you can't help but feel anxious yourself about the monumental task you have ahead: the responsibility of getting her safely through the operation.

You help the patient out of bed and into the wheelchair for transport. You think you are about to make a clean break for the operating room, but wait. The family and their pastor start to close in around you and the patient. They ask, "Please, doctor, join us in prayer." You all join hands and pray for the patient, her surgery, and her safe recovery. Hugs abound, and it is now just you and the patient heading for the operating room.

Just as you are about to cross the red line, you hear "wait, wait, is that her?" in the distance behind you. The patient states that that is her mother, and she would like to see her before her surgery, if possible. Her mother was hoping to be there earlier but just got out of work. You wheel the patient back into the postanesthesia care unit (PACU) and give her the chance to see her mother before going back to the OR. After an emotional parting, you finally arrive outside the OR, only to hear that the surgeons are behind schedule and the operation is delayed. The patient is visibly disheartened. You then begin the long trip back to her room to play the waiting game. The patient and her family are concerned that the operation may be canceled again.

After the delay, the patient returns to the OR 2 hours later and undergoes a successful double lung transplantation.

Patient care

Residents must be able to provide patient care that is compassionate, appropriate, and effective for the treatment of health problems and the promotion of health.

> Communicate effectively and demonstrate caring and respectful behaviors when interacting with patients and their families.

In dealing with such a major operation, it is critically important to take your time and *communicate* with the patient and his or her family the full spectrum of anesthetic risks that coincide with such a major surgery. It is essential that they have realistic expectations so that they may be better able to cope with any unexpected (bad) outcomes. The patient and her family should be allowed ample time to ask any questions they may have, and you should listen with undivided attention. Turn off that cell phone and answer only emergency pages. This is the time to instill confidence in the patient and her family. You must show that the patient is the number one thing on your mind, and you are prepared to vigilantly guide her through undoubtedly the biggest, scariest event in her life. In our case, the family asked us to join in prayer with them before taking their loved one to the operating room. No matter what your religion, all walls are taken down in such an instance, and we felt like part of her family.

> Gather essential and accurate information about their patients.

A double lung transplant is a complex case, with many opportunities for things to go awry. Therefore it is important to know your patient's medical history like the back of your hand and be prepared as to how her medical problems and resultant cardiac, pulmonary, and renal physiology may influence your anesthetic or resuscitative efforts.

> Make informed decisions about diagnostic and therapeutic interventions based on patient information and preferences, up-to-date scientific evidence, and clinical judgment.

We need to come up with an anesthetic plan tailored for this patient and her specific needs. She is fairly anxious, so an IV premedication would likely be helpful for anxiolysis and amnesia prior to taking her back to the operating room. Given the severity of the operation, extensive invasive monitoring will be necessary. She will need an arterial line, large-bore central IV access, and pulmonary artery pressure monitoring to assess left heart pressures. Postoperatively, she will need a plan for pain control as the "clam-shell" incision is quite large. Placement of a postoperative thoracic epidural should be discussed with the patient preoperatively, and her preference should be honored after explaining the risks, benefits, and alternatives for postoperative pain control.

> Develop and carry out patient management plans.

Once discussed with the patient, you must proceed as planned. Deviations from the plan should only be entertained when emergencies or patient safety issues arise based on your clinical judgment.

> Counsel and educate patients and their families.

As mentioned earlier, the patient and her family should be counseled extensively prior to the operation. This includes preparing the family for seeing the patient in the ICU after the surgery. Seeing their loved one intubated, sedated, and fully monitored, surrounded by endless "spaghetti" tubing seeming to come from every bodily orifice, would be disconcerting to anyone, especially those not in the medical field. It is important to educate the family about the postoperative course, including seeing their loved one immediately after surgery in the ICU.

> Use information technology to support patient care decisions and patient education.

From the physician's perspective, you will want to look at the patient's labs, echocardiogram, electrocardiogram, and cardiac catheterization results prior to the procedure.

From the patient's perspective, the Internet is a fountain of knowledge, many times to the dismay of the physician. However, it can prove very useful by providing visual imagery of any or all parts of the procedure, although some patients may take the stance that "the less information, the better." From lung anatomy to the process of placing an epidural, some patients may be put at ease if they have an understanding of the procedures involved.

> Perform competently all medical and invasive procedures considered essential for the area of practice.

Perform all procedures (arterial lines, central lines, IVs) under sterile conditions. Take your time and accurately identify the pulse for the arterial line and anatomical landmarks for your central lines; you will make life easier for yourself, and your patient will appreciate fewer skin puncture holes, all of which have the possibility to cause complications (infection, hematoma, pneumothorax). All procedures must be done according to the standard of care.

> Provide health care services aimed at preventing health problems or maintaining health.

Prophylactic administration of antibiotics is crucial in a transplant operation. You must give antibiotics within 1 hour of incision and vigilantly at repeated time intervals, according to the standard of care.

> Work with health care professionals, including those from other disciplines, to provide patient-focused care.

It is important to constantly communicate with the surgeons in this case, especially at critically important times such as coming off bypass and reperfusion of the transplanted organs.

Medical knowledge

Residents must demonstrate knowledge about established and evolving biomedical, clinical, and cognate (e.g., epidemiological and social-behavioral) sciences and the application of this knowledge to patient care.

Demonstrate an investigatory and analytic thinking approach to clinical situations.

The patient with primary pulmonary hypertension is likely to be one of the most cardiovascularly compromised patients you will encounter to anesthetize. [1] An evidence-based approach to the anesthetic management is not possible because the disease is quite rare and large studies are thus not possible. Sound anesthetic management is therefore necessarily based on a broad understanding of the pathophysiologic consequences of the primary pathology, with clear and accurate maintenance of hemodynamic goals during induction, maintenance, and emergence. Furthermore, the impact of the procedure on these hemodynamic goals needs to be understood so they may be attenuated, or at least predicted. Historical anesthetic management has been based on case studies, and in general, the outcome of these patients undergoing noncardiac surgery is notoriously poor. This is because these patients live on the edge, and any small hemodynamic alteration could lead to instability and a downward spiral. Thus ultimate vigilance and preoperative assessment and planning are critical in these patients, as is a sophisticated understanding of the underlying pathophysiology.

Reperfusion after CPB and ischemic injury to the pulmonary vasculature of the transplanted lungs increases endothelial permeability and may result in pulmonary edema. Therefore fluid management after lung transplantation is a fine balance between minimizing pulmonary edema and preserving adequate cardiac function. It is ideal to keep the pulmonary capillary wedge pressure as low as possible after surgery, without compromising preload and cardiac output [2].

Know and apply the basic and clinically supportive sciences that are appropriate to their discipline.

Primary pulmonary hypertension (PPH) is a rare disease that causes a progressive increase in pulmonary vascular resistance (PVR), which ultimately results in right heart failure and death. Although other treatment modalities aimed at attenuating and reversing vascular remodeling and pulmonary vasoconstriction (Ca2+ channel blockers, phosphodiesterase-5 inhibitors, prostacyclin analogues, and endothelin antagonists) are helpful, lung or heart lung transplantation is the only curative procedure. Three pathologic features considered to be the hallmarks of PPH include vasoconstriction, intimal proliferation, and thrombosis. As a result of the progressive narrowing of the distal pulmonary arteries, there is increasing PVR. This, in turn, leads to RV hypertrophy and, ultimately, decompensation, dilatation, and RV failure. RV hypertrophy leads to an increase in oxygen demand for the RV as a result of an increase in preload and RV end diastolic pressure. Thus a decrease in systemic pressure, which may have little effect in RV perfusion in a normal heart, leads to myocardial ischemia and further decompensation and failure in PPH patients. In addition, the dilation and hypertrophy of the RV causes displacement of the interventricular septum, which limits LV filling (thus the disappearing ventricle) and stroke volume, further compromising blood pressure. This is a classic scenario of supply and demand imbalance: inadequate myocardial blood supply coupled with increased cardiac oxygen demands. Progressive myocardial ischemia can rapidly deteriorate to cardiac arrest, from which successful resuscitation is rare. Cardiopulmonary bypass may be the only option. In rare cases, unresponsive RV failure may respond to an atrial septostomy, in which arterial saturation is compromised (right to left shunt) in favor of LV filling, stroke volume augmentation, and blood pressure.

In addition to the underlying pathobiologic consequences for anesthetic management of patients with pulmonary hypertension, lung transplantation is associated with significant alteration and extremes of physiology. These might include single-lung ventilation in an already pulmonary compromised patient with resultant hypoxia and hypercarbia and an increase in airway pressure. The acute problems associated with lung transplantation in the perioperative period include acute graft failure as a result of reperfusion injury. There is some evidence that inhaled NO (nitric oxide) might attenuate this early graft dysfunction. If graft failure occurs and is fulminant, the patient may need a period of cardiopulmonary support such as extracorporeal membrane oxygenation. Long-term complications of transplantation include bronchiolitis obliterans (small airway narrowing and inflammation with graft failure) as well as infection associated with immunosupression.

Professionalism

Residents must demonstrate a commitment to carrying out professional responsibilities, adherence to ethical principles, and sensitivity to a diverse patient population.

Demonstrate respect, compassion, and integrity; a responsiveness to the needs of patients and society that supersedes self-interest; accountability to patients, society, and the profession; and a commitment to excellence and ongoing professional development.

No one would disagree – this is a major operation. It is important to respect the patient's wishes at all times, including inconvenient ones. In our case, we could see the bright lights of the operating theater, when suddenly the patient's mother was heard down the hallway. It was quite clear that it would mean a lot to the patient to see her mother prior to her surgery. "*Screech*!" The wheelchair came to a sudden halt as we made a 180° turn back to the PACU. Dramatic, but true, this may be the last time the patient sees her mother.

Demonstrate a commitment to ethical principles pertaining to provision or withholding of clinical care, confidentiality of patient information, informed consent, and business practice.

Because the patient is surrounded by her family, make sure she is comfortable discussing her care with everyone present. This should be done with subtlety and in such a way that does not offend her family. Confidentiality should be maintained even after the case. It would be inappropriate to discuss the "really cool case" you did on call last night while riding in the elevators.

Demonstrate sensitivity and responsiveness to patients' culture, age, gender, and disabilities.

As mentioned earlier, you must be sensitive to the patient's cultural background, including religious beliefs.

Interpersonal and communication skills

Residents must be able to demonstrate interpersonal and communication skills that result in effective information exchange and teaming with patients, their patients' families, and professional associates.

Create and sustain a therapeutic and ethically sound relationship with patients.

For anesthesiologists, this can be a particular challenge. I mean, would you want to put your life in the hands of someone you just met a few hours or sometimes minutes prior to surgery? Patients have to be extremely trusting in your abilities, and this can be facilitated by establishing a good relationship with the patient from the onset. Communicate effectively and in terms the patient understands. Be prepared to thoughtfully and knowledgeably answer all questions. In our case, it was particularly difficult as we had to gain the trust of the patient and her 10 eager family members!

Use effective listening skills and elicit and provide information using effective nonverbal, explanatory, questioning, and writing skills.

Again, listen thoughtfully to the patient's concerns and address them accordingly. Obtain a thorough, accurate history from the patient and her family, if she wishes them to be present. Sometimes the patient may not think to mention something "small," like the persistent expulsion of purulent phlegm balls she has been hacking up for the past week. A family member may pick up on this and chime in when you are eliciting your history.

Work effectively with others as a member or leader of a health care team or other professional group.

In our case, it was important to keep all lines of communication open between the nurses, the surgeons, the anesthesiologists, the patient, and her family, especially given the surgery delay, both in terms of being prepared at the appropriate time (patient in room, intubated, all lines placed) to minimize organ ischemic time and also to help ease the anxiety the delay generated with the patient.

Systems-based practice

Residents must demonstrate an awareness of and responsiveness to the larger context and system of health care and the ability to effectively call on system resources to provide care that is of optimal value.

Understand how their patient care and other professional practices affect other health care professionals, the health care organization, and the larger society and how these elements of the system affect their own practice.

Satisfactory graft function can be obtained after an ischemic time of 6–8 hours. Timing is crucial, as the less ischemic time, the better. Therefore communication between the harvesting team and the team in the operating room is extremely important. Once the lungs are determined to be transplantable, the OR team should be made aware and patient preparation begun. From the anesthesiology standpoint, the patient should be brought back into the OR and general anesthesia induced. All appropriate vascular access lines should be placed, in addition to the TEE. Every effort should be made to minimize the organ ischemic time.

References

1. Rubin LJ. Primary pulmonary hypertension. N Engl J Med 1997;336:111–117.

2. Heerdt PM, Triantafillou A. Perioperative management of patients receiving a lung transplant. Anesthesiology 1991;75:922–923.

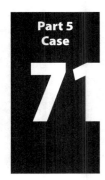

**Part 5
Case**

71

Contributions from Johns Hopkins Medical Institutions under Deborah A. Schwengel

Exit procedure – twins!

Gillian Newman and Eugenie Heitmiller

The case

A 44-year-old, gravida 4 para 0120 woman with gestational hypertension and a dichorionic, diamniotic twin pregnancy was referred to our center at 21 weeks' 5 days' gestation for congenital high airway obstruction syndrome (CHAOS) in Twin B; diagnosis was confirmed by ultrasound. After multidisciplinary consultation and discussion with the patient, all parties agreed that the ex utero intrapartum treatment (EXIT) procedure was the best option. Weekly sonograms confirmed that fetal hydrops did not develop. Fetal magnetic resonance imaging (MRI) was performed to better delineate Twin B's fetal anatomy.

Before delivery, a multidisciplinary planning session was held that included physician and nursing teams from maternal and fetal medicine, pediatric otolaryngology, neonatology, and anesthesiology (pediatric and obstetric). Two days before the procedure, the team conducted a walk-through in the operating room (OR).

The patient was admitted to the hospital at 36 weeks' gestation. Ultrasound showed a vertex position for the normal Twin A and a superior, anterior breech for the affected Twin B. The surgical plan thus included intraoperative sonogram and intra-abdominal/extrauterine version of Twin B to allow for the delivery of Twin A before the EXIT procedure was performed on Twin B.

Delivery was planned for 3 days after admission. Before the patient's arrival to the OR, a team briefing took place, during which all personnel identified themselves and their roles. The case plan was reviewed; equipment, drug supplies, and blood availability were verified. The patient was brought into the OR and placed in the supine, left uterine displacement position. Standard monitors and external fetal monitors were applied, and the patient was preoxygenated prior to a rapid sequence induction with 100 mg lidocaine, 200 mg propofol, and 120 mg succinylcholine and was easily intubated. A second, large-bore peripheral intravenous line and a radial arterial line were placed after induction. To facilitate uterine relaxation, deep inhalational anesthesia was established with desflurane. Vecuronium was used to maintain muscle relaxation. A nitroglycerin infusion was titrated to achieve additional uterine relaxation, while a phenylephrine infusion was titrated to maintain maternal blood pressure and uteroplacental perfusion. Twenty-six minutes after induction, anesthetic conditions were appropriate to allow the obstetricians to start the surgery.

A vertical skin incision was made and low uterine exposure was achieved. Intra-abdominal/extrauterine version of Twin B was successfully performed, and this position of Twin B was maintained by an obstetrician. Hysterotomy was made, preserving intact membranes. Fetal vertex presentation was reconfirmed with ultrasound, and membranes for Twin A were ruptured. Twin A was delivered without difficulty and was passed to the neonatal intensive care unit (NICU) team. She was intubated, weighed (2,500 g), and transported to the NICU. Apgar scores were 2, 4, and 6 at 1, 5, and 10 minutes, respectively. The neonate was extubated and breathing room air within hours of delivery.

Throughout delivery of Twin A, Twin B was monitored with a sterile ultrasound probe. After delivery of Twin A, Twin B's head was manually guided to the uterine incision by the obstetrician, and the fetus was situated for the EXIT procedure. Once positioned, membranes were ruptured, and the head, neck, and right upper extremity were exteriorized. Warmed normal saline was infused into the uterus to maintain uterine volume.

The pediatric anesthesia team administered a single injection of 5 mcg/kg fentanyl, 0.2 mg/kg atropine, and 1.5 mg/kg rocuronium into the right deltoid muscle of Twin B. A pulse oximetry probe was placed around the neonate's right hand; a single attempt at a peripheral IV was unsuccessful.

The otolaryngology team performed rigid bronchoscopy, followed by tracheostomy with release of clear fluid from the lungs. Twin B's airway was then suctioned, and a size 3.0 neonatal Shiley tracheostomy tube was secured. Ventilation of Twin B commenced via Ambu-bag with confirmation of bilateral breath sounds and end-tidal CO_2. Delivery was completed 20 minutes after delivery of Twin A.

Twin B was weighed (1,910 g) and then transported to the NICU; her Apgar scores were 2, 4, and 4 at 1, 5, and 10 minutes, respectively. During the EXIT procedure, fetal heart rate was 140–160 beats per minutes, and fetal O_2 saturation was 40% to 50%. The placenta did not separate from the uterus, and uterine contractions were not present. One hour after surgery start time, the EXIT procedure was complete, and both babies were stable in the NICU.

The mother remained stable throughout the EXIT procedure, and the desflurane, phenylephrine, and nitroglycerin were discontinued after delivery of Twin B. She was then given 5 mg of midazolam and begun on an oxytocin infusion. In total, 20 units of oxytocin were given. Over the course of the closure, the patient received 100 mg propofol, 1.2 mg hydromorphone, 4 mg ondansetron, and 3 mg/0.6 mg neostigimine/glycopyrrolate. After smooth emergence and extubation, the patient's PACU (postanesthesia care unit) course was uneventful. She was discharged to home on postoperative day 4.

Patient care

Residents must be able to provide patient care that is compassionate, appropriate, and effective for the treatment of health problems and the promotion of health.

Communicate effectively and demonstrate caring and respectful behaviors when interacting with patients and their families.

Obviously, this day was full of emotion for the patient and her family – the joy of childbirth coupled with the fear of losing a child. It was important to share in the happiness of the day, while addressing all the patient's and her family's concerns. Before proceeding to the operating room, all anesthesia providers met with the patient to discuss the plan as well as to provide support for this rare delivery.

Gather essential and accurate information about their patients.

For this case, we were providing care for three patients: the mother and her twins. It was imperative to know all the mother's medical history as well as the important history of the twins. This allowed us to prepare an in-depth anesthetic plan for the mother and her children.

Make informed decisions about diagnostic and therapeutic interventions based on patient information and preferences, up-to-date scientific evidence, and clinical judgment.

Since the EXIT procedure is a rarely performed procedure, the anesthetic team prepared in the days leading up to the surgery by reading articles, searching the literature, and discussing the case with experts in the field from our own institution as well as outside institutions. Having this information and experience allowed us to give the highest possible care to this patient.

Develop and carry out patient management plans.

An anesthetic plan was needed for the mother and her infants. Because this is a rare procedure with very few reported cases of EXIT procedures in twin gestation, it was even more important to have a detailed knowledge of both the surgical and anesthetic requirements for the case. This plan was worked out with nurses and physicians from multiple specialties; a rehearsal prior to the day of the procedure helped identify any problems with the management plan. All aspects of the procedure were carried out as planned and without incident.

Counsel and educate patients and their families.

The anesthesia, obstetric, and neonatology team members discussed the preoperative, intraoperative, and postoperative course with the patient and her family in a manner that they could easily understand; allowed for multiple opportunities to ask questions; and discussed options and possible outcomes without causing unnecessary alarm and distress.

Use information technology to support patient care decisions and patient education.

We used literature databases to find relevant articles and case reports detailing EXIT procedures to guide our anesthetic plan[1–3].

Perform competently all medical and invasive procedures considered essential for the area of practice.

Prior to induction, we secured one large-bore intravenous line, trying to minimize the stress and anxiety of the patient. Once in the operating room, it was important to quickly and effectively secure the airway of the patient to provide optimal care for her and the twins. Following airway management, we quickly established a second intravenous line as well as an arterial line. It was important in this case to perform these procedures competently and quickly to minimize anesthetic exposure to the twins.

Work with health care professionals, including those from other disciplines, to provide patient-focused care.

One of the most important points of this case was working in conjunction with maternal and fetal medicine, pediatric otolaryngology, neonatology, and anesthesiology (pediatric and obstetric) as well as operating room staff to provide the best care possible for this patient. Interdisciplinary meetings were held prior to the operative day. In addition, before induction, every member of the intraoperative team introduced themselves and specified their role in the day's events. The communication and teamwork of everyone involved was a key part of the successful management of this case.

Medical knowledge

Residents must demonstrate knowledge about established and evolving biomedical, clinical, and cognate (e.g., epidemiological and social-behavioral) sciences and the application of this knowledge to patient care.

Demonstrate an investigatory and analytic thinking approach to clinical situations.

This case required a detailed preoperative investigatory approach – while it was not necessary for the anesthesia team involved to determine the cause of Twin B's pathology, it was important for us to investigate the proper management of this case prior to entering the operating room. Fortunately, there were no intraoperative complications, but it is also important to be able to think analytically in the operating room. For instance, if the mother experienced an episode of hypoxia, it would be necessary to quickly formulate a differential diagnosis for the hypoxia, while simultaneously treating the patient.

Know and apply the basic and clinically supportive sciences that are appropriate to their discipline.

Anesthesiology is a field that bridges basic and clinical sciences very smoothly. In this case, it was important to understand the pharmacological mechanisms of all drugs administered, while knowing the clinical implications. For example, in this case, it was necessary to maintain uterine relaxation using nitroglycerin. However, nitroglycerin is a potent venous vasodilator, causing iatrogenic hypotension. To counteract this hypotension, phenylephrine, an alpha-1 agonist, was employed to maintain blood pressure. Thus a thorough understanding of pharmacology and physiology was necessary, but more important, it was essential to be able to apply these clinical sciences to the clinical case at hand.

Practice-based learning and improvement

Residents must be able to investigate and evaluate their patient care practices, appraise and assimilate scientific evidence, and improve their patient care practices.

Analyze practice experience and perform practice-based improvement activities using a systematic methodology.

Following this case, we held a debriefing, which allowed us to assess our management of this case. If a debriefing is held after each case, especially between the resident and the attending, this provides for a systematic way in which to improve practice-based activities.

Locate, appraise, and assimilate evidence from scientific studies related to their patients' health problems.

As previously discussed, a major part of this case was the preoperative preparation. We searched the literature not only for information to prepare for the EXIT procedure, but we also needed to prepare for management of Twin B intraoperatively. The entire team of anesthesiologists involved with the case read case reports prior to the operating room and discussed the case with each other beforehand.

> Use information technology to manage information, access online medical information, and support their own education.

Informatics is a rapidly expanding and important part of the daily practice of medicine. In this case, I used PubMed to search for relevant literature to teach myself the important points of an EXIT procedure. I also learned about Twin B's pathology, CHAOS syndrome, and the clinical implications of this disease. Being able to use online material both pre- and intraoperatively is an important skill to learn and definitely helped in the preparation for such a rare procedure as EXIT.

Professionalism

Residents must demonstrate a commitment to carrying out professional responsibilities, adherence to ethical principles, and sensitivity to a diverse patient population.

> Demonstrate respect, compassion, and integrity; a responsiveness to the needs of patients and society that supersedes self-interest; accountability to patients, society, and the profession; and a commitment to excellence and ongoing professional development.

In this case, a 44-year-old mother is giving birth to twins, one of which has a life-threatening disorder. This is the first and, most likely, last pregnancy for this mother. It was very important in this case to show respect to this patient and her family and to try to empathize with the situation. Imagine the possibility of one of the happiest days of this patient's life (childbirth) turning into one of the saddest (the loss of a child). It is always important to provide compassionate health care, and this case allowed me to realize how significant this compassion is for patients.

> Demonstrate a commitment to ethical principles pertaining to provision or withholding of clinical care, confidentiality of patient information, informed consent, and business practice.

For this case, the most applicable core competency value is the informed consent. It was important to hold

a detailed discussion with the patient about the implications of anesthesia for both her and her twins.

> Demonstrate sensitivity and responsiveness to patients' culture, age, gender, and disabilities.

Again, this patient was 44 years old and giving birth for the first time. It was very important to respect this patient's age, realizing that she may not have another opportunity for pregnancy.

Interpersonal and communication skills

Residents must be able to demonstrate interpersonal and communication skills that result in effective information exchange and teaming with patients, their patients' families, and professional associates.

> Create and sustain a therapeutic and ethically sound relationship with patients.

For me, one of the most important parts of being an effective physician is being able to communicate and empathize with patients. As an anesthesiologist, there is a very brief window of time in which to form a rapport with the patient for whom you will be caring. Thus it is important to develop good interpersonal and communication skills to facilitate a trusting relationship with patients.

> Use effective listening skills and elicit and provide information using effective nonverbal, explanatory, questioning, and writing skills.

In this case, this learning point came prior to the case itself. While discussing the anesthetic risks and benefits with the patient and her family, I listened to every concern and answered every family member in turn. I was not impatient and did not try to rush this interview. There are many days when, as an anesthesiologist, you feel rushed to get the patient to the operating room. However, it is more important to assuage patient and family concerns prior to starting a case, and if this requires a 5-minute delay to the operating room, then the delay is necessary.

> Work effectively with others as a member or leader of a health care team or other professional group.

The biggest piece of this case was working with other physicians and nurses to provide a health care team. In this EXIT procedure, we had to coordinate with obstetrics, neonatology, otolaryngology, obstetric and pediatric anesthesiology, and operating room support nurses and staff. This was a very large group, all coming together to provide outstanding care for mother and infants. The most satisfying aspect of this case was the way in which the group came together to provide this care.

Systems-based practice

Residents must demonstrate an awareness of and responsiveness to the larger context and system of health care and the ability to effectively call on system resources to provide care that is of optimal value.

> Understand how their patient care and other professional practices affect other health care professionals, the health care organization, and the larger society and how these elements of the system affect their own practice.

In this case, our anesthetic management affected the ability of the obstetricians to perform the EXIT procedure as well as the ability of the otolaryngologists to care for Twin B. Our ability to maintain uterine relaxation without compromising blood flow was essential for a successful surgery, not only for the patient, but also for her children.

> Practice cost-effective health care and resource allocation that does not compromise quality of care.

In anesthesiology, there are areas in which we can provide cost-effective health care. This includes selecting volatile anesthetics that are less expensive to produce (such as isoflurane over desflurane) and using generic medications, when possible, to cut down on costs (e.g., ondansetron instead of Zofran). Being aware of cost-effectiveness applies to almost every case.

> Know how to partner with health care managers and health care providers to assess, coordinate, and improve health care and know how these activities can affect system performance.

As previously discussed in detail, the way in which many health care providers came together to provide outstanding clinical care for this patient demonstrates how important it is to assess and coordinate the anesthetic plan with other providers prior to each and every case. Ongoing communication in the operating room is an essential part of anesthesia and was the key piece of this complicated and rare case.

References

1. Kiyoshi Y, Takeuchi M, Nakayama M, Suehara N. Congenital cervical rhabdomyosarcoma arising in one fetus of a twin pregnancy. Fetal Diagn Ther 2005;20:291–295.

2. Liechty KW, Crombleholme TM, Weiner S, et al. The ex utero intrapartum treatment procedure for a large fetal neck mass in a twin gestation. Obstet Gynecol 1999;93,:824–825.

3. Stevens GH, Schoot BC, Smets MJW, et al. The ex utero intrapartum treatment (EXIT) procedure in fetal neck masses: a case report and review of the literature. Eur J Obstet Gynecol Reprod Biol 2002;100:246–250.

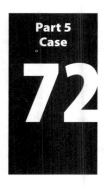

Contributions from Johns Hopkins Medical Institutions under Deborah A. Schwengel

OMG, that's the RV!

Christine L. Mai and Robert S. Greenberg

The case

A 44-year-old male with a history of pectus excavatum status post minimally invasive pectus excavatum repair and multiple chest reconstructions presented for removal of the pectus bar due to irritation and ongoing pain. The patient and his family were anxious in the preop holding area. He had been through multiple surgeries and wanted to relay to the surgeon and anyone who was listening the irritation in his chest from the pectus bar and wires.

After a smooth intravenous induction, a laryngeal mask airway (LMA) was placed with ease, and the surgeon was given the green light to remove the annoying pectus bar. Incision was made, and after 10 minutes of dissection, the surgery resident commented about a pulsatile mass that he was meticulously trying to avoid. Avoid, he did not! Gushing through the chest incision was dark, venous blood. OMG (Oh, my God), Houston, I think we hit a large venous structure!

Patient care

Residents must be able to provide patient care that is compassionate, appropriate, and effective for the treatment of health problems and the promotion of health.

Communicate effectively and demonstrate caring and respectful behaviors when interacting with patients and their families.

The patient and his family members had concerns and anxiety in the preoperative holding area and wanted to relay their worries to the anesthesiologist and the surgeon. You are communicating with an operating room frequent flier. It is best to spend the extra time listening to his concerns, addressing these issues, and being his advocate. Who knows, the trust you build with the patient and his family members may help you in the future.

Gather essential and accurate information about their patients.

Pectus excavatum, or funnel chest, is a congenital anomaly of the anterior chest wall. The excavatum defect is characterized by a depression of the lower sternum, with the deepest area at the junction of the chest and the abdomen. The defect can compress thoracic structures, causing restrictive pulmonary function, shortness of breath, or chest pain [1]. Preoperative evaluation of patients undergoing pectus excavatum repair or pectus bar removal includes a thorough history and physical exam, focusing on the extent of the chest wall compression on pulmonary and cardiovascular function. Previous surgical history in the chest might suggest scarring adhesions, and anesthetic history could indicate any difficulties with vascular access or airway difficulties. Lab studies include preoperative hemoglobin and a type and screen. Special studies could include a pulmonary function test, computed tomogram (CT) scan, body image survey, and exercise stress test to evaluate the extent of compression on the thoracic structures [2].

Develop and carry out patient management plans.

The gush of venous blood indicated that we had a catastrophe at hand and that we needed to step up to stay ahead of the game. Timing was crucial in this case. An emergency was declared, and a call for help brought in all the right players, including a cardiothoracic surgeon, a cardiac anesthesiologist, and additional anesthesia staff members, who were summoned to man their stations for an imminent large-fluid resuscitation. In an emergency situation, a team leader needs to effectively communicate and organize division of patient care.

A cardiothoracic surgeon miraculously walked through the operating room door within minutes, scrubbed in, and declared that the right ventricle (RV) had been lacerated. Continuous communication between the surgeons and the anesthesiology team was key. Once the surgeons were able to identify the source of bleeding and temporarily control hemostasis, the anesthesiology team dove underneath the sterile drapes to secure a definitive airway. The patient's airway was carefully exchanged from an LMA to an endotracheal tube under direct laryngoscopy. Ventilation was confirmed with bilateral breath sounds and end-tidal CO_2. Circulation (i.e., be ready to give blood – and lots of it) had to be managed expeditiously: two large-bore IVs were placed expectantly, and warm crystalloid was given rapidly through pressurized bags (a means to reduce the workload of hand squeezing). An arterial line was placed to monitor hemodynamic beat-to-beat variability, and a blood gas was sent stat to determine the starting hemoglobin and acid-base balance so as to permit allowable blood loss expectations. Two units of type and crossed blood were called for immediately. As the cardiothoracic surgeon worked on repairing the heart, continuous fluid management with balanced salt solution was given to stay ahead of the blood loss. A cardiac anesthesiologist performed an intraoperative transesophageal echo to assess for wall motion abnormalities, preload, and right ventricular and left ventricular function and to determine the extent of the damage to the heart. A heads-up was called to the central intensivist (ICU) to arrange for postoperative care.

Counsel and educate patients and their families.

Now, aren't you glad you had spent the extra time developing rapport with the patient and his family, discussing the risks and benefits of anesthesia?

Use information technology to support patient care decisions and patient education.

The patient's history profiles were in the medical records because he had been a frequent flier in the hospital. A review of electrocardiograms, echocardiograms, stress tests, CT scans, and pulmonary function tests could indicate the extent of his cardiovascular status and restrictive lung disease. During the emergency, the intraoperative transesophageal echocardiogram provided valuable information regarding the patient's cardiac function, ejection fraction, filling pressures, and potential violation to the myocardium. This information, in addition to the review of cardiac and pulmonary function tests, could provide an indication of the patient's exercise tolerance and how he would handle the insult.

Perform competently all medical and invasive procedures considered essential for the area of practice.

For a standard pectus bar removal, all procedures, including starting an IV, induction, securing an airway with an LMA (this usually works just fine) or endotracheal tube, maintaining the anesthetic, and waking up the patient, must be done according to standards of care. In the light of an emergency such as this case, additional invasive monitors, such as an arterial line, a possible central line, and a transesophageal echocardiogram, had to be performed expeditiously. Remember, this stuff had to be done under drapes, with the surgeons establishing control of the bleeding chest.

Provide health care services aimed at preventing health problems or maintaining health.

Because the risks of a pectus excavatum bar removal involved blood loss, and possible perforation to the chest wall cavity and organs, a type and screen for blood must be available prior to the surgery. We were happy this happened in the preop area. To prevent infection, antibiotics are given at least 30 minutes to an hour prior to incision. Had the procedure lasted longer, redosing would be required at regular intervals.

Work with health care professionals, including those from other disciplines, to provide patient-focused care.

This was a multidisciplinary effort to expeditiously manage the catastrophe. An emergency was declared, and the different services responded immediately, including the cardiothoracic surgeon, the cardiac anesthesiologists, the nursing staff, the critical care lab, the blood bank, and the intensive care unit. Key to such teamwork was a cool, focused, organized tone set in the OR when this happened. Everyone had his or her job and did it. Maintaining that steely-eyed control kept everyone on task. And it worked!

Medical knowledge

Residents must demonstrate knowledge about established and evolving biomedical, clinical, and cognate (e.g., epidemiological and social-behavioral) sciences and the application of this knowledge to patient care.

Demonstrate an investigatory and analytic thinking approach to clinical situations.

You must be able to acknowledge, respond to, and adapt to the change in pace of the situation. We went from a stable patient undergoing an elective procedure to remove a pectus bar in a controlled setting to a critical emergency with a massive bleed and a laceration to the heart. You must declare an emergency – yup, say it – and call for help. Not just for anyone, but rather, you must call for the right source of help – in this case, the cardiothoracic surgeon and the cardiac anesthesiologist. The perfusionist (in case we needed to go on bypass, if the rent was big enough) was next on our list.

And how was the patient during all this? Just fine. Sure there was blood coming out, but the crystalloid supported blood pressure, the heart rate stayed normal, and oxygenation remained fine.

Know and apply the basic and clinically supportive sciences that are appropriate to their discipline.

Anticipatory fluid resuscitation was key in this case. But what fluid should be given? Since the crystalloid was there, it went in first. There wasn't any particularly good reason to give colloid. There are plenty of debates as to what's best, crystalloid versus colloid, and how much to give [3]. Too little would reveal the tachycardia of hypovolemia, while too much could lead to dilutional anemia and may even lead to congestive heart failure (not ideal for a heart that was already damaged). Allowable blood loss (ABL) = estimated blood volume (EBV) × (hematocrit initial – hematocrit final)/hematocrit initial. Our calculated allowable blood loss was much more than what the patient lost; therefore blood product was not given. There wasn't any hemodynamic change that would prompt giving blood empirically – at least as a clinical test. Basically, we tried to balance doing good from doing harm. Keep the patient right where he is, and keep watching.

Practice-based learning and improvement

Residents must be able to investigate and evaluate their patient care practices, appraise and assimilate scientific evidence, and improve their patient care practices.

Analyze practice experience and perform practice-based improvement activities using a systematic methodology.

After all was said and done, it was time to think. What actually happened? Could we have predicted or prevented it? How did we think we responded? Was there something to learn? Sure enough, we surprised ourselves in how we looked in the mirror.

In retrospect, perhaps the history of multiple chest procedures might have suggested the risk of adhesions to the heart and lungs. The patient had undergone a minimally invasive pectus excavatum repair (Nuss procedure), which has late complications of pectus bar migration, resulting in thoracic pain. Perhaps we could have been more alert and prepared for a possible difficult extraction of the bar. But one thing was for certain: the organized approach in the OR that afternoon did the trick. Dividing and conquering of tasks made things happen superfast and efficiently.

Obtain and use information about their own population of patients and the larger population from which their patients are drawn.

Correction of pectus excavatum can be done via two approaches: the Ravitch approach and the minimally invasive surgical repair (Nuss procedure). The Ravitch procedure involves the placement of a steel bar behind the sternum after mobilizing the deformed cartilages around the sternum. The Nuss procedure involves the placement of a large, curved bar through small incisions on the chest wall. The bar is rotated into position using thoroscopy to guide bar placement [1,4]. A review of the literature shows that a laceration to the heart from removal of a pectus bar is very rare, with three cases of cardiac perforation reported in the literature. Fortunately, severe, life-threatening hemorrhages from perforation of the heart, lung, and diaphragm are very rare in the literature. Common early postoperative complications from pectus excavatum repair include pneumothorax, hemothorax, wound infections, seroma, rib fractures, and acute and chronic pain. Later complications include contour overcorrection, bar displacement, and bar migration [1,5].

Use information technology to manage information, access online medical information, and support their own education.

A search through PubMed and Ovid provided multiple resources and literature on minimally invasive pectus excavatum repair and its complications. Thank goodness for the Internet!

Professionalism

Residents must demonstrate a commitment to carrying out professional responsibilities, adherence to ethical principles, and sensitivity to a diverse patient population.

Demonstrate respect, compassion, and integrity; a responsiveness to the needs of patients and society that supersedes self-interest; accountability to patients, society, and the profession; and a commitment to excellence and ongoing professional development.

For frequent fliers to the operating room, it is important to demonstrate respect and compassion. They have spent much of their lives in the hospital and have experienced an array of bedside manners from doctors, nurses, and hospital staff. The patient knows best and can tell you what has worked for him in the past. Care and compassion in interactions with the family members also need to be addressed. The family has been with the patient for years during his struggle; they can also provide information that would help with caring for the patient.

Demonstrate a commitment to ethical principles pertaining to provision or withholding of clinical care, confidentiality of patient information, informed consent, and business practice.

When you are obtaining the history and physical and informed consent in the holding area, confirm the site of surgery and review the risks and benefits of anesthesia with the patient. Observe all HIPAA regulations (don't talk about the case in public venues such as the cafeteria or elevator and don't reveal any confidential patient information).

(*First author's note*: This must be the millionth time you were reminded to keep your yaps shut in the elevators. I hope everyone who reads this book realizes what a "HIPAA violation hotspot" the darned elevator is!)

Demonstrate sensitivity and responsiveness to patients' culture, age, gender, and disabilities.

The patient is a 44-year-old male with pectus excavatum repair and multiple chest reconstructions with scarring. You may have never seen a patient with pectus excavatum before, but please refrain from pointing out his chest deformity in public or talking about it in a disparaging way. Many patients come to the hospital with obvious or subtle medical conditions that might be striking to the eyes. Refrain from pointing, gawking, and making weird gestures. Act professionally and be respectful of the patient's age, gender, and disabilities.

Interpersonal and communication skills

Residents must be able to demonstrate interpersonal and communication skills that result in effective information exchange and teaming with patients, their patients' families, and professional associates.

Create and sustain a therapeutic and ethically sound relationship with patients.

During your preoperative visit with the patient, it is important to be professional, to build rapport, and to address the potential risks and benefits of the anesthetic management for this particular patient. When emergencies arise intraoperatively, family members will need to be informed of what has happened and what is being done to manage the crisis. Continuity of care continues into the postoperative period with a visit to the patient to follow up with the intensive care management. In this case, the patient was effectively resuscitated intraoperatively and maintained hemodynamic stability overnight in the ICU. He was extubated on postop day 1 in stable condition. A postoperative check on the patient demonstrates continuity of care and a true test of your interpersonal and communication skills in explaining the intraoperative complications and what had been done to manage the situation.

Use effective listening skills and elicit and provide information using effective nonverbal, explanatory, questioning, and writing skills.

As an anesthesiologist, effective listening skills are key because you have a limited amount of time in the holding area to take a focused history and physical, analyze the labs and special studies, and formulate an anesthetic plan. By listening to the patient and his family members' accounts of his previous anesthetic history, you can fast-track to a more tailored plan. Document that you have obtained informed consent and that the risks and benefits of anesthesia have been discussed. A signature is just a signature, but written documentation that the patient has been informed and agrees to proceed with the anesthetic plan demonstrates that both you and the patient are aware of the potential risks, should these risks arise.

Work effectively with others as a member or leader of a health care team or other professional group.

When an emergency arises in the operating room, effective communication with the surgeon and operating room staff is crucial. An emergency was declared, and a call for help brought in multidisciplinary services immediately, including the cardiothoracic surgeon, the cardiac anesthesiologists, the nursing staff, the critical care lab, the blood bank, and the intensive care unit. It is important to organize division of care. The general surgeon immediately realized that he had a problem, and a call to the cardiothoracic surgeon and cardiac anesthesiologist helped the surgeon in his efforts to locate and control the bleed and repair the heart. The anesthesia team rapidly mobilized to divide and conquer in securing the airway with an endotracheal tube, obtaining large-bore IV access for fluid resuscitation, and obtaining an arterial line to monitor hemodynamic variability. Through effective communication and expeditious mobilization of health care resources, the patient remained hemodynamically stable throughout the right ventricle repair. He received 6 L of crystalloid and did not require a blood transfusion, even though blood was available in the operating room. His family members were informed of the emergency and were reassured that the patient was hemodynamically stable. A call to the ICU was made, and the patient was transported to the ICU for postoperative recovery.

Systems-based practice

Residents must demonstrate an awareness of and responsiveness to the larger context and system of health care and the ability to effectively call on system resources to provide care that is of optimal value.

Understand how their patient care and other professional practices affect other health care professionals, the health care organization, and the larger society and how these elements of the system affect their own practice.

Effective communication, organized division of care, and strong team leadership were key elements in this case to expedite care during an emergency. Involving other experts early on for help, such as the cardiothoracic surgeon, cardiac anesthesiologist, blood bank, and intensive care unit, demonstrated rapid, efficient access of the hospital system.

Practice cost-effective health care and resource allocation that does not compromise quality of care.

Fluid resuscitation involved choosing between crystalloid, colloid, and blood products. We initially started with crystalloid because it was readily available and cheap. There was no real indication for colloid, so it was not given. The amount of blood loss, though brisk, was well below the calculated allowable blood loss, and the patient remained hemodynamically stable; therefore excessive blood transfusions were not utilized. An invasive monitor that made a difference in this case was the arterial line to monitor beat-to-beat variability and obtain blood gases. Two large-bore IVs were placed; hence a central line was not needed for access. Overall, the management of this case was very cost-efficient because excessive resources were not utilized.

Advocate for quality patient care and assist patients in dealing with system complexities.

In addition to the patient, the family members also need support and assistance in dealing with an intraoperative emergent complication:
- Tell the family members the facts and how you are handling the situation.
- Address family member questions.
- Allow time for family members to vent their emotions.

The nursing staff was very supportive and gave the family intermittent updates to reassure them that the patient had been resuscitated and would be recovering in the ICU. Building a good rapport with the family preoperatively helped with continuity of care postoperatively and assured the family that you were providing care not only to the patient, but also to the family as a whole.

Know how to partner with health care managers and health care providers to assess, coordinate, and improve health care and know how these activities can affect system performance.

An expeditious call for help not only to the anesthesia team, but also to the nursing staff, blood bank, and intensive care unit set the wheels in motion for backup help, blood availability, and bed space in the unit. Without the quick response of the health care managers and ancillary staff, the patient's resuscitation effort could have lasted longer, with more blood loss and hemodynamic instability. This was a team effort and a team victory!

References

1. Tahmassebi R, Ashrafian H, Salih C, Deshpande R, Athanasiou T, Dussek J. Intra-abdominal pectus bar migration – a rare clinical entity: case report. J Cardiothorac Surg 2008;3:39.

2. Kelly R, Shamberger R, Mellins R, et al. Prospective multicenter study of surgical correction of pectus excavatum: design, perioperative complications, pain, and baseline pulmonary function facilitated by Internet-based data collection. J Am Coll Surg 2007;205:205–216.

3. O'Malley C, Bennett-Guerrero E. Does the choice of fluid matter in major surgery? In: Evidence-based practice of anesthesiology. Fleisher L, editor. Saunders/Elsevier. Philadelphia; 2004: 136–144.

4. Nuss D. Minimally invasive surgical repair of pectus excavatum. Semin Pediatr Surg 2008;17:209–217.

5. Leonhardt J, Kubler J, Feiter J, Ure B, Petersen C. Complications of the minimally invasive repair of pectus excavatum. J Pediatr Surg 2005;40:E7–E9.

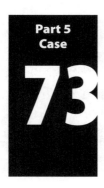

73 Aborted takeoff

Emmett Whitaker and Deborah A. Schwengel

Any landing you walk away from is a good one.
– anonymous pilot wisdom

The case

A 12-year-old white female with idiopathic scoliosis, but an 85° curve, comes to the operating room (OR) for anterior-posterior (AP) spinal fusion. She is obese, weighing 100 kg at 5 feet 1 inch, but was thought to be otherwise healthy. She had limited exercise ability due to back pain but was reportedly able to swim six laps without difficulty. She had donated three autologous units and came to the OR with a hematocrit of 34%. Her other preoperative laboratory values were normal. The electrocardiogram (ECG) showed inverted *T*-waves in leads III and AVF. Preoperative vital signs were as follows: blood pressure 138/74, P 118, R 20, and SaO_2 98% on room air. She reported being nil per os (NPO) since 10 o'clock the night before surgery.

The airway exam was consistent with a Mallampati I classification, the lungs were clear, and the heart sounds were normal. A peripheral IV was started and monitors were placed. Induction of anesthesia was achieved with midazolam 5 mg, fentanyl 250 mcg, lidocaine 40 mg, and propofol 100 mg, and after mask ventilation was assured, pancuronium 6 mg was given. Isoflurane of approximately 1% was administered while neuromuscular blockade was established. The patient was nasally intubated with a full, grade I view of the vocal cords. No end-tidal CO_2 was returned and ventilation was difficult, so the patient was extubated and reintubated with the same results. She was again extubated, the isoflurane was increased to 5%, an oral airway was placed, and the patient was successfully mask ventilated, but with difficulty. Compliance was definitely abnormal but gradually improved. Oxygen saturation fell during this episode but returned to 100% in approximately 2 minutes. She was subsequently reintubated, and both end-tidal CO_2 and bilateral breath sounds were confirmed and the chest was

observed to rise. Breath sounds were rhonchorous, with some indistinct wheezes heard primarily over the right lung field. The endotracheal tube was suctioned for a small amount of blood-tinged mucus. Ten puffs of albuterol were given, along with 200 mg Solu-Medrol IV. Oxygenation was maintained while on the ventilator, but the patient quickly desaturated when disconnected from the ventilator. Compliance was not normal, and peak inflating pressures of 38 were required to achieve a normal tidal volume. During this time, a left radial arterial catheter and right internal jugular central line were atraumatically placed. An arterial blood gas was obtained on 100% oxygen with the following results: pH 7.28, pCO$_2$ 57, paO$_2$ 179, and HCO$_3$ 26. Owing to the patient's respiratory problems on induction, high peak inflating pressures, and large A-a gradient, a chest X-ray was obtained. The radiograph showed a loop of colon in the right chest and a moderate component of atelectasis on the right and poor inflation of the chest overall. Aha! A diagnosis! How did we even get into the operating room with this patient?

The findings were made known to the surgeon, who was very upset that the anesthesiologists wanted to cancel his case; after all, the patient had donated three autologous blood units and a whole operating room day had been reserved for this AP fusion. It would take months to reschedule!

Patient care

Residents must be able to provide patient care that is compassionate, appropriate, and effective for the treatment of health problems and the promotion of health.

Communicate effectively and demonstrate caring and respectful behaviors when interacting with patients and their families.

Of course, there's no family in the room after induction, so it's easy to concentrate on saving the patient's life. There is no doubt, however, that caring and respectful behaviors will go a long way in informing this child and her parents of the complication and cancellation of the surgery. Full disclosure is an important part of maintaining trust in the patient-doctor relationship.

Gather essential and accurate information about their patients.

Identify and execute appropriate tests and consults. Verification of all findings, in particular, the radiological studies, is essential here. Put a few more Benjamins in your friendly neighborhood radiologist's pocket and get an official read. Consults and a chest CT are a good place to start, but consider other investigations as those don't necessarily constitute what you will need to adequately get the information you need.

And then, if you order a test, you must follow up to get the results. This patient had preoperative films with a radiologist's reading that said the patient had evidence of a foramen of Morgagni hernia! Presumably both the orthopedic surgery team and the anesthesiology team had reviewed the film reports before the day of the case, and no one from radiology called to alert the ordering physician of the presence of an unusual and unexpected finding.

Make informed decisions about diagnostic and therapeutic interventions based on patient information and preferences, up-to-date scientific evidence, and clinical judgment.

In the middle of the crisis, evaluate all components of the oxygen delivery system, the airway, and then the patient's lungs. There are many causes of perioperative hypoxia, and it's important for you to develop a differential diagnosis and then narrow it! Arriving at a (correct) diagnosis will help this patient's recovery.

Experience and judgment also help in the crisis and afterward when making decisions about when to cancel the case. Cancellation was not a difficult choice in this case because of unexpected and persistent wheezing, significant A-a gradient, and abnormal pulmonary compliance – all of this in the setting of a patient due to have an all-day surgical procedure for a severe scoliosis and a new diagnosis of diaphragmatic hernia!

Develop and carry out patient management plans.

Can you say think fast? Endotracheal intubation was easy, but esophageal tube placement is always a possibility. After the reintubation, the lack of end-tidal CO_2, poor compliance, and no chest rise, differential diagnosis included mechanical obstruction or bronchospasm. The circuit and endotracheal tube (ETT) were not the culprits. So how do you treat life-threatening bronchospasm in the operating room? Mask ventilation is a good place to start, but anticipate that reintubation will likely be necessary because a longer-acting neuromuscular blocker had been given and the hypoxemia and poor compliance might become difficult to manage by mask ventilation. In the meantime, turn up your agent as far as it will go, get on 100% oxygen if you aren't already, and administer a beta agonist and possibly steroids. If the bronchospasm does not abate with volatile anesthetics, consider giving magnesium sulfate or epinephrine. Always have in the back of your mind that you may need assistance.

Counsel and educate patients and their families.

It is hoped that you've discussed the potential risks of general anesthesia with this young girl and her patients. Education is important so that families have realistic expectations, and it's also important to protect you from a legal standpoint. Exercise compassion, patience, and humility when disclosing the event to this patient's parents! Be forthright and don't place blame on anyone. Everything that happened in this case was unexpected; further investigate the medical history for any suggestion of past breathing problems.

Use information technology to support patient care decisions and patient education.

Information technology is only useful if a person enters the history or data and if the next person reads what is there. If there is good transfer of information to supplement a history and physical examination, patient care decisions should be safer and more effective.

Perform competently all medical and invasive procedures considered essential for the area of practice.

Before anesthetizing a patient for this procedure, a careful anesthesiologist would establish adequate intravenous access (if appropriate for the child) and would be planning an arterial line, and possibly central venous access. In this case, the circumstances of the immediate postinduction period may preclude the routine placement of an arterial line. After stabilization, most would agree that an arterial line is compulsory and would consider central access for vasoactive drug administration. Don't forget sterile technique!

Provide health care services aimed at preventing health problems or maintaining health.

Stabilization is the key here. We're no longer worried about fixing this child's scoliosis; rather, we just aim to get back to where we started.

Work with health care professionals, including those from other disciplines, to provide patient-focused care.

In such a crisis, the Partridge Family approach is essential. You'll need help from other anesthesiologists, nursing staff, and potentially the surgeon, as well. Remember that the patient is the most important person in the room.

Medical knowledge

Residents must demonstrate knowledge about established and evolving biomedical, clinical, and cognate (e.g., epidemiological and social-behavioral) sciences and the application of this knowledge to patient care.

Demonstrate an investigatory and analytic thinking approach to clinical situations.

While hypoxia is a common problem in the operating room, in this case, it was sudden, severe, and coupled with failed ventilation, and the etiology was unknown. That being said, the child became hypoxemic and difficult to ventilate for a reason. As mentioned before, you need to put on your thinking cap and come up with a differential diagnosis, and fast! Think about what would cause hypoxemia and difficulty with ventilation in a child with no known lung disease. Always start with the basics – make sure you're on supplemental oxygen, ensure that there's not a mechanical problem with your anesthesia machine, and verify patency of airway. It can't hurt to listen to the chest, either. Once you have a thought about what is causing the problem (in this case, bronchospasm), start treatment.

On the issue of the diaphragmatic hernia, perhaps the resident reading the preoperative radiology report didn't know what a Morgagni hernia was? It is sometimes necessary to open a book, search the literature, or even search the Internet when you don't know a definition or diagnosis. That day, we simply Googled the word "Morgagni," and the second item returned was the following Wikipedia entry on congenital diaphragmatic hernia (CDH): "This rare anterior defect of the diaphragm is variably referred to as Morgagni's, retrosternal, or parasternal hernia. Accounting for approximately 2% of all CDH cases, it is characterized by herniation through the foramina of Morgagni which are located immediately adjacent to the xiphoid process of the sternum. The majority of hernias occur on the right side of the body and are generally asymptomatic; however newborns may present with respiratory distress at birth similar to Bochdalek hernia. Additionally, recurrent chest infections and gastrointestinal symptoms have been reported in those with previously undiagnosed Morgagni's hernia" [1].

Know and apply the basic and clinically supportive sciences that are appropriate to their discipline.

As an anesthesiologist, airway management and the physiology of oxygen-carbon dioxide exchange are your bag, baby! You need to be able to anticipate a difficult airway and know what to do when you don't expect a difficult airway but you find one nonetheless. Immediate postintubation hypoxemia happens, and you may only have seconds to correct it. Your automatic internal checklist in this situation should include the following:

1. Check your machine. Are you delivering oxygen at an appropriate partial pressure? Is the ventilator on? Is your circuit connected to the machine? Are you achieving appropriate tidal volumes? Are your airway pressures sky high or too low? Are you reading sustained end-tidal CO_2?
2. Check the patient. Is he or she blue or a nice shade of pink? Is the chest rising symmetrically? Are all connections between the ETT and the circuit intact? Is there a significant leak around the cuff of the ETT, and if so, is your cuff adequately inflated? Is the patient biting down on the tube?

3. Listen to the air bags. Do you have bilateral breath sounds? Does the patient sound ronchorus, crackly, or wheezy?

Practice-based learning and improvement

Residents must be able to investigate and evaluate their patient care practices, appraise and assimilate scientific evidence, and improve their patient care practices.

> Analyze practice experience and perform practice-based improvement activities using a systematic methodology.

From your vast experience, you know that prolonged hypoxemia can become full-blown cardiorespiratory arrest. You need to act fast. After the acute event has passed, regardless of the outcome, root cause analysis is indicated to evaluate how you can better respond to such an event in the future. Ask yourself, could we have anticipated this problem? Was our preoperative assessment appropriately diligent? Did we respond appropriately to the crisis? Did we ensure adequate aftercare once the patient was stabilized?

> Locate, appraise, and assimilate evidence from scientific studies related to their patients' health problems.

You don't have time to do this during the crisis, but after the patient is safely delivered to the postanesthesia care unit, you can reflect on the events and discuss them with the rest of the team. Debriefings are meant to lead to solutions to problems and learn how we might have handled the situation differently. Then, search the relevant literature.

Professionalism

Residents must demonstrate a commitment to carrying out professional responsibilities, adherence to ethical principles, and sensitivity to a diverse patient population.

> Demonstrate respect, compassion, and integrity; a responsiveness to the needs of patients and society that supersedes self-interest; accountability to patients, society, and the profession; and a commitment to excellence and ongoing professional development.

It is a given that patients always come first during a crisis and in the operating room. They also always deserve our full attention during preparation for a case and full vigilance during the case, whether simple or complex. We then have to be accountable for the time during which we are caring for the patient. When a complication occurs, it is our professional duty to fully disclose the event.

For patients, the distinctions between the terms errors, adverse events and unexpected complications are not important. Patients experience harm, and regardless of how members of the health care community and legal profession wish to classify it, patients who have suffered harm expect and deserve a timely, supportive and informative conversation about their concerns. [2, p. 1236]

Interpersonal and communication skills

Residents must be able to demonstrate interpersonal and communication skills that result in effective information exchange and teaming with patients, their patients' families, and professional associates.

> Create and sustain a therapeutic and ethically sound relationship with patients.

Listen, listen, listen, and disclose what happened. When an error or unexpected outcome occurs, identify it and take responsibility for the care of the patient. Even if it was only a minor problem, you must still give the patient and his or her family adequate time to ask questions. Each event is different, so your conversation and how you identify the causes of the problem will be unique to each situation. When serious events occur, it is natural to feel uncomfortable with the conversation. Take another team member with you so that the disclosure is complete and you have support. The Australian Commission on Safety and Quality in Health Care has published the following guidelines for managing an error [3]; these are further discussed in other publications [4]:

> **How to manage a medical error [3]**
>
> - Identify that an error has occurred.
> - Take responsibility for the error, apologize, and explain what happened to the patient and his or her support people.

- Explain how further similar errors will be prevented.
- Provide appropriate care.
- Adjust the response to the severity of the error: A clinician can handle minor incidents on his (or her) own, while a team should be involved in major incidents.
- Consider financial compensation.

Examples of words to use – initial discussion with patient

from: http://www.health.gov.au/internet/safetv/publishing.nsf/Cbntent/6B75B6A3EM3CH)FD\2571D50001E19D/$Rle/hlth careprofhbk.pdf

- These are examples of phrases that may assist in the disclosure process. However, they should be used as a guide only and not be read out verbatim.
- Area of discussion examples

1. Expression of regret
   - "I am very sorry this has happened."
   - "I realize it has caused great pain/distress/anxiety/worry."

2. Known clinical facts
   - "We have been able to determine that…"
   - "Unfortunately…has happened."
   - "We are not sure exactly what happened at present; however, we will be investigating the matter further and will give you more information as it becomes available."

3. Patient questions/concerns
   - "How do you feel about this?"
   - "Do you have any questions about what we have discussed?"
   - "What do you think might have happened?"
   - "You must be feeling pretty disappointed/angry/upset/distressed about this."
   - "I think I would feel the same way too."

4. Discussion of ongoing care
   - "I have reviewed what has occurred and this is what I think we need to do next."
   - "I'll be with you every step of the way as we get through this and here is what I think we need to do now."

5. Any side effects to look out for
   - "You may at some later time experience.…In this event you should.…"

Work effectively with others as a member or leader of a health care team or other professional group.

Discuss with the surgeons the need to cancel and then arrange for consultations after the patient is awake and delivered to the postanesthesia care unit (PACU).

Systems-based practice

Residents must demonstrate an awareness of and responsiveness to the larger context and system of health care and the ability to effectively call on system resources to provide care that is of optimal value.

Understand how their patient care and other professional practices affect other health care professionals, the health care organization, and the larger society and how these elements of the system affect their own practice.

A systems defect occurred that resulted in scheduling this patient for major spine surgery without acknowledging the findings of a foramen of Morgagni hernia with bowel in the chest. The preparations for the spinal fusion, including autologous blood donation, should not have occurred. The radiologist and surgeon should have known about the Morgagni hernia weeks before the scheduled surgery, and the anesthesia team should have learned of it the day before.

Practice cost-effective health care and resource allocation that does not compromise quality of care.

It was not cost-effective to cancel this case, but it was not safe to proceed. The best options in this case, after cancellation, included the following:

- workup of the reactive airway disease
- design of a treatment plan to optimize lung function
- meticulous planning for the surgery to correct the diaphragmatic hernia

References

1. http://en.wikipedia.org/wiki/Congenital_diaphragmatic_hernia

2. Flemons WW, Davies JM, MacLeod B. Disclosing medical errors. CMAJ 2007;177:1236.

3. Australian Commission on Safety and Quality in Health Care. Open disclosure: health care professional's handbook. Canberra: Commonwealth of Australia; 2003. Available from: http://www.safetyandquality.org/internet/safety/publishing.nsf/Content/6B75B6A3eA43Ce0FCA2571D50001e19D/$File/hlthcareprofhbk.pdf.

4. Calvert JF, Hollander-Rodriguez J, Atlas M. What are the repercussions of disclosing a medical error? Available from: http://www.jfponline.com/Pages.asp?AID=5919.

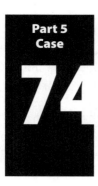

Contributions from Johns Hopkins Medical Institutions under Deborah A. Schwengel

Revenge of the blue crab cake

Samuel M. Galvagno Jr. and Theresa L. Hartsell

The case

A 26-year-old moderately obese woman presented to the emergency department (ED) with progressive abdominal pain and nausea. She was found to have tenderness over a preexisting 4-cm-diameter umbilical hernia and was posted to the operating room (OR) for an exploratory laparotomy and repair of likely incarcerated hernia. She denied any medical problems or allergies.

Despite the curious aroma of Old Bay seasoning, the patient vehemently denied having had anything to eat or drink for 2 days! "Couldn't even get out of bed! I promise!" she said. Hmmm…Her sister and several friends who had accompanied her to the ED exchanged a few anxious glances before agreeing – nothing to eat or drink within the past 48 hours.

In the OR, she underwent a standard intravenous induction, followed by easy mask ventilation. Then the inevitable occurred. Before the trachea was intubated, the patient vomited copious amounts of undigested food. What a mess! Trying hard not to swear under your breath, you manage to place an endotracheal tube after aggressively suctioning and manually clearing her oropharynx. Hoping that the worst of it is over, you patiently wait for the beep of the pulse oximeter to return to normal. Unfortunately, her SpO_2 remains in the 85% to 90% range, despite now being on 100% oxygen and increased positive end-expiratory pressure (PEEP). You call for a bronchoscope and take a look; you see large amounts of particulate matter, clearly recognizable as…*crab cake*?

In the meantime, the surgeon has already proceeded with incision. You tell her to make quick work of things, and in a stroke of good luck, the patient's bowel is found to be normal. The incision is closed and you bring her to the intensive care unit for further care. In the waiting room, the patient's sister and her friends reveal that, never one to miss the excitement, your patient had insisted on stopping for crab cakes and beer in Baltimore's Inner Harbor before heading to the emergency room.

Patient care

Residents must be able to provide patient care that is compassionate, appropriate, and effective for the treatment of health problems and the promotion of health.

Communicate effectively and demonstrate caring and respectful behaviors when interacting with patients and their families.

Hmmm. Sounds like a seemingly healthy patient, but the real question, is she really nil per os (NPO)? You know the American Society of Anesthesiology (ASA) guidelines for perioperative fasting specifically state that a patient may have a *light* meal 6 hours before general anesthesia, but by *light*, they mean *light*. Not one Big Mac instead of two Big Macs. Toast, crackers, and clear liquids are probably fine, but anything else may prolong gastric emptying time and increase gastric volume. Deep-fried boardwalk-style crab cakes, smothered with tartar sauce and Old Bay seasoning, don't qualify. It's up to you to rapidly gain the trust of both the patient and her family in an effort to obtain the correct information required to keep her safe.

Gather essential and accurate information about their patients.

Did she or did she *not* eat? You want the truth, and you can handle the truth! A discussion about the consequences of not being NPO, done in a professional and nonthreatening manner, is called for here. You can't place an endoscope to prove that she's lying; good old-fashioned history-taking skills are what it takes to get the job done.

Make informed decisions about diagnostic and therapeutic interventions based on patient information and preferences, up-to-date scientific evidence, and clinical judgment.

Obviously, confirmation of a full stomach drastically changes your plans. The standard of care for such cases is a rapid sequence induction (RSI) and intubation. That, or an informed discussion with the surgeon about the risks involved with proceeding emergently to the OR versus waiting for a few hours. Of course, you could certainly argue that with an incarcerated hernia (heck, maybe she even has a bowel obstruction!), you would assume high aspiration risk *regardless* of her NPO time and proceed with a rapid sequence induction anyway. Unfortunately, there's no solid evidence to guide you here, just a fair bit of "standard of care" stemming from physiologic reasoning.

Ultimately, it comes down to your clinical judgment. What does your "Spidey sense" tell you about her aspiration risk? Are you able to effectively treat the consequences if you're incorrect? You'll obviously need to take her airway and pulmonary status into consideration, as you might just realize that a rapid sequence induction has minimal risk and may, potentially, have quite a bit of benefit.

Develop and carry out patient management plans.

Have her chug some Bicitra (sodium citrate) and consider administering an H2-blocker before going back to the OR. Metoclopramide, in the face of a potential bowel obstruction, is relatively contraindicated. Once in the OR, execute an RSI with cricoid pressure (keeping the pressure in place until tube placement is confirmed). Keep in mind, though, that cricoid pressure is meant to protect against passive reflux of stomach contents. If she does experience an active emetic event, you're best off with a plan that includes tipping the table into Trendelenburg (to let gravity move gastric contents up and away from the glottic opening) and a very large bore suction device!

Counsel and educate patients and their families.

The damage is done. The patient has aspirated and has landed herself a bed in the intensive care unit (ICU) with a stormy postoperative course lying ahead. Are you going to stomp out into the waiting room, red-faced and irate, letting her family members know that it is "their fault that this happened" because they lied

to you? That won't help matters. What is done is done. Better to use this as an opportunity to explain to the family why accurate information about her NPO status might have been important. Explain how you and your ICU team are now going to do everything possible to take care of this patient's aspiration pneumonitis, and let them know what to expect in the hours and possibly days to come. Managing the complications of anesthesia is part of the job, and this includes communication with the patient and her family and friends.

Use information technology to support patient care decisions and patient education.

There isn't much here that would have helped you in your decision making. You had all the objective information that you needed while doing your assessment in the ED. Should a nasogastric tube have been placed beforehand? Should she have had an upper endoscopy? It's easy to play the Monday morning quarterback in cases like this, but the bottom line is that no amount of preexisting information other than a more detailed history would have been likely to help you in this case. Nevertheless, we are always obligated to learn as much as we can about our patients, so the responsibility of going over previous charts, studies, labs, and electronic records with a fine-toothed comb falls squarely on your shoulders.

However, with increasing information available to patients via the Internet and other health portals, we as anesthesiologists can work to educate the public as much as possible on issues important to our care. Making sure that we, as a group, take advantage of such media as well as making sure that misinformation is not propagated will be part of our job, now and in the future. This can carry over into resources that we use in our own clinical setting. For example, perhaps a pamphlet in the preop area or emergency room about fasting guidelines and aspiration risk would have been an additional way to inform your patient about risks? She might have been more receptive to your questions. Many hospitals are starting to use television or computer screens in strategic places to give patients and visitors key pieces of information – this, too, could be harnessed to help inform your patients.

Perform competently all medical and invasive procedures considered essential for the area of practice.

417

After ensuring adequate intravenous access and appropriate preoperative medication, you preoxygenate the patient with 100% oxygen. In a moderately obese female, her functional residual capacity is already decreased, and with her underlying pathophysiology of a potential bowel obstruction, general anesthesia, and the supine position, she might be near her closing capacity. But all physiologic babble notwithstanding, her lack of pulmonary reserve will be self-evident as you hear the steadily descending tones (blip-blip-blip) of the oxygen saturation monitor should you try to intubate her without preoxygenating first. Cricoid pressure, despite the possibility that you might obscure your laryngoscopic view, is still regarded as a standard of care. Hold it until the tube is in. You can choose any drug you want for induction – as long as you know how to use it. Propofol or thiopental are usual first choices. Adding a bit of fentanyl might help blunt the hemodynamic changes associated with your laryngoscopy. In terms of paralytics, succinylcholine is still the fastest, so push it and wait at least a full 30 seconds before proceeding with direct laryngoscopy. Performing the rapid sequence induction and intubation is just one procedure you'll be doing tonight. Being facile with bronchoscopy to evaluate and clear the airways, particularly with her clinical status pushing you to be both fast and accurate, will be important here. You'll also probably want to place an arterial line, both for measurement of arterial blood gases now and in the ICU and to keep an eye on her blood pressure, which may be fine now but may not stay that way for long!

Provide health care services aimed at preventing health problems or maintaining health.

There's not much you'll be able to do at this point about preventing health problems. Sticking to the established guidelines for perioperative antibiotics, perioperative fasting, and standard anesthetic techniques will certainly go a long way toward maintaining this patient's health.

Work with health care professionals, including those from other disciplines, to provide patient-focused care.

An RSI and intubation truly require a team approach. You will be intubating and pushing drugs. Get the surgeons and nurses in the OR involved. Show them how to correctly perform cricoid pressure and have them do it. If you need to push the drugs, have the surgeon, nurse, or surgical resident hold the mask over the patient's face (but make sure they do not bag the patient; there is no need to insufflate the stomach while doing an RSI). Once the patient has aspirated, inclusion of the other team members becomes even more important. You will not have enough hands to simultaneously intubate, suction, bronch, reposition, and do whatever else it takes to keep the patient alive. Directing the other team members helps them feel involved and allows you to maintain control of a bad situation.

Medical knowledge

Residents must demonstrate knowledge about established and evolving biomedical, clinical, and cognate (e.g., epidemiological and social-behavioral) sciences and the application of this knowledge to patient care.

Demonstrate an investigatory and analytic thinking approach to clinical situations.

There's not much to investigate during a critical crisis such as obvious aspiration, and the analytic thinking approach should have happened long before you encountered a situation like this in the OR. Being prepared beforehand by thinking and talking through problems like this is the way to go. In aviation parlance, pilots "chair fly" the next day's flight to make sure they get everything right. Get into a habit of "chair flying" your cases for the next day as well as other emergency cases that you might have read about but have not yet encountered. Critical action procedures that should already have been learned and memorized for this case are as follows:

- 100% oxygen
- head down at least 30°, allowing gastric content to drain
- apply cricoid pressure
- suction the oropharynx
- intubate the trachea
- suction through the ET tube quickly
- maintain 100% oxygen
- provide PEEP
- apply in-line bronchodilators, as needed
- place an orogastric tube
- continue positive pressure ventilation

Know and apply the basic and clinically supportive sciences that are appropriate to their discipline.

Aspiration of gastric contents into the lung, as described in Mendelson's classic 1946 paper, is associated with much badness [1]. Respiratory distress is imminent, followed by bronchospasm, hypoxemia, and severe dyspnea. The critical pH for aspiration of gastric contents has been described as 2.5, the level at which the bronchioles become severely reactive to hydrochloric acid and clamp spasm in response. A paltry 25 mL of gastric contents with low pH, when injected into the lungs, is all it takes to cause massive pulmonary damage – aspiration pneumonitis [2].

But what about prophylactic antibiotics? How about steroids? They prevent inflammation, and a pneumonitis is, by definition, an inflammatory process, right? Aspiration *pneumonitis* is *not* the same as aspiration *pneumonia*. Once a secondary infection is established, antibiotics might be acceptable, but they should not be otherwise administered routinely, especially not so early in the course. The same goes for steroids. While it might intuitively make sense, steroids are not recommended [3–5]. We're not making this up. All of this has been rigorously studied!

Now that the event has happened and the patient is in the throes of hypoxia, knowledge of pulmonary physiology and the evidence surrounding treatment of severe hypoxia are key. Although she may not yet meet the full criteria for adult respiratory distress syndrome, you may decide to use some of the information we have about therapy and outcomes in that syndrome to guide your management prophylactically. This is where some knowledge of how your ventilator works, knowledge of the risks associated with barotrauma and volutrauma, and a working familiarity of some of the ARDSNet studies would be helpful.

Practice-based learning and improvement

Residents must be able to investigate and evaluate their patient care practices, appraise and assimilate scientific evidence, and improve their patient care practices.

Analyze practice experience and perform practice-based improvement activities using a systematic methodology.

As with most cases in this book, this case should be presented at a multidisciplinary morbidity and mortality (M&M) conference. Furthermore, cases like this should be exactly what we practice in the simulator or in other simulated environments.

After the dust has settled and as the patient is cooling off in the ICU, you should gather the team members involved and have a debriefing. An analysis of what went right and what could have been done better may singularly be one of the most productive learning opportunities during your residency.

Locate, appraise, and assimilate evidence from scientific studies related to their patients' health problems.

You already know the pathophysiology of aspiration pneumonitis after having read the major anesthesia texts and all the other review articles on the subject (Paul Marik's 2001 review article in the *New England Journal of Medicine* is particularly good [2]). Now it is your responsibility to integrate the clinical evidence into your practice. Sometimes after reading the literature, you might end up with more questions than answers:

- Does an H2-blocker help decrease acidic gastric contents?
- Are you absolutely sure I shouldn't give antibiotics right away?
- How about "neutralizing" the acidic contents by injecting some bicarb during the bronch?
- Why shouldn't I try to wash out some of the acid with saline?

Patients with aspiration pneumonitis will be incredibly ill, and you will find yourself wanting to do more for them to get them better. The bottom line with aspiration pneumonitis is that supportive care is the only way to go. The H2-blocker that you gave in the preop area won't do much during this short case but may help lower gastric pH down the line. You have to remember that pneumonitis is not the same animal as pneumonia [2]. Supportive ICU care, including mechanical ventilation and PEEP, are the cornerstones [6,7]. Irrigating the bronchial tree with saline is not indicated, nor is the instillation of bicarbonate, even though both therapies might intuitively make sense. Adding funky ventilator modes *may* be indicated, however, as part of your supportive strategy. The patient in this case eventually required high-frequency oscillatory ventilation for a day after becoming more hypoxemic on an ARDSNet protocol. It did the trick; she was extubated 3 days after the event and had an excellent recovery.

Obtain and use information about their own population of patients and the larger population from which their patients are drawn.

The risk factors for aspiration pneumonitis include extremes of age, neurologic dysphagia, disorders of the gastroesophageal junction, general anesthesia, and other anatomic abnormalities. Drug overdoses are another likely cause, and knowing your patient population may help you identify and act on these risk factors. In this case, there was little you could do for this seemingly healthy (yet deceitful) patient.

Apply knowledge of study designs and statistical methods to the appraisal of clinical studies and other information on diagnostic and therapeutic effectiveness.

Getting back to the steroid and antibiotic issue, you'll run across this again. The surgeon will be shouting across the curtain with instructions for you to start steroids, antibiotics, and other agents that you know will simply not work. This is where knowing the literature comes into play. Politely, but firmly, tell the surgeon to "read 'em and weep." In the world of anesthesiology, 1974 was a big year for publications on the effect of steroids for aspiration pneumonitis. Two large studies, one by Downs and colleagues and one by Dudley and colleagues, showed that they don't really work [3,4]. Experiments done in the lab by Lowrey a few years later confirmed this [5]. Several other studies have since shown that the issue is, at best, still controversial. Supportive care is fairly well backed up by the literature, and knowing this not only helps you provide better care for your patient, but also establishes you as a subject area expert – as you should be.

Use information technology to manage information, access online medical information, and support their own education.

Although a simple Google search is frowned on in most academic circles, you'll find Marik's paper among your first hits if you do so. PubMed, Ovid, STAT!Ref, and many other online resources are only a point and a click away. The days of trying to get away with the excuse of being "computer illiterate" have long passed. Managing the vast amount of clinical information available is just one of the many challenges for our generation of anesthesiologists.

Professionalism

Residents must demonstrate a commitment to carrying out professional responsibilities, adherence to ethical principles, and sensitivity to a diverse patient population.

Demonstrate respect, compassion, and integrity; a responsiveness to the needs of patients and society that supersedes self-interest; accountability to patients, society, and the profession; and a commitment to excellence and ongoing professional development.

"Liars!" Chastising the patient, her friends, and her sister is not the right move. Use the situation as an opportunity to let them know about the importance of providing an accurate medical history. Should any of them be faced with a similar problem again, it is likely that the problem can be avoided. Keep in mind that, regardless of what they did or didn't do that impacted the case, they now have a loved one who is critically ill and are in need of support and nonjudgmental explanation to help navigate this crisis.

"Well, it's not my fault. The surgeons insisted that this was an emergency case." Likewise, pointing fingers at the surgeons will get you nowhere. Part of your job will *always* include building relationships with other medical professionals. Again, a debriefing provides a great opportunity for everyone to vent, and by organizing this and leading the discussion, you will also be establishing yourself as a leader and expert in perioperative medicine.

Demonstrate a commitment to ethical principles pertaining to provision or withholding of clinical care, confidentiality of patient information, informed consent, and business practice.

Still miffed and steaming after the case, while in the elevator with a colleague, you say, "Can you believe that they lied to me? Oh well, she's in the ICU now, sick as a dog. Guess she got what she deserved." Sure, you'll be very angry having exposed a patient to unnecessary risk in the context of having received misinformation, but HIPAA violations and privacy are taken very seriously nowadays. No matter how tempted you might be, save it for the debriefing or for M&M. Even if you're retelling the story for an educational purpose, just to help the listener learn from your mistake, the elevator and the lunchroom are not the appropriate places for this conversation.

Thinking back to the concept of informed consent, you wonder whether you could have used this as a communication tool when your gut instinct told you your patient may not be sharing all the pertinent information. Perhaps your taking a moment from your usual consent spiel and discussing the risks of aspiration in patients with food in their stomach would have made the difference in this case. Perhaps not. But it makes sense to be sure to include this as a risk when you consent your next patient!

Demonstrate sensitivity and responsiveness to patients' culture, age, gender, and disabilities.

In this situation, there's not much more to this than common sense. You don't know what was underlying her decision not to be truthful with you, or her decision to stop by the crab shack on the way to the emergency room in the first place. However, this is not the opportunity to let any inner bias show, particularly when her friends and family come clean and give you their reasons for the impromptu dinner party and for not letting you know about it at the appropriate time.

Interpersonal and communication skills

Residents must be able to demonstrate interpersonal and communication skills that result in effective information exchange and teaming with patients, their patients' families, and professional associates.

Create and sustain a therapeutic and ethically sound relationship with patients.

If you figure that an ounce of prevention is worth a pound of cure, then getting this patient to be honest with you up front about her NPO status and other potential issues would be one of the key moments of the night. How often do we rush through preoperative evaluations in a very doctor-centered manner, aiming to get all the vital pieces of information we need, while being so goal oriented that we forget to notice the patient on the other side of the conversation? Of course, we don't act that way all the time, but sometimes the pressure to get a case started, or

that argument with your significant other earlier today, carries over to the patient. Often we have just a few moments to gain our patients' trust so that they'll be open and honest – no small feat, given that many may assume we'll be judgmental about certain areas. Of course, communication isn't just about verbal language – learning to read a patient's expressions and body language can be very helpful in deciding what areas may need some more gentle probing to get the information you need to form a safe anesthetic plan.

What about once the case is over? The damage done? Of course, once you've turned the patient's care over to your colleagues in the ICU, you'll need a moment to collect your thoughts and rest. But remember, the patient is still sick from what happened! You've spoken to the family extensively after the case, using your best nonconfrontational and supportive language, but your responsibility doesn't end there. You were still the patient's physician in the OR. Stay on the case. Get updates from the ICU team and continue to communicate with the family. As the patient recovers, she may want to know what happened to her. There is no better person to give her that information than someone like you, with the front seat view.

Use effective listening skills and elicit and provide information using effective nonverbal, explanatory, questioning, and writing skills.

This is what it's all about in this case – how to listen effectively and use all our skills to deliver information to our patient and her family and friends in a way in which they can understand and become willing partners in the health care process. Your communication with the patient beforehand needs to convey through both verbal and nonverbal techniques that her well-being is your first concern and that you will treat all the information she gives you in a nonjudgmental and professional manner. Depending on her level of understanding, careful explanation of risks specifically tuned to her vocabulary is needed. Afterward, the same is true as you explain the circumstances to her family and friends. Perhaps a diagram of the aerodigestive tract is called for here to explain the pathophysiology of aspiration to the family. Certainly give a careful and sensitive explanation of what they can expect when they walk into the ICU and see her for the first time!

Finally, keeping in mind that this patient is extremely ill and will have multiple caregivers as well as multiple people reviewing her chart, possibly for legal reasons, carefully worded documentation of your discussions with her, what happened in the OR, and what you did in response will be exceedingly important. An additional note in the chart, as opposed to just on your anesthesia data record, may be helpful for both the ICU team and for the primary surgical team. In today's world of postgraduate medical education and duty hour restrictions, it is rare that one group of individuals can maintain a continuous stream of information about patients without a legible written record. Provide the future teams of residents, interns, and attending with an accurate written description of what happened.

Work effectively with others as a member or leader of a health care team or other professional group.

As discussed earlier, there are ample opportunities in a case like this to distinguish yourself as a leader and a concerned, conscientious physician. First of all, as in most intraoperative crises, your role in leading the team to stabilize and treat the patient is crucial. This is why they train us in "crisis *resource* management" – sometimes how you communicate with and enlist others for help is as important, if not more so, than the patient care you deliver yourself. Here the specifics of how you communicate with the surgical team and the other anesthesia providers who come to your aid will go a long way toward effectively treating the patient as well as avoiding the finger-pointing that sometimes occurs later on. You'll keep your cool and demonstrate authority with a sense of urgency, but also of control, making sure the surgeons know what you need from them (waiting before proceeding, stopping as soon as they are safely able) and assigning roles to others who arrive to help.

Systems-based practice

Residents must demonstrate an awareness of and responsiveness to the larger context and system of health care and the ability to effectively call on system resources to provide care that is of optimal value.

Understand how their patient care and other professional practices affect other health care professionals, the health care organization, and the larger society and how these elements of the system affect their own practice.

As anesthesiologists continue to gain the respect and trust they deserve from the medical community, it is important to remember that our job continues well beyond the confines of the operating room. Establishing protocols (for fasting in this case), training programs (simulation exercises, knowledge of critical action procedures), follow-up care (making sure postoperative checks get done), and means for effective communication are skills that are now within the realm of anesthesiologists as perioperative medical specialists.

In this case, your understanding of the system can be very helpful in coordinating the best care for your patient. Knowing what level of care can be provided in the recovery room versus the intensive care unit, and realizing that her care needs (critical care bed, specialty ventilator equipment, and increased levels of nursing support) may take some time to set up, will allow you to address her postoperative needs even before the surgery is complete and provide for as seamless a transition of care as possible. Efficiently obtaining needed resources is an important part of your role, in addition to your hands-on patient care. Knowing who to call, and what issues may exist regarding scarce resources (ICU beds, ventilators, etc.), allows you to advocate for your patient from a systems standpoint. This is crucial for this situation, in which you have a single, critically ill patient, but will become all the more important as we begin to consider needs for resource management during disasters or epidemics.

Practice cost-effective health care and resource allocation that does not compromise quality of care.

This is linked to the evidence for providing the proper supportive care for a patient with aspiration pneumonitis. Starting antibiotics, steroids, or other non-evidence-based therapies just so you or the surgeons will "feel better" does not help the patient and, in aggregate, may impose considerable cost to the health care system as a whole. Individual therapies, such as the high-frequency oscillator or inhaled nitric oxide, are expensive in their own right, and so taking into consideration the realities of whether they will help your patient is important before making treatment decisions.

Advocate for quality patient care and assist patients in dealing with system complexities.

As described earlier, your job does not start and stop at the doors to the OR. A case like this demonstrates multiple opportunities for you to stay involved, while helping your patient and her family through a critical event. Even small things like showing your patient's sister to the ICU waiting room or walking her in to introduce her to the nurse and helping explain some of what is going on will help cement your role as a patient and family advocate.

Know how to partner with health care managers and health care providers to assess, coordinate, and improve health care and know how these activities can affect system performance.

First of all, once you've had a chance to rest briefly, grab a drink, and let your own heart rate come back down to normal, you need to have a quick debriefing session with others involved in the incident. We know that moments of terror are part of the anesthesiology workday, but it's important to make sure that while everyone's memory is still fresh, you allow folks to reflect on their performance, give positive and constructive feedback, and discuss if there was anything that could have been done better. In particular, discuss whether there were any equipment or system issues that need to be improved or fixed. Were you able to get the bronchoscope in a timely fashion? Was everything in working order? Did you know who to call to get that emergency ICU bed? Were the surgeons responsive to your patient care needs, and did they give you the time and support to stabilize the patient before proceeding? Don't forget, also, to ask whether there is anyone who is so upset by the circumstances that he or she may need some extra support?

Later on, look-backs in the form of morbidity and mortality conferences, departmental "difficult case" files, simulator curricula, or problem-based learning sessions are some of the opportunities that you, as a leader in the field of perioperative medicine, can support or institute in an effort to improve quality and safety in your department. Cases like this one, in which there are clear teaching points – both in up-front decision making and in crisis management – are some of the best examples to use in these conferences. Take advantage of multidisciplinary opportunities, as well: don't be surprised if 1 year later, you are called back by an OR nurse manager to give a lecture on fasting guidelines or aspiration pneumonitis. Alternatively, some of the best learning that takes place during residency comes from resident-to-resident teaching. A conversation about the case, preferably in a confidential setting (and not over lunch!), may prove to be invaluable for your colleagues in their own future care.

References

1. Mendelson CL. The aspiration of stomach contents into the lungs during obstetric anesthesia. Am J Obstet Gynecol 1946;52:191–205.

2. Marik PE. Aspiration pneumonitis and aspiration pneumonia. New Eng J Med 2001;344:665–671.

3. Downs JB, Chapman RL Jr, Modell JH, Hood CI. An evaluation of steroid therapy in aspiration pneumonitis. Anesthesiology 1974;40:129–135.

4. Dudley WR, Marshall BE. Steroid treatment for acid-aspiration pneumonitis. Anesthesiology 1974;40:136–141.

5. Lowrey LD, Anderson M, Calhoun J, Edmonds H, Flint LM. Failure of corticosteroid therapy for experimental acid aspiration. J Surg Res 1982;32:168–172.

6. Girard TD, Bernard GR. Mechanical ventilation in ARDS: a state-of-the-art review. Chest 2007;131:921–929.

7. Chan KP, Stewart TE, Mehta S. High-frequency oscillatory ventilation for adult patients with ARDS. Chest 2007;131:1907–1916.

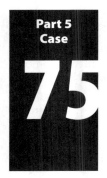

75

Contributions from Johns Hopkins Medical Institutions under
Deborah A. Schwengel

Mind, body, and spirit

Christina Miller and Adam Schiavi

The case

A 31-year-old African American with Down's syndrome developed end-stage renal disease 8 years ago and has been maintained on peritoneal dialysis (PD) since then. He lives with his parents, who are quite devoted and lovingly care for all his needs at home. He does well with PD, but it is cumbersome and time consuming. Several years ago, the patient was evaluated for a kidney transplant and placed on the transplant list.

The parents are Jehovah's Witnesses, and the family is quite active in the religious community. They consider their son to be a Jehovah's Witness, as well. He participates in church activities and gets great pleasure from singing in church and his involvement in the community. He has limited cognitive ability and has the intellectual capacity of a young school-aged child. During his perioperative evaluation, he is watching *Sesame Street*.

On initial evaluation by the transplant team, the family is clear that their son is unwilling to accept blood products. The transplant team assures them that "bloodless" kidney transplants are done routinely and that this will not be a problem. The options of preoperative hemoglobin supplementation with intravenous iron or erythropoietin are never discussed. The team tells the parents that they will need legal papers establishing guardianship of their son because of his adult status.

They obtain a short statement from the court indicating that they are the guardians of their son; however, it does not elaborate specific circumstances, including medical decision making. At the time of the initial evaluation, the transplant team contacts the legal department about the issue via e-mail. Legal is concerned about the complexity of the situation and recommends a formal ethics consult. The transplant team never pursues this.

Several years after the initial evaluation, a cadaveric donor kidney match is found, and the patient is scheduled for surgery. The transplant team tells the anesthesia team that the patient has refused blood products, that the case has been cleared with the Hopkins ethics and legal teams, and that there is court documentation of the parents as guardians who will be making medical decisions.

The patient proceeds to surgery. Intraoperatively, the patient suffers acute blood loss and a period of hypotension after reperfusion with blood pressures in the 80s/50s for several minutes. He is treated with vasopressors and resuscitated with crystalloid. The patient comes to the surgical intensive care unit (SICU) in the evening postoperatively with hemoglobin of 6. The transplanted kidney is not making urine. The morning after his arrival, a new SICU attending comes on service and an ethics consult is called with the question of whether it is permissible to transfuse this patient against his family's wishes in the event that his anemia becomes life threatening.

The parents remain adamant that they do not want their son to be transfused, even if it means that he will die. They maintain that they never would have proceeded with the transplant had they known that there was a possibility that their son would be transfused against their wishes, and they feel that they were promised that this would not be the case. They feel that transfusion would be an assault tantamount to rape. However, if the medical team goes against their wishes and transfuses the patient, they do not believe that God or the Jehovah's Witness community will reject the patient because he will be viewed as the victim of a crime.

When the patient is questioned regarding his beliefs (postoperatively, with a hemoglobin of 5), he says that he does not want a blood transfusion because that would be "bad." He answers affirmatively to the question "are you a Jehovah's Witness?" and then proceeds to answer the same way to "are you Jewish?" "Are you Muslim?" and "are you Hindu?"

Patient care

Residents must be able to provide patient care that is compassionate, appropriate, and effective for the treatment of health problems and the promotion of health.

Communicate effectively and demonstrate caring and respectful behaviors when interacting with patients and their families.

As a member of the ICU team, you have been put in a difficult position. Let's first consider this family's situation. They agreed to a "bloodless" kidney transplant with the intention of helping their son, thereby freeing him from dependence on dialysis. Their religious beliefs and refusal of blood products were clearly communicated to the surgical team. They followed the team's instructions and obtained legal guardianship of their son. They now find themselves after the operation with a son who has a tenuous kidney graft and life-threatening anemia, and a new ICU team is telling them that the treatment plan they agreed on may not be valid and that their son could be transfused against their wishes to save his life.

At this point, it is crucial that the ICU team communicate effectively and demonstrate behaviors that are caring and respectful. One must maintain an open dialogue with the patient's parents about his health issues and the deliberation regarding whether the ICU team will override the parents' refusal to transfuse the patient. It is reasonable for the patient's family to feel confused, betrayed, and angry. The ICU team members must demonstrate their concern for and commitment to the well-being of this patient. They must be respectful of this family's religious beliefs and cognizant of the enormous emotional burden this family must feel when making life or death decisions for their son. They must gain the trust of this family and quickly demonstrate that they have the patient's best interest at heart. As a member of this team, you have about a minute to do all of this. Good luck.

Gather essential and accurate information about their patients.

Information gathering from a variety of sources is essential. The ICU team must determine the patient and his family's understanding of the gravity of the situation, the details of the agreement the patient's family had with the transplant team, the specifics of the legal documentation the family obtained, the religious

beliefs of the patient's family, their specific wishes for their son's medical treatment, the patient's comprehension of the beliefs of the Jehovah's Witnesses, and the patient's level of competency. Each of these things can significantly impact the team's decision regarding whether to transfuse if the anemia becomes a threat to the patient's life.

Make informed decisions about diagnostic and therapeutic interventions based on patient information and preferences, up-to-date scientific evidence, and clinical judgment.

This is the crux of the issue. In this case, the patient's parents' preferences are at odds with the standard therapeutic intervention for anemia, a blood transfusion. The ICU team must take each conflicting priority and weigh it carefully to come to a decision. The first issue is whether the team ought to transfuse for life-threatening anemia. If they decide to transfuse, they must determine their transfusion threshold by balancing the risks and benefits. In this case, the patient's hemoglobin is critically low, and he is showing hemodynamic pathophysiology associated with anemia. However, the risks of transfusion for this patient are distinct, beyond the standard risks associated with receiving blood. The patient risks being spiritually marred in the eyes of his parents and his community by a transfusion. This has the potential to distance him from his community and may impact his parents' relationship with their community if they do not successfully prevent their son from being transfused. Exercising clinical judgment becomes even more difficult when there is no up-to-date scientific evidence to support or refute one's position; in medical ethics literature, there is no precedent for how to treat an adult who has never had the capacity to make health care–related decisions yet has family that wishes him to refuse blood products based on faith. Decisions must be made with the utmost care, with the understanding that they could impact how these issues are dealt with in the future.

Develop and carry out patient management plans.

In this case, the ICU team felt that this complex case warranted a consult from the hospital ethics committee. The ethics team determined that the patient's family had his best interest at heart and were acting lovingly on behalf of their son. After this, they carefully weighed the conflicting responsibilities involved in the ICU team's care of the patient, which involved not only preservation of life, but also preservation of that patient's self-image and his relationship with his parents and community. On deliberation, the ethics committee decided that it would be ethically permissible either to transfuse the patient to save his life or to honor his parents' wishes and allow him to die of anemia. Either alternative was ethically defensible, and it was left to the judgment of the ICU team to make the ultimate decision. The ICU team discussed the issue extensively and decided by a slim margin to transfuse the patient in the event that the patient became hemodynamically unstable and was refractory to all alternative treatments in a precode situation. In the end, the patient was able to survive a tenuous period of severe anemia with no such imminently fatal events. He was transferred out of the ICU and recovered his red cell counts without allogeneic blood cell products. After many months of delayed graft function, his transplanted kidney recovered, and he was taken off hemodialysis.

Counsel and educate patients and their families.

Once the ICU team had reached a plan for patient management, this needed to be communicated in a candid and sensitive way to the patient and his family. It was very important to express to the family how difficult it was for the team to reach this decision and the great lengths the team would take to exhaust alternative options before deciding to transfuse. The family has refused blood based on their religious beliefs as members of the Jehovah's Witness faith. Many Jehovah's Witnesses adhere to Watchtower Doctrine, which specifically prohibits allogeneic and preoperative autologous transfusion of four blood fractions: red cells, white cells, platelets, and plasma. However, official doctrine discourages, but does not specifically prohibit, other "minor fractions," which include human blood derivatives such as albumin, cryoprecipitate, immunoglobulin, and so on. Other options include erythropoietin, chemically modified bovine hemoglobin, and recombinant factor VII. Beyond the product itself is the manner in which it is utilized; hemodilution, cell salvage, cardiopulmonary bypass, dialysis, and plasmapheresis are a few examples [1]. Medical science presents myriad specific options that patients may not have considered in the past; it is up to the care team to explain each of the relevant options to the patient and counsel him or her about the risks and benefits so that the patient can make decisions consistent with his or her beliefs.

Use information technology to support patient care decisions and patient education.

Technology has developed several blood alternatives, some approved for routine use and some products that are still experimental but may be approved for compassionate use. Awareness of these alternative therapies and their associated risks is important to helping this patient and his family make decisions consistent with their wishes. As the medical professional, you must use your resources to gather this information in a timely manner, integrate it into the overall treatment plan, and present these options to the family.

Perform competently all medical and invasive procedures considered essential for the area of practice.

Intensive care involves a number of medical and invasive procedures. There are several challenges with this patient. First, he is an adult patient with developmental delay, which can make painful invasive procedures like lab draws a challenge. Second, every effort must be made to minimize blood sampling, while still monitoring crucial labs like kidney function and levels of potentially toxic antirejection drugs. It is also important to gain peripheral access quickly and with minimal blood loss, when necessary. This patient doesn't have much blood left to lose.

Provide health care services aimed at preventing health problems or maintaining health.

In a patient with severe anemia, for whom transfusion would only be considered in the most critical situation, care must be taken to avoid unnecessary blood loss or anything that could perturb hemodynamic stability. Every effort must be made to avoid hypoxemia and maintain oxygen delivery with judicious use of supplemental oxygen. Volume status, blood pressure, and heart rate are of great importance; the patient needs to be adequately resuscitated with crystalloid after a large intraoperative blood loss to perfuse vital organs, including the new kidney graft. However, despite the transplant, the patient remained anuric postoperatively and was still requiring dialysis for volume and electrolyte management. Other aspects of ICU care postoperatively include maintaining normoglycemia, deep venous thrombosis prophylaxis, treatment of postoperative pain, and maintenance of the patient's immunosuppression regimen.

> Work with health care professionals, including those from other disciplines, to provide patient-focused care.

Care of the medical issues of any transplant patient requires members from the ICU, transplant surgery, anesthesia, nursing, nutrition, physical therapy, and social work to work collaboratively. The ethical issues in this specific case also required the involvement of the hospital ethics and legal teams. Communication between each of these groups is important to present a unified plan to the patient and family. During these deliberations, it is crucial that the staff maintain open lines of communication with the family. It should be continuously reinforced that each team is working in the best interest of the patient because the family may feel that their trust has been betrayed.

Medical knowledge

Residents must demonstrate knowledge about established and evolving biomedical, clinical, and cognate (e.g., epidemiological and social-behavioral) sciences and the application of this knowledge to patient care.

> Demonstrate an investigatory and analytic thinking approach to clinical situations.

From an ethics standpoint, this is a complex and difficult case, and it deserved careful consideration prior to surgery. The patient has Down's syndrome with associated mental retardation; he has never been competent enough to make complex medical decisions. If he were a minor, the medical team would not permit his parents to refuse life-saving treatment on his behalf, but he is a disabled adult, and there is no clear precedent on what to do in this case. The transplant was done with insufficient investigation into these ethical dilemmas. The anesthesia team in the OR proceeded with the operation with the assurance of the transplant team that everything had been "cleared" with the ethics committee, when, in fact, it had not. Once the surgery and the irreversible acute blood loss had occurred, the ICU team was presented with the case. This illustrates the important lesson that you cannot blindly trust information that you are given. There was no ethics consult preoperatively, and the legal documentation was cursory and did not pertain to the spe-

cific situation. At this point, a thorough discussion was held with the patient and his parents, and the ethics committee was consulted to investigate the matter further; this led to consultation with the hospital legal team, and a search for ethical and legal precedents in this situation began. With no prior cases of this complex nature, it is up to the ethics committee and ICU team to balance conflicting ethical principles and formulate a plan.

> Know and apply the basic and clinically supportive sciences that are appropriate to their discipline.

The optimal goal of the postoperative period is to keep the patient alive, healthy, and with good functional capacity, without having to transfuse blood products (in a perfect world, with a working kidney, as well). This requires specific knowledge of the pathophysiology of anemia and kidney failure to understand how and to what extent the body is able to compensate for these deficiencies. Tachycardia, for instance, is a compensatory mechanism, and in a 31-year-old with no heart disease, it could be devastating to attempt to treat this compensation with beta-blockade. It is also important to understand where the limit of compensation lies – the point at which only red cells can prevent the situation from deteriorating into an arrest [2,3]. With a hemoglobin of 5 and absence of kidney function, homeostasis is much more precarious. Specific knowledge of pharmacology, including being able to identify drugs that may exacerbate anemia or hemodynamic instability, have prolonged or toxic effects in kidney failure, or jeopardize the newly transplanted organ is key to the care of this patient.

Practice-based learning and improvement

Residents must be able to investigate and evaluate their patient care practices, appraise and assimilate scientific evidence, and improve their patient care practices.

> Analyze practice experience and perform practice-based improvement activities using a systematic methodology.

Once the ICU team began investigating how the surgery had been performed without a prior ethics consult, we began to identify problems in the system that had prepared the patient for surgery. Our patient was evaluated several years prior to the surgery, when his family first considered transplant as an option. At this time, one of the transplant nurses who saw the family e-mailed the story to the ethics committee; there was obvious concern that further workup was needed, and the ethics committee suggested a formal consult. From an ethics standpoint, the patient was lost to follow-up and several years elapsed. When the patient had risen on the transplant list and surgery in the near future was likely, the case should have been revisited. First, the case needed to be evaluated from an ethics perspective, and second, the patient needed to be optimized from a medical standpoint prior to surgery. The patient's starting hemoglobin was 11. This patient could have benefited from preoperative erythropoietin therapy to increase his hemoglobin. Intraoperative cell salvage could have been arranged, if the family was willing to accept this therapy. The key is to determine the optimal time to do this based on the patient's position on the list: too early and the patient endures unnecessary therapy; too late and these details are lost in the excitement to rush to transplant once an organ becomes available and the clock starts ticking.

> Locate, appraise, and assimilate evidence from scientific studies related to their patients' health problems.

From the medical perspective, there is literature on the optimization of Jehovah's Witness patients before surgery that involves boosting the starting hemoglobin. Helm et al. [4] published a report of 100 consecutive coronary artery bypass graft operations without transfusion utilizing a comprehensive multimodal blood conservation strategy, which included preoperative erythropoietin, iron, folate, and vitamins B12 and C. In terms of ethics literature, there is strong precedent for allowing competent adult Jehovah's Witnesses to refuse blood products and for not permitting parents to refuse life-saving therapy on behalf of their minor children. What is not clear is what to do with a never-competent adult whose guardians refuse on his behalf. The Americans with Disabilities Act does offer some guidance that adults who are mentally disabled should be treated as adults and not according to their "age" mentally.

> Obtain and use information about their own population of patients and the larger population from which their patients are drawn.

Transplants in Jehovah's Witnesses are not uncommon at our institution. The idea of accepting a solid organ transplant but not a transfusion of blood products may seem incongruous. However, it is important to respect the autonomy of these patients. In the case of competent adults, one must discuss what interventions and products the patient will accept or refuse in a life-threatening event prior to surgery and then respect those decisions. The important point is that each Jehovah's Witness has individual beliefs, and it is crucial that we discuss each option with each patient in detail preoperatively so that there is no ambiguity about what treatments are available in an emergency situation.

> Apply knowledge of study designs and statistical methods to the appraisal of clinical studies and other information on diagnostic and therapeutic effectiveness.

Ethics literature consists almost exclusively of case reports and editorials. Precedent may be firmly established after multiple legal cases reach similar conclusions, but this is not a field that lends itself to formal studies and statistical analysis of data.

> Use information technology to manage information, access online medical information, and support their own education.

While there are mostly case reports, legal verdicts, and editorials in medical ethics literature, these references can be quite helpful in guiding one's thought process when considering an ethical dilemma. These papers are available through online ethics journals, and the vast array of sources can be manipulated with search engines like PubMed. Our hospital legal department has access to similar search engines, such as Westlaw or LexisNexis, which permit identification of landmark cases and judicial opinions.

Professionalism

Residents must demonstrate a commitment to carrying out professional responsibilities, adherence to ethical principles, and sensitivity to a diverse patient population.

> Demonstrate respect, compassion, and integrity; a responsiveness to the needs of patients and society that supersedes self-interest; accountability to patients, society, and the profession; and a

commitment to excellence and ongoing professional development.

The patients we see come from a wide variety of ethnic, religious, cultural, and socioeconomic backgrounds that are likely distinct from our own. Understanding the belief systems of our patients, how they view health and disease and end-of-life issues, enables us to gain perspective into their decisions and helps us assist them in making decisions that are consistent with their beliefs. The ICU team members, although they did not share the family's beliefs regarding blood transfusions, fully supported the parents' autonomy to refuse a transfusion for themselves. What was not clear was whether they had the right to refuse a life-saving transfusion for their adult son. Ultimately, the team was accountable to the patient. While the ICU team valued maintaining the patient's positive self-image (the patient understood that it was wrong to accept blood) and the patient's relationship with his community, it is more difficult to say that these considerations would prevail over protecting the patient from the harm of death from an easily treatable condition. When acting on behalf of this vulnerable patient, one has to weigh the merits of life at the expense of spiritual harm and backlash from the patient's support system.

Demonstrate a commitment to ethical principles pertaining to provision or withholding of clinical care, confidentiality of patient information, informed consent, and business practice.

The ethical issues are paramount in this case. The complexity of the issues makes the answer unclear. Withholding blood products is consistent with the wishes of the family and community who have loved and supported this patient for 31 years. If the patient was competent to consciously choose a religion for himself, most likely, he would be a Jehovah's Witness, a community in which he already actively participates, and he may have views on transfusion that are similar to his parents' views. However, there is an array of practices among Jehovah's Witnesses, and many do not adhere to Watchtower Doctrine in this regard. Provision of a transfusion is consistent with a medical community and concerned society that aims to protect disabled and vulnerable patients from harm. Ultimately, the ethics committee decided that neither option was ethically objectionable and that either argument could be substantiated. The process of informed consent for

transplant in this patient was more complex than usual and may have been oversimplified in some respects; the issue of who was authorized to make medical decisions for this patient was not clearly delineated prior to transplant. After the surgery was complete, the patient's parents both said that they never would have agreed to transplant if they had thought that there was any chance their son would be transfused against their will. These were details that would have been better addressed prior to surgery.

Demonstrate sensitivity and responsiveness to patients' culture, age, gender, and disabilities.

The ICU team had an incredibly hard task. It is difficult to convey respect for the family's religious beliefs and yet violate them by transfusing the patient. The team made it clear that they would comply with the family's wishes up until the point at which the patient could imminently die from anemia. We asked the family to talk openly about their belief and consulted with elders from their community. Additionally, the patient was a 31-year-old man with developmental delay, functioning at the intellectual level of a young school-aged child. During rounds on the first postoperative day, the patient was watching *Sesame Street*. The team did everything possible to alleviate the fear and uncertainty associated with being in an ICU. We explained our role in caring for the patient in an intellectual-age-appropriate manner and limited painful procedures as much as possible. We discussed with the patient his views about being part of the Jehovah's Witness community and his thoughts about receiving blood. In some respects, he received treatment as an adult would, but in others, he was protected similar to the way a pediatric patient would be.

Interpersonal and communication skills

Residents must be able to demonstrate interpersonal and communication skills that result in effective information exchange and teaming with patients, their patients' families, and professional associates.

Create and sustain a therapeutic and ethically sound relationship with patients.

The ICU team interacted with this patient in a caring and compassionate manner. Every attempt was made to keep medical care consistent with the family's beliefs and longtime practices, to which the patient was accustomed. At the same time, we were candid with the family about our ethical duty to protect the patient from harm and our intent to transfuse him in a truly life-threatening situation. Our honesty and consistency as a team was essential because the family had dealt with so many care teams throughout this process and had received conflicting promises with respect to transfusion.

> Use effective listening skills and elicit and provide information using effective nonverbal, explanatory, questioning, and writing skills.

It was critical that the patient's parents had the opportunity to express their beliefs and wishes to a concerned and attentive team. Regardless of the team's decision to transfuse, if the family felt that an indifferent team of doctors who did not respect them was overriding their will, it would have been damaging to the therapeutic relationship. In addition, it was important for the family to feel that they had done everything to defend their son from what they considered to be an assault. Interviewing the family about how they would feel toward their son if he received a transfusion, how the community would treat the patient and his parents, what they felt this meant for his spiritual future, and how they would handle his death if it occurred as a result of refusing blood added nuance to this complicated discussion. This sensitive and sophisticated interview helped to shape the team's decision on how to act (or not act), if required to do so.

> Work effectively with others as a member or leader of a health care team or other professional group.

The care of this patient required the coordinated effort of multiple teams, including transplant surgery; the ICU team; and nursing, ethics, and legal teams. Each team had different priorities for how best to care for the patient, and within each team, there were widely differing opinions on how the situation should be addressed. This required a great deal of calm and controlled communication in a situation in which it would have been easy to point blame at others. The ICU team consulted the ethics committee to clarify the pertinent issues and facilitate discussion between the various teams and the family. The final clinical decision rested on the ICU attending of record, who made a judgment based on multiple solicited opinions from all levels of training within the various teams.

Systems-based practice

Residents must demonstrate an awareness of and responsiveness to the larger context and system of health care and the ability to effectively call on system resources to provide care that is of optimal value.

> Understand how their patient care and other professional practices affect other health care professionals, the health care organization, and the larger society and how these elements of the system affect their own practice.

The involvement of the ethics and, ultimately, the legal teams in this case was of key importance. The ICU team identified a potential problem but was hindered by the responsibility for many important aspects of clinical care and a position that seemed at odds with the parents' position. The team consulted the ethics committee, which was able to bring skill and expertise in dealing with this manner of dilemma and which acted as a neutral, nonthreatening third party that was able to facilitate a difficult discussion between parties that were not in agreement. As a result, a forum was created, in which members from the various care teams and the parents could express their concerns with mediation by the consult team. The involvement of these resources not only helped to clarify the issues in this particular case, but may also help to shape hospital and, potentially, societal policy on how to address similar cases.

> Practice cost-effective health care and resource allocation that does not compromise quality of care.

The goal of minimizing near-code situations and minimizing duration spent in the ICU are certainly in accordance with the practice of cost-effective health care. Proper ethical and legal consultation as well as maintaining open, honest communication with the patient and family minimizes litigious behavior, which is extremely costly to the hospital and to society and detrimental to the doctor-patient relationship. Resource allocation is particularly relevant in this case because solid organs are relatively scarce. One might ask whether organs should be transplanted into patients who are unwilling to accept resources such as blood products to support the graft. Patients may be judged to be poor stewards of a donated organ if they are unwilling to take immunosuppressive drugs or unable to come for follow-up appointments. This may be a valid reason for taking them off the transplant list. Would a patient who promises to do everything possible to support the donation be more deserving of the organ?

Advocate for quality patient care and assist patients in dealing with system complexities.

By the time the patient reached the ICU, he had partially navigated the complex health care system. However, at that point, it was appropriate to reevaluate the prior agreement the family had with the transplant team to ensure that a plan was in place to pro-vide optimal patient care for the physical and spiritual needs of the patient. It was important to reassess the previous plan, rather than unconsciously following it for the sake of continuity.

Know how to partner with health care managers and health care providers to assess, coordinate, and improve health care and know how these activities can affect system performance.

This case identifies a flaw in the transplant preoperative evaluation system. The failure to involve the ethics team prior to the surgery might point to a lack of training in identifying this scenario as a potential problem, a lack of awareness regarding the resources the ethics committee could provide, or a problem in accessing these resources. Communication by providers back to health care managers can prompt an evaluation of this process, with a targeted assessment of how to improve the system.

References

1. Remmers PA, Speer AJ. Clinical strategies in the medical care of Jehovah's Witnesses. Am J Med 2006;119:1013–1018.

2. Carson JL, Noveck H, Berlin JA, Gould SA. Mortality and morbidity in patients with low postoperative Hb levels who decline blood transfusion. Transfusion 2002;42:812–818.

3. Tobian AA, Ness PM, Noveck H, Carson JL. Time course and etiology of death in patients with severe anemia. Transfusion 2009;7:1395–1399.

4. Helm RE, Rosengart TK, Gomez M, et al. Comprehensive multimodality blood conservation: 100 consecutive CABG operations without transfusion. Ann Thorac Surg 1998;65:125–136.

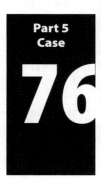

**Part 5
Case**

76

Contributions from Johns Hopkins Medical Institutions under Deborah A. Schwengel

He's not dead yet!

Veronica Busso and Mark Rossberg

The case

A 5-year-old boy is taken from the emergency department (ED) to the operating room (OR) for an emergency ventricular peritoneal shunt revision for a proximal ventriculoperitoneal (VP) shunt obstruction. The patient is transported with his mother by a neurosurgeon and an ED nurse and is monitored with pulse oximetry, electrocardiogram, and noninvasive blood pressure (NIBP). He is receiving oxygen by face mask and has a heart rate of 54, a blood pressure of 120/54, and an O_2 saturation of 99%. He is obtunded. His intravenous (IV) is infiltrated.

The child is a former 24-week premature infant who had had an intracranial bleed with subsequent hydrocephalus, which was treated with a VP shunt insertion in infancy. The child awakened this morning with a headache. Over the course of the day, he developed nausea, vomiting, and lethargy. His mother was worried and brought him to the ED this evening. The child also has a history of chronic lung disease and asthma.

Patient care

Residents must be able to provide patient care that is compassionate, appropriate, and effective for the treatment of health problems and the promotion of health.

Gather essential and accurate information about their patients.

This child is symptomatic from increased intracranial pressure. He demonstrates evidence of Cushing's reflex, indicative of brain-stem ischemia. (Cushing's reflex is the hypertension often seen as part of Cushing's triad: hypertension, bradycardia, and irregular respirations.) This is a late sign of increased intracranial hypertension. To safely take care of this child in an optimal fashion, a pertinent history should be obtained rapidly from the parent and the ED and neurosurgeon. This includes a brief report of history, physical findings, and treatment given. A history of problems with anesthesia should be probed, as should a family history of life-threatening reactions to anesthesia. Other pertinent information includes vital signs, cardiovascular stability, vomiting/aspiration, and other medical conditions. This should be done while transferring the monitors and moving the patient to the OR table so as not to delay anesthetic induction and surgery to quickly relieve the shunt obstruction.

Make informed decisions about diagnostic and therapeutic interventions based on patient information and preferences, up-to-date scientific evidence, and clinical judgment.

We concur with the emergent nature of this situation, and then we must quickly protect the brain. The major risks to this patient are as follows:

1. Increased intracranial pressure (ICP) is present, which compromises cerebral perfusion, worsens cerebral ischemia, and increases the risk of impending herniation.
2. Increased risk of pulmonary aspiration is present. This is secondary to delayed gastric emptying from elevated ICP, vomiting from the same, and possible diminished ability to protect the patient's airway secondary to altered mental status.
3. Potential for intraoperative bronchospasm with hypercarbia and hypoxia further worsening elevated ICP and cerebral ischemia.

Develop and carry out patient management plans.

This is an absolute emergency!

1. Ensure that all placed monitors are functional.
2. Check the suction and laryngoscope.
3. If the patient does not already have an IV, place one and have the parents escorted to the waiting room with the exiting ED team.

4. Preoxygenate with 100% FiO_2.

5. Request some quiet in the room.

6. Perform modified rapid sequence induction (RSI) of general endotracheal anesthesia (GETA) with cricoid pressure. After loss of consciousness, we choose to ventilate the patient's lungs while applying cricoid pressure until successful tracheal intubation has been confirmed. This is done to decrease ICP through hyperventilation, while protecting the airway from passive regurgitation during anesthetic induction.

7. Use anesthetic agents that are going to provide rapid intubating conditions while either decreasing ICP or at least without increasing ICP. Direct laryngoscopy and endotracheal intubation cause an increase in intracranial pressure, the mechanism of which is unclear.

   a. Atropine is useful to prevent worsening of bradycardia or precipitation of asystole with induction and intubation.

   b. Ketamine should be avoided (increases ICP).

   c. Thiopental and propofol both decrease ICP and are effective for RSI. Propofol is preferable to thiopental in this patient because it will blunt airway reflexes, and thiopental can trigger asthma.

   d. We will avoid succinylcholine here because it increases ICP. Other problems with the use of succinylcholine in this patient include the risk of malignant hyperthermia and the potential for exaggerated potassium release if this child has a yet to be diagnosed muscular dystrophy.

   e. Rocuronium will be our paralytic of choice 1 mg/kg for intubation. It does not increase ICP. It does not cause histamine release, which could trigger bronchospasm, but it does provide the most rapid onset of paralysis after succinylcholine.

   f. Fentanyl 1 mcg/kg will be given with induction to blunt the noxious effects of direct laryngoscopy.

   g. Lidocaine 1–1.5 mg/kg will also be given prior to intubation to decrease the likelihood of bronchospasm. Lidocaine has been demonstrated to be useful for this purpose. Its mechanism of bronchospasm prevention has been speculated to include blockade of histamine-related bronchospasm as well as blockade of parasympathetic smooth muscle

contraction. It is interesting to note that the administration of intravenous lidocaine is often used to attenuate ICP increases that occur with direct laryngoscopy and endotracheal intubation; however, there is little evidence to support this intervention [1,2].

8. Successfully intubate the trachea.

9. Quickly position for surgical intervention.

10. Mildly hyperventilate the patient's lungs to help decrease ICP until it is relieved surgically.

Counsel and educate patients and their families.

A cursory conversation about risks with attention to pulmonary aspiration and asthmatic exacerbation should take place if time permits. Remember that this child is hypertensive, bradycardic, and lethargic. We don't want him to herniate while we discuss the nuances of risks that only increase if we delay.

Perform competently all medical and invasive procedures considered essential for the area of practice.

Intubate the trachea!

Work with health care professionals, including those from other disciplines, to provide patient-focused care.

We obtained necessary information from the neurosurgeon and the ED staff. We had an orderly transfer of care. We informed the family, the OR nurses, and the neurosurgeons of our plans. We politely reestablished order and quiet in the room and refocused everyone on the patient for a safe neuroprotective general endotracheal anesthetic.

Medical knowledge

Residents must demonstrate knowledge about established and evolving biomedical, clinical, and cognate (e.g., epidemiological and social-behavioral) sciences and the application of this knowledge to patient care.

Know and apply the basic and clinically supportive sciences that are appropriate to their discipline.

While a complete discussion of the pathophysiology of increased intracranial pressure is beyond this exercise, some understanding of ICP is central to the management of a patient with a VP shunt obstruction. Once the fontanelles of a child close, an increase in volume in any intracranial compartment – brain, cerebral blood volume, or cerebrospinal fluid – will cause a displacement of one of the other intracranial compartments. There is little room within the rigid cranial vault, and small increases in intracranial volume can cause significant increases in intracranial pressure. Normal ICP measurements are 5–15 mmHg in adults and 3–7 mmHg in children. Maintenance of adequate cerebral blood flow (CBF) is critical to the prevention of cerebral ischemia [3]. Cerebral autoregulation maintains CBF constant over a range of cerebral perfusion pressures (CPP) of 50–150 mmHg (in adults without chronic hypertension). CPP is the difference between mean arterial pressure and ICP:

$$CPP = MAP - ICP.$$

The hallmark of anesthesia management for patients with VP shunt obstructions is to maintain CPP and decrease ICP. Strategies employed include the avoidance of hypotension to avoid decreases in MAP and CPP, hyperventilation to decrease CBF and ICP, and the use of drugs, such as intravenous agents (except for ketamine) and inhaled isoflurane, that decrease cerebral metabolic rate ($CMRO_2$).

Practice-based learning and improvement

Residents must be able to investigate and evaluate their patient care practices, appraise and assimilate scientific evidence, and improve their patient care practices.

Analyze practice experience and perform practice-based improvement activities using a systematic methodology.

After the case is over, reflect on what went well and what you would do differently next time. Consult the literature, if needed.

Professionalism

Residents must demonstrate a commitment to carrying out professional responsibilities, adherence to ethical principles, and sensitivity to a diverse patient population.

Demonstrate respect, compassion, and integrity; a responsiveness to the needs of patients and society that supersedes self-interest; accountability to patients, society, and the profession; and a commitment to excellence and ongoing professional development.

If, after an uneventful induction, the case is proceeding well and the child is stable with the relief of the shunt obstruction, a member of the anesthesia team may choose to go out to the waiting room to reassure the family that things are OK.

Interpersonal and communication skills

Residents must be able to demonstrate interpersonal and communication skills that result in effective information exchange and teaming with patients, their patients' families, and professional associates.

Create and sustain a therapeutic and ethically sound relationship with patients.

After the case, we apologize to the parents for the rushed, cursory history and physical and preop discussion and explain that our urgency to proceed with the case was with the best interests of their child in mind. We reassure the parents and answer any lingering questions.

Work effectively with others as a member or leader of a health care team or other professional group.

This patient presents to the hospital and then to the operating room in critical condition. It is important that the patient care team form quickly and work together effectively. There should be no unnecessary delay in starting this case. Handoff of this patient to the anesthesia team should be done in a rapid, organized fashion, with a report given during movement of the patient to the OR table and replacement of monitors.

In the event of further deterioration of the patient's condition with worsened bradycardia, atropine and epinephrine should be administered, as needed, and surgery to relieve ICP should proceed immediately. Should cardiac arrest ensue in this child, the anesthesiologist should take charge of the resuscitation, provide airway management, administer drugs, and continue monitoring. The anesthesiologist should assign someone from the nursing or surgical team to do chest compressions and should discuss with the surgeon the best way to proceed with relieving the increased intracranial pressure.

Systems-based practice

Residents must demonstrate an awareness of and responsiveness to the larger context and system of health care and the ability to effectively call on system resources to provide care that is of optimal value.

> Understand how their patient care and other professional practices affect other health care professionals, the health care organization, and the larger society and how these elements of the system affect their own practice.

Make sure your emergency response system is functional so that a critically ill patient like this can be cared for without delay.

References

1. Hamill JF, Bedford RF. Lidocaine before endotracheal intubation: intravenous or laryngotracheal? Anesthesiology 1981;55:578–581.

2. Robinson N, Clancy M. In patients with head injury undergoing rapid sequence intubation, does pretreatment with intravenous lignocaine/lidocaine lead to an improved outcome? A review of the literature. Emerg Med J 2001;18:453–457.

3. Bershad EM, Humphries WE III, Suarez JI. Intracranial hypertension. Semin Neurol 2008;28:690–702.

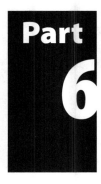

Part 6

Contribution from the Medical College of Wisconsin under Elena J. Holak

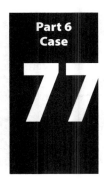

Contribution from the Medical College of Wisconsin under
Elena J. Holak

The Four Horsemen of Notre Dame or the Four Horsemen of the Apocalypse?

The story of how horses tried to ruin
my first night on call

Elena J. Holak and Paul S. Pagel

The case

It's my first night on call alone, all by myself. I've finally relinquished the puppy-call leash that tethered me to a supervising senior resident since the beginning of my anesthesiology residency training. Of course, I'm scared out of my mind! I'm armed with every medication and portable airway device known to man; I look like I'm about to be deployed to Fallujah, Iraq. I sincerely regret my complete lack of weight training at the Highlander Elite Tennis and Racket Club. It's not that all the heavy equipment provided me with any legitimate sense of self-confidence. To the contrary, I'm watching the clock, quietly counting the minutes until the night is over, and praying that I won't accidentally kill anyone with my lack of experience, which has never been more blatantly obvious (at least to me). My prayers go unanswered, and my night doesn't pass silently. I conclude that God doesn't exist when I receive a stat page to the gastroenterology (GI) laboratory at the convenient time of 3:00 A.M. It probably goes without saying that I wasn't sleeping anyway. A female voice screams into my pager, "We need you *now* in GI room 3."

Able to leap tall buildings in a single bound, I appear in the GI lab within mere seconds of the page, thereby proving some evidence, at least, that my health club cardio training was beneficial, or alternatively, that epinephrine is a truly miraculous substance. I'm immediately confronted by a disoriented, combative, 42-year-old, 205-kg, 165-cm male in a semirecumbent position being physically restrained by several nurses, residents, and medical students. Clearly the concept of restraint is not easily achieved when the weight (in kilograms) to height (in centimeters) ratio is greater than 1. In the emergency department, the patient claimed to have taken a "small" bite of a

roasted chicken, which became lodged in his esophagus and caused complete obstruction. He was not a healthy man, as his past medical history of essential hypertension, non-insulin-dependent diabetes mellitus, tobacco abuse, and morbid obesity (shock and awe) indicated. The staff gastroenterologist had not yet graced the scene with his beatific presence, and the GI fellow had begun performing an esophagoscopy without supervision. The patient received intravenous midazolam (3 mg) and fentanyl (200 μg), and the GI fellow had been pulling shreds of chicken from the patient's esophagus for over 45 minutes, when I was summoned to provide assistance with further conscious sedation and possible airway management.

The body habitus of this unfortunate man was highly reminiscent of the *Star Wars* villain Jabba the Hutt. Considering the patient's penchant for fast food, Jabba the Pizza Hut seems like a perfect moniker for the current report. While in the GI lab, I kept hearing hoofbeats (it wasn't schizophrenia as I had taken my Prolixin earlier in the day); I was hoping for help from the Four Horsemen of Notre Dame (Stuhldreher, Miller, Crowley, and Layden) to provide brute strength, but instead, I believed that the Four Horsemen of the Apocalypse (Famine, Pestilence, War, and Death) may be arriving at any minute. That piece of chicken in Jabba's esophagus was certainly the Red Horse – War! I was at war with an intrusive invader of the esophagus and the airway problems created by Jabba's obesity combined with too much conscious sedation. It was obvious that the patient didn't believe in the Black Horse – Famine. He also hadn't heard of Weight Watchers or Jenny Craig (who doesn't own a horse of any color, at least to my knowledge). While we were all struggling with the patient and trying to formulate a plan, the staff gastroenterologist (just call him

"Dr. X the Absent") finally arrived and harshly admonished the GI fellow for failing to complete the procedure. He complained indignantly that someone with an ancient Toyota Corolla had taken his favorite parking spot near the hospital entrance, forcing him to park his new (gull-wing doored, Grigio Antares metallic) Lamborghini Murcielago in a less convenient location. Dr. X openly criticized every aspect of the patient's care in front of the struggling man, while completely ignoring him, but instead of assisting or instructing the GI fellow, he went straight to the computer to check the status of a pair of ostrich boots advertised on CraigsList. His nickname "X the Absent" was well earned as he typically assists with most procedures for only 5 to 10 minutes and then retires in glorious triumph over his personal conquest of disease and his salvation of mankind. Of course, he always leaves the patient with the impression that he alone performs all procedures billed under his name. In his profound narcissism, he is, of course, the only person who possibly could have provided care, but I'm thinking that he is one totally bogus dude, to paraphrase *Bill and Ted's Excellent Adventure*.

My dilemma: how was I going to sedate this gigantic man while protecting his airway from aspiration, preserving oxygenation, and maintaining adequate ventilation? I'm beginning to think that I've lost my mojo.

Patient care

Residents must be able to provide patient care that is compassionate, appropriate, and effective for the treatment of health problems and the promotion of health.

Communicate effectively and demonstrate caring and respectful behaviors when interacting with patients and their families.

Dealing with a partially sedated, combative patient in the wee hours of the morning is not optimal for effective communication. Nevertheless, demonstrating a respectful, caring approach to the patient is of paramount importance. However difficult the circumstances, the physician must use the tone of voice and general demeanor necessary to engender a feeling of trust. Social scientists indicate that one of the most primitive actions for which humans strive is connection, that is, an insatiable inner need for meaningful interaction with others. Thus each patient should be cared for the same way that you would like a member of your family treated when seeking health care. A patient may remember a particular good or bad experience for the rest of his or her life. In the information age, a physician's name and reputation certainly have the potential to appear in an Internet chat room in very positive or negative light, depending on an individual patient's experience. This is a very sobering thought indeed.

Gather essential and accurate information about their patients.

In the current case, the very limited information was available from the medical record. The procedure was deemed a medical emergency because the esophageal obstruction prevented the patient from swallowing saliva. As a result, he was urgently transported to the GI lab after a very cursory initial evaluation. Laboratory analysis demonstrated a blood glucose concentration of 250 mg/dL (non-insulin-dependent diabetes and recent chicken consumption), but no other abnormalities were observed. The arterial oxygen saturation measure using pulse oximetry was 89% with the patient breathing room air. The electrocardiogram was normal. The patient received lisinopril and metformin for treatment of hypertension and diabetes, respectively. In the emergency department, the patient denied a history of obstructive sleep apnea, but he lived alone and was unaware whether he snored on a regular basis. A complete history and physical examination is essential to modern anesthesia practice, but I was unable to obtain any historical information from the patient because he was sedated and combative.

On physical examination, a Mallampati class III airway, poor dentition, and a small mouth opening were readily apparent. His cervical range of motion was quite limited. The patient also had a bushy beard that was clearly hiding micrognathia. With the beard and generous abdominal girth, Jabba the Pizza Hut could have easily passed as the bass player for ZZ Top (whose name happens to be Dusty Hill, for readers who are students of rock and roll history). I couldn't help but wonder how he'd managed to shovel down all that food, enabling him to achieve the size of three grown men. He was literally wearing his addiction to food. I kept these thoughts to myself, of course, as one day, I, too, may become a Hostess Twinkies addict, thereby transforming myself from a svelte figure into a walking water bed.

Develop and carry out patient management plans.

The patient needed oxygen, oxygen, and more oxygen, which is the other big "O" (and I'm *not* referring to *Othello*, *Oliver Twist*, the Cirque du Soleil show, or the large Internet retailer Overstock.com). Administration of oxygen by face mask increased the patient's arterial oxygen saturation to 95%. An indwelling 20-gauge peripheral intravenous catheter was secured and standard American Society of Anesthesiology (ASA) monitors were applied. A second suction set was obtained to allow the patient to suction his own saliva, thereby providing him with a modicum of control over his predicament. I had to immediately address the type and conduct of anesthesia for the remainder of the procedure. Dr. X the Absent and his pathetically compliant GI team favored additional conscious sedation, but this strategy was unacceptable to me because the airway was unsecured and the patient remained at high risk of aspiration. It was at this very moment that X the Absent exclaimed, "Damn, think I may get those boots!" How nice for an awake patient in acute distress to hear this comment! Note to self: look for mojo in the morning, or is it a cup of Joe? Because Jabba was conscious and maintaining adequate arterial oxygen saturation, I had time to provide topical local anesthesia before securing his airway using a fiber-optic bronchoscope. After successful nasal endotracheal intubation using this approach, I planned to provide additional sedation, thereby allowing Dr. X and his inadequate GI fellow to be more aggressive in their retrieval of the chicken playing chicken.

Perform competently all medical and invasive procedures considered essential for the area of practice.

The key component to any successful fiber-optic intubation is excellent topical anesthesia. Intravenous glycopyrrolate is usually administered as an antisialogogue before topical aerosolized 4% lidocaine is used to provide pharyngeal and hypopharyngeal anesthesia. However, glycopyrrolate was not used in this case because there was inadequate time for the medication to take effect. In addition, the anticholinergic side effect of reduced GI peristalsis was not desir-

able. This adverse effect may provide succor to the Red Horse in his struggle to win the Battle of Chicken. The nares were pretreated with oxymetazoline 0.05% spray (a vasoconstrictor that reduces the risk of intranasal hemorrhage), followed by a nebulized treatment of 4% lidocaine mixed with phenylephrine. Five milliliters of 2% lidocaine jelly were then placed in the right nares, and a series of red rubber dilators were used to facilitate passage of the endotracheal tube (ETT). The tube passed easily through the nares, but unfortunately, a small area of the patient's hypopharynx had not been rendered insensate by inhaled, nebulized lidocaine. Of course, the ETT stimulated this precise location, and this irritation by the ETT incited the most violent, bombastic cough recorded in human history. The Big Bad Wolf couldn't hold a candle to Mr. Jabba's F-5 tornadic wretch emanating deep from the diaphragm. Perhaps he was an opera singer and not a founding member of ZZ Top in a former life. In any case, the cough was forceful enough to bring up the remainder of the roaster chicken, which had happily resided, minding its own business, in the patient's lower esophagus. The shear volume of chicken was astounding; if this were Jabba's idea of a little bite of chicken, I'd hate to see what he considered a large morsel. For an instant, I thought that he'd swallowed an entire 25-pound Butterball Thanksgiving turkey, complete with stuffing and gravy. Another thought crossed my mind: could the anesthesiology department bill for the GI procedure since I was solely responsible for dislodging the esophageal chicken? I, and I alone, drove off the Red Horse and won the war. With all due respect to your 580-horsepower, V-12 Lamborghini, ostrich boots, and massive ego, Dr. X you are a total loser! Res ipsa loquitur.

Provide health care services aimed at preventing health problems or maintaining health.

The high risk of aspiration was critically important in the management of this patient, and every precaution was taken to prevent this potentially catastrophic event. After the chicken had been deesophagized (*First author's note*: "deesophagized" is the coolest word in this entire book. We kept the best for last!), the aspiration risk was no longer an acute concern. However, the patient clearly required a dietary referral for portion control and a sensible, easy-to-follow weight-loss regimen. A lower body-mass index may resolve or at lease substantially improve his comorbid conditions. A psychiatric evaluation should also be strongly considered for assessment and definitive treatment of a compulsive eating disorder.

Work with health care professionals, including those from other disciplines, to provide patient-focused care.

During the acute event, two major medical services (gastroenterology and anesthesiology) were needed to care for the patient. All members of the health care team participated in caring for this morbidly obese man who just consumed half a chicken in one bite, but the contributions of the GI attending physician, Dr. X were less than ideal. It is very important for the attending physician to communicate with the team and actually participate in the care of the patient.

Medical knowledge

Residents must demonstrate knowledge about established and evolving biomedical, clinical, and cognate (e.g., epidemiological and social-behavioral) sciences and the application of this knowledge to patient care.

Demonstrate an investigatory and analytic thinking approach to clinical situations.

I knew I was in deep kimchi when confronted by the combative, drooling Jabba the Pizza Hut and his difficult airway. My mind reflexively recited the ASA difficult airway algorithm in four different languages, but instead of following such a similar, well-established strategy, many physicians have relied on dogma, anecdote, and tradition to guide patient care. A sensible plan for patient care is generated that provides the most ideal possible care for the patient and uses the best available resources. The ASA difficult airway algorithm was the template I followed in this case, albeit with somewhat unexpected results.

Know and apply the basic and clinically supportive sciences that are appropriate to their discipline.

Medical information alone is not the only prerequisite for compassionate, effective patient care. The history of medicine is full of examples in which dogma and tradition were later proven false. Trephination, bloodletting, and laser face-lifts represent only three examples. Thus, along with solid communication abil-

ities, a competent anesthesiologist must be an excellent historian capable of performing a comprehensive, careful physical examination; possess a deep understanding of the patient's family and community; have the empathy to understand the patient's beliefs and values; and recognize the availability of resources in the community. The anesthesiologist should rapidly be able to identify precise, clearly defined goals and formulate a detailed plan and timetable for achieving them for each patient.

Practice-based learning and improvement

Residents must be able to investigate and evaluate their patient care practices, appraise and assimilate scientific evidence, and improve their patient care practices.

Analyze practice experience and perform practice-based improvement activities using a systematic methodology.

Analyzing practice experience is a multistep process. The right questions require formation, and the relevance and validity of appropriate information need to be examined before the information can be applied to each patient's clinical condition. Dr. Evil (of *Austin Powers* fame) used these principles, and Mini-Me quickly incorporated them. The patient, and not pathophysiologic reasoning or a specialty-specific approach, is the center of all care decisions within the guidelines of conscientious, explicit, and judicious use of current best evidence.

Locate, appraise, and assimilate evidence from scientific studies related to their patients' health problems.

The ASA difficult airway algorithm clearly delineates the appropriate strategy for successful management of the patient with a difficult airway. Nevertheless, case reports, diagnostic dilemmas, and review articles expand the breadth of knowledge and expertise in this highly technical area. Evidence-based medicine also encourages a culture of inquiry. Anesthesiologists may have clear evidence to support current medical practice in many circumstances, but extrapolation of research data or anecdotal experience may be required when little other information is available to guide care. Remember when duodenal ulcers were treated with a bland diet? Who would have ever thought that a bacterium was responsible for ulcer disease? Blood-letting was used as a cure for centuries, but President George Washington probably expired as a result of hypovolemic shock after too much bloodletting. Oops.

Apply knowledge of study designs and statistical methods to the appraisal of clinical studies and other information on diagnostic and therapeutic effectiveness.

Medically useful information has three attributes: it must be correct, easily accessible, and immediately relevant. Dr. X the Absent was a genius at the easy part and little else. When evaluating a study in the literature, the anesthesiology resident should verify that the reference standard was applied to all patients, assess for appropriate blinding and inherent study design bias, and evaluate whether the authors tested a clear hypothesis. The reader should critically assess whether the conclusions reached by the authors are consistent with the data. Systematic reviews and meta-analyses can be powerful tools, but such studies should contain only the results of randomized, controlled clinical trials.

Use information technology to manage information, access online medical information, and support their own education.

The Internet is a very powerful tool. Google will reveal millions of hits on the vast majority of medical subjects, which may initiate further questions. Two particularly useful Web sites are the Cochrane Library (http://www.updateuse.com/clibhome/clib.htm) and the Agency for Healthcare Research and Quality (AHRQ) (http://ww.ahrq.gov). Readers are always encouraged to check sources for validity.

Professionalism

Residents must demonstrate a commitment to carrying out professional responsibilities, adherence to ethical principles, and sensitivity to a diverse patient population.

Demonstrate respect, compassion, and integrity; a responsiveness to the needs of patients and society that supersedes self-interest; accountability to patients, society, and the profession; and a commitment to excellence and ongoing professional development.

Professionalism is an elusive, intangible concept that may be easier to identify than define. The American Board of Internal Medicine was the first to delineate the tenets of professionalism, which include altruism, accountability, excellence, duty, honor and integrity, and respect for others. These noncognitive behaviors and habits are not easily taught in traditional ways and require a new pedagogy. In 1925, Abraham Flexner described scientific medicine in America as young, vigorous, and positivistic. Unfortunately, he felt that medicine was sadly deficient in cultural and philosophical background. Of note, Jordan Cohen, president emeritus of the American Association of Medical Colleges felt that a deficiency in professionalism would result in the loss of autonomy in our interactions with patients, self-regulation, public esteem, and a rewarding career. His personal sentiment was that professionalism was the basis of medicine's contract with society and thus, the keystone in the future of medicine.

The Hippocratic Oath and HIPAA are all over this one. How pleasantly ironic is it that *Hippocrates* and *HIPAA* both start with *H-I-P*? So does *hippopotamus*, which might also apply to the current case. HIPAA clearly delineates the principles of patient confidentiality. This patient's story should not be fodder for chats in the break room, regardless of how interesting, funny, difficult, or entertaining it may be. The Hippocratic Oath clearly states, "I will prescribe regimens for the good of my patients, according to my ability and judgment and never do harm to anyone." Patient confidentiality is addressed as well: "all that may come to my knowledge in the exercise of my profession or in daily commerce with men, which ought not to be spread abroad, I will keep secret and never reveal." Does anyone remember agreeing to "being free of mischief and in particular of sexual relations with both female and male persons be they free or slaves"? This part of the Hippocratic Oath somehow escaped the authors' attention when they graduated from medical school. Neither of us realized that we were committed to a life of celibacy on graduation.

Demonstrate sensitivity and responsiveness to patients' culture, age, gender, and disabilities.

It is certainly not sensitive or professional for the authors to nickname the patient "Jabba the Pizza Hut" because of his rather large size. The fact that he attempted to consume one half a roaster chicken in a single bite should also not be a source of amusement.

These examples were used only in this chapter to illustrate the irony of a tragic situation, that is, a frightened, morbidly obese man with multiple chronic medical problems in acute distress resulting from an esophageal impaction. Professional behavior entails showing respect for patients, colleagues, and oneself. The need for empathy and compassion at all times cannot be overemphasized. This behavior was one termed *bedside manner*, admirably displayed by the quartet of famous television characters Ben Casey, Dr. Kildare, Marcus Welby, and Benjamin Franklin "Hawkeye" Pierce.

Interpersonal and communication skills

Residents must be able to demonstrate interpersonal and communication skills that result in effective information exchange and teaming with patients, their patients' families, and professional associates.

> Create and sustain a therapeutic and ethically sound relationship with patients.

This objective proved to be a very difficult task with Jabba the Pizza Hut as he was relatively hypoxemic, sedated, and combative. Obviously, the current case is not the ideal situation in which to demonstrate this Core Clinical Competency. A sound relationship is predicated on the principle of respect. The physician must listen to the patient and develop an understanding of the patient, family, and culture, but an anesthesiologist may not be able to accomplish this objective in a 5- to 10-minute preoperative evaluation. Instead, stronger, more sincere efforts should be made to imbue a sense of mutual trust, respect, and rapport. Radar O'Reilly, from the old television series $M*A*S*H$, was portrayed with an excellent set of communication skills. He was attuned to the needs of others before being asked for a particular item, favor, or skill and even completed the thoughts and sentences of friends and coworkers. Given the time and experience, many physicians are able to develop similar insights into their patients.

> Use effective listening skills and elicit and provide information using effective nonverbal, explanatory questioning, and writing skills.

It bears repeating that conversations with patients and their families should be approached from a perspective that they are able to clearly understand. Medical jargon that is unintelligible is useless and does nothing but alienate, confuse, and frighten the patient. Translators, sign language interpreters, and pictures should be liberally used with patients who do not speak English, are deaf, or cannot read, respectively. The use of such tools should be clearly documented in the operative consent and continued into the postoperative period.

> Work effectively with others as a member or leader of a health care team or other professional group.

The anesthesiologist is a member of the operating health care team whose critical functions are to keep the patient alive and out of harm's way. The surgeon may claim that he or she is the captain of the ship – as Walt Whitman wrote, "Oh Captain! My Captain! Our fearful trip is done / the ship has weather'd every rack, the prize we sought is won / the port is near, the bells I hear, the people all exulting" – but the anesthesiologist is the admiral who decides whether and how the ship sails in the first place. Dr. Surgeon may feel that good old Walt personally wrote the poem for him or her, but every member of the operative team contributes to the successful outcome of the patient. Surgery truly is a team sport, and there is no *I* in *team*, only in *amide local anesthetics*.

Systems-based practice

Residents must demonstrate an awareness of and responsiveness to the larger context and system of health and the ability to effectively all on system resources to provide care that is of optimal value.

> Understand how their patient care and other professional practices affect other health care professionals, the health care organization and the larger society and how these elements of the system affect their own practice.

Anesthesiologists are often focused on limited specialty-specific ideologies that may adversely affect our ability to acknowledge the viewpoint of other medical specialties. Recognition of this potential source of distraction from patient-centered care is an important component of systems-based practice. Mastery of skills used in the service of others, compliance with a code of ethics, and dedication to continuous education of colleagues, residents, and medical studies within the framework of a professional culture are also essential goals of systems-based practice. In the current case, a sensible, nonconfrontational conversation between the gastroenterologists and the anesthesiologist, in which the advantages of airway control were compared with additional conscious sedation, opened a line of communication between the physicians involved in Jabba's care. This approach allowed the gastroenterologists to understand the anesthesiologist's specialty-specific needs, without jeopardizing patient safety.

Practice cost-effective health care and resource allocation that does not compromise quality of care.

The supplies (oxygen, topical lidocaine, oxymetazoline, and phenylephrine) used in the care of the current patient were very cost-effective. A fiber-optic bronchoscope is a very durable product that can be used for years after a simple cleaning procedure, thereby recouping the initial cost of the device. Expensive sedatives were not used in this case. Perhaps Ivana Trump would not care for this approach, but she isn't a physician!

Advocate for quality patient care and assist patients in dealing with system complexities.

All physicians are dedicated to providing excellent patient care. This should be job number 1, not Mission Impossible. Our motto: treat every patient as if he or she were a family member. System complexities may be difficult to navigate, but proper counsel, support, and assistance from ancillary staff facilitate the journey. It is always the small acts of kindness that people remember the most.

Know how to partner with health care managers and health care providers to assess, coordinate, and improve health are and know how these activities can affect system performance.

In this case, the anesthesiologist partnered with gastroenterology as a team to explain to the patient the course of events, immediate treatment, and the potential mechanisms by which a future recurrence may be avoided. Referrals may be made to other specialists who are able provide assistance with the patient's plethora of medical problems. Should he avail himself of these opportunities, his general overall state of health may improve, thereby making him a happier, healthier person and reducing the burden on the health care system.

Additional reading

1. Robins LS, Braddock CH, Fryer-Edwards KA. Using the American Board of Internal Medicine's "Elements of Professionalism" for undergraduate ethics education. Acad Med 2002;77:523–530.

2. Stern DT, Papadakis M. The developing physician – becoming a professional. N Engl J Med 2006;355:17.

3. Lattore P, Lumb P. Professionalism and interpersonal communications: ACGME Competencies and core leadership development qualities – why are they so important and how should they be taught to anesthesiology residents and fellows? Sem Anesth Perioper Med Pain 2005;24:134–137.

4. Baker DP, Salas E, King H, Battles J, Barach P. The role of teamwork in the professional education of physicians: current status and assessment recommendations. J Qual Patient Safety 2005;31.

5. Council on Ethical and Judicial Affairs. Code of medical ethics: current opinions. American Medical Association; 1992.

6. Lema MJ. Professionalism and the anesthesiologist: I'll know it when I see it. ASA Newsl 2003;67(9):1, 30.

7. Medical professionalism in the new millennium: a physician charter. Ann Int Med 2002;136:243–246.

8. Sackett DL, Haynes RB, Guyatt GH, Tugwell P. Clinical epidemiology: a basic science for clinical medicine. 2nd ed. Boston: Little, Brown; 1991.

9. Amalberti R, Auroy Y, Berwick D, Barach P. Five system barriers to achieving ultrasafe health care. Ann Intern Med 2005;31:756–764.

10. Sise MJ, Sise CB, Sack BA, Goerhing M. Surgeons' attitudes about communicating with patients and their families. Curr Surg 2006;63:213–18.

11. Sloan PD, Slatt LM, Ebell MH, Jacques LB, Smith MA. Essentials of family medicine. In: Information mastery: basing care on the best available evidence. 5th ed.: Lippincott, Williams, and Wilkins; 2007: 85–96.

Summary

You can think what you like about the Core Clinical Competencies. You can slice them, dice them, julienne them. But you still have to teach them (if you're an attending) and learn them (if you're a resident). This little foray attempted to make the Core Clinical Competencies – if not delectable – at least digestible.

Bon appétit!

And keep quiet in the elevators!

Index

459